THE DIGITAL PATIENT

Wiley Series in
Modeling and Simulation
A complete list of the titles in this series appears at the end of this volume.

THE DIGITAL PATIENT

Advancing Healthcare, Research, and Education

Edited by

C. DONALD COMBS
Eastern Virginia Medical School

JOHN A. SOKOLOWSKI
Old Dominion University

CATHERINE M. BANKS
Old Dominion University

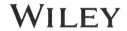

Library of Congress Cataloging-in-Publication Data:

The digital patient : advancing healthcare, research, and education / edited by C. Donald Combs,
John A. Sokolowski, Catherine M. Banks.
    p. ; cm.
  Includes bibliographical references and index.
  ISBN 978-1-118-95275-7 (paperback)
I. Combs, C. Donald, editor. II. Sokolowski, John A., 1953– , editor.
III. Banks, Catherine M., 1960– , editor.
[DNLM: 1. Patient Care Management. 2. Individualized Medicine–methods.
3. Patient-Specific Modeling. W 84.7]
RA971.6
362.10285–dc23
                                              2015029789

Cover image courtesy of Hector M. Garcia

Set in 10/12pt Times by SPi Global, Pondicherry, India

Printed in the United States of America

10 9 8 7 6 5 4 3 2 1

1 2016

CONTENTS

LIST OF CONTRIBUTORS

Sun Joo (Grace) Ahn, PhD
Department of Advertising
and Public Relations
Grady College of Journalism
and Mass Communication
University of Georgia
Athens, GA, USA

Mona Alimohammadi, PhD
Department of Mechanical Engineering
University College London
London, UK

Koray Atalag, PhD, MD
Bioengineering Institute
University of Auckland
Auckland, New Zealand

Catherine M. Banks, PhD
Virginia Modeling, Analysis and
Simulation Center
Old Dominion University
Suffolk, VA, USA

Scarlett R. Barham, MPH
School of Health Professions
Eastern Virginia Medical School
Norfolk, VA, USA

Eric B. Bauman, PhD, RN
Clinical Playground LLC
Madison, WI, USA

Jim Blascovich, PhD
Department of Psychological
and Brain Sciences
University of California
Santa Barbara, CA, USA

C. Donald Combs, PhD
Vice President and Dean
School of Health Professions
Eastern Virginia Medical School
Norfolk, VA, USA

Jessica E. Cornick, BA
Department of Psychological
and Brain Sciences
University of California
Santa Barbara, CA, USA

Bernard de Bono, PhD, MD
Bioengineering Institute
University of Auckland
Auckland, New Zealand

Saikou Y. Diallo, PhD
Virginia Modeling, Analysis and
Simulation Center
Old Dominion University
Suffolk, VA, USA

Vanessa Díaz-Zuccarini, PhD
Department of Mechanical Engineering
University College London
London, UK

Barry C. Ezell, PhD
Virginia Modeling, Analysis and
Simulation Center
Old Dominion University
Suffolk, VA, USA

Hector M. Garcia, PhD
Virginia Modeling, Analysis and
Simulation Center
Old Dominion University
Suffolk, VA, USA

Jörg Hähner, PhD
Organic Computing Institute
University of Augsburg
Augsburg, Germany

Robert L. Hester, PhD
Department of Physiology and Biophysics
University of Mississippi
Jackson, MS, USA

Peter J. Hunter, PhD
Bioengineering Institute
University of Auckland
Auckland, New Zealand

Christian Jacob, PhD
Department of Biochemistry and
Molecular Biology and Department of
Computer Science
University of Calgary
Calgary, Alberta, Canada

Christopher J. Lynch, MS
Virginia Modeling, Analysis and
Simulation Center
Old Dominion University
Suffolk, VA, USA

David P. Nickerson, PhD
Bioengineering Institute
University of Auckland
Auckland, New Zealand

V. Andrea Parodi, PhD, RN
Virginia Modeling, Analysis and
Simulation Center
Old Dominion University
Suffolk, VA, USA

César Pichardo-Almarza, PhD
Department of Mechanical Engineering
University College London
London, UK

William A. Pruett, PhD
Department of Physiology and Biophysics
University of Mississippi
Jackson, MS, USA

Albert Rizzo, PhD
Institute for Creative Technologies
University of Southern California
Los Angeles, CA, USA

Richard M. Satava, MD
Department of Surgery
University of Washington
Seattle, WA, USA

Stefan Schellmoser, M Sc
Organic Computing Institute
University of Augsburg
Augsburg, Germany

Peter M. A. Sloot, PhD
Department of Computational
Science
University of Amsterdam
Amsterdam, the Netherlands

John A. Sokolowski, PhD
Virginia Modeling, Analysis and
Simulation Center
Old Dominion University
Suffolk, VA, USA

Victor M. Spitzer, PhD
Center for Human Simulation
University of Colorado-Denver
Aurora, CO, USA

Thomas Talbot, MD
Institute for Creative Technologies
University of Southern California
Los Angeles, CA, USA

Joseph A. Tatman, PhD
Innovative Decisions, Inc.
Vienna, VA, USA

Andreas Tolk, PhD
Simulation Engineering Department
The MITRE Corporation
Hampton, VA, USA

Sebastian von Mammen, PhD
Organic Computing Institute
University of Augsburg
Augsburg, Germany

Seth H. Weinberg, PhD
Virginia Modeling, Analysis and
Simulation Center
Old Dominion University
Suffolk, VA, USA

PREFACE

Understanding in detail and with certainty what is going on within one's own body has been an elusive quest. Partial glimpses and general understanding are the best we have been able to do with the data we have at our disposal and with the limitations of population-normed theories of what the data mean for diagnosis and treatment of individuals. In the not-too-distant future, however, that will change as the Digital Patient platform is developed. The capacity to measure one's personal physiological and social metrics, compare those metrics with the metrics of millions of other humans, personalize needed therapeutic interventions, and measure the resulting changes will realize the vision of personalized medicine. Incorporating all of this rich data in simulations will have significant impacts on medical research, education, and healthcare systems around the world, as more interventions are simulated and assessed *in silico* prior to their use in therapy.

So, what exactly is the Digital Patient? The most commonly referenced definition of the Digital Patient is that provided through the European Union's *DISCIPULUS project: a technological framework that, once fully developed, will make it possible to create a computer representation of the health status of each citizen that is descriptive, interpretive, integrative and predictive.* Not explicitly stated, but implied, is that this framework will include behavioral, social, temporal, and spatial dimensions.

Major technological advancements in recent years have paved the way for more systematic approaches to modeling, simulation, and visualization of biological and social processes that make the realization of the Digital Patient possible. Modeling now encompasses high degrees of complexity and holistic methods of data representation. Various levels of simulation capability allow for improved outputs and analysis of discrete and continuous events. Simulation complements both natural language and mathematical and statistical analysis by introducing new ways of thinking. Simulation also provides tools to build understanding and generate insight into complex biological systems and processes, thus allowing much more comprehensive human models.

In the past, biologists sought to understand living things largely by examining their constituent parts. They studied individual genes, proteins, or signaling molecules to learn everything they could about the structure and function of a single and largely isolated biological entity. The emerging scientific strategy adds a new dimension to this traditional approach. Researchers now seek to understand both each constituent of a biological network *and* how all of a network's constituents function together. They use cutting-edge technologies to gather as much information as they can about a biological system. They then use this information to build mathematical and graphical models that account for the behavior of the system. They test these models by gathering additional data, often by perturbing a system through genetic or environmental changes. In this way, they build an understanding of biological systems that can be used, for example, to explore what goes wrong when a biological system becomes diseased and how to treat or prevent that disease.

The Digital Patient will not be constructed based solely on new information from all the "omics" fields, from the various efforts to model the human physiome and represent it virtually, from systems analysis, or from Big Data. It will only be realized through the purposeful collaboration of researchers (whether they are patients or scientific, clinical, or policy researchers) on both their research and the framework into which their research will fit. The Digital Patient will continue to depend on the efforts of a wide variety of individual researchers and modelers across many disciplines worldwide. It is inevitably an emergent phenomenon, governable only by sustained cooperation among those with an interest in its development and with guiding principles of openness, flexibility, rigorous validation and reliability processes, and respect for personal privacy.

People will ultimately be able to have personalized genetic codes and medical imaging stored in a cloud database, along with charts of vital signs and detailed nutritional analysis of everything they consume. They can then compare this data with data on millions of other similarly monitored bodies across the world, resulting in a colossal database (now widely referred to as Big Data) mined by software that can utilize the data to provide specific, personalized guidance regarding diet, vitamins, supplements, sleep, exercise, medication, treatments, social interactions, and overall health. That, simply stated, is the overarching goal of the Digital Patient.

The text is divided into four parts. To begin the discussion, **Part 1—The Vision**—makes the case for engaging the Digital Patient in all facets of healthcare: research and development, education, and practice (Chapter 1). A brief review of some of the most significant efforts in the development of the Digital Patient is presented (Chapters 2 and 3) as well as a discussion of the challenges of modeling a complex system such as the human body (Chapter 4).

Part 2—State of the Art—presents the corpus of research cataloging and analyzing the progress that has been made in developing a Digital Patient during the past decade. Since the Visual Human Project of the 1990s that focused on developing models of male and female anatomy based on dissection, substantial progress has been made in the development of physiological, anatomical, and social models and simulations. Chapters 5 through 14 present the various projects underway across the world; these contributions address anatomical modeling, facial and expressive modeling, and social and cultural modeling of humans.

Part 3—Challenges—attends to the substantial challenges of assimilating the various "parts" of the Digital Patient to make it whole. Chapters 15 through 17 address issues with the integration of all (modeled) components, interoperability of all models, and reliability and contextualization of the composite Digital Patient. Also included is Chapter 17 as the means to calibrating or refining the Digital Patient specific to an individual patient.

Part 4—Potential Impact—looks to the future of medicine and the usefulness of enabling the Digital Patient. Chapters 18 and 19 present the potential impact of the Digital Patient in research and experimentation in medical devices and technology, biologic development and testing, medical education and training, and, of course, patient care. Chapter 20 provides a closing word on the potential impact of the Digital Patient in medicine and healthcare vis-à-vis an increasing global population, lengthening life spans, and a mounting demand for medical care. Chapter 21 proposes a research and policy agenda aimed at fully constructing the Digital Patient: that is, why and how this needs to take place at an all-encompassing level.

EDITORS' NOTE

The editors stress that this text has set the topic of discussion within the reasonable bounds of the research and development currently underway. Thus, we make no claims that this is an exhaustive study of model development, simulation design, and applications of modeling and simulation in the structuring of the Digital Patient; rather, the text provides sufficient examples to present the breadth and depth of research in the field, speaks to the need for an overarching process to assimilate these projects, and suggests the means to do this in the form of a research and policy agenda. The intent of the agenda is twofold: (i) bring together these resources in a holistic approach for completing the Digital Patient and (ii) fully utilize the Digital Patient in the medical community for research, education, and practice.

PART 1

THE VISION: THE DIGITAL PATIENT—IMPROVING RESEARCH, DEVELOPMENT, EDUCATION, AND HEALTHCARE PRACTICE

1

THE DIGITAL PATIENT

C. Donald Combs

School of Health Professions, Eastern Virginia Medical School, Norfolk, VA, USA

Whatever we do together is pure invention,
The maps they gave us were out of date by years.

—Adrienne Rich, *21 Love Poems*

"Men's courses will foreshadow certain ends, to which, if persevered in, they must lead," said
Scrooge. "But if the courses be departed from, the ends will change."
—Charles Dickens, *A Christmas Carol*

It is, perhaps, odd to begin a book about a highly technical subject, the Digital Patient, with quotations from a poem and a book that, in very different ways, confront the vagaries of relationships. Then again, perhaps it is not so odd after all. Rich identifies the reality that relationships change and head in unexpected directions and that, often, what we thought was settled turns out to be in flux. Dickens describes the inevitable intertwining of past, present, and future in a hopeful homily. Imagine if we could all, without the ghosts, have the opportunity to revisit our past, understand clearly how it affects the present, and realize that the future can be changed into a more rounded, healthier human experience. In its essence, that is what the Digital Patient entails—the development of an evolving foundation for a better future in terms of personal and population health, in the validity of biological and social research, and in the development of more effective drugs and devices.

Dickens' story is a useful metaphor because it invokes the passage of time and describes that passage within a social context. Incorporating those two factors, time and social context, into the discussion of the Digital Patient foreshadows the emergence of an infinite array of applications that will advance our understanding of health and the factors affecting its realization. This introductory chapter provides some historical context for the concept

The Digital Patient: Advancing Healthcare, Research, and Education, First Edition.
Edited by C. Donald Combs, John A. Sokolowski, and Catherine M. Banks.
© 2016 John Wiley & Sons, Inc. Published 2016 by John Wiley & Sons, Inc.

of a Digital Patient, refines the definition to reflect explicitly the impact of the emerging fields of systems biology and computational physiology, and provides a rationale for the chapters that follow. The chapter draws heavily from the writings of Vanessa Díaz-Zuccarini, Peter Hunter, Robert Hester, Leroy Hood, Richard Satava, Peter M. A. Sloot, and other chapter authors. It draws as well from the research conducted by hundreds of international researchers who address topics important to the Digital Patient as diverse as Big Data, the human physiome, systems biology, human behavior, multiscale modeling and simulation, ontologies in healthcare, and Bayesian analysis.

HEALTH, THE GOAL

The most widely accepted definition of health is the one developed by the World Health Organization: *Health is a state of complete physical, mental and social well-being and not merely the absence of disease or infirmity* [1]. The definition applies to individuals and to populations. From a societal perspective, achieving the goal of health, both individually and as a whole, is why we fund (through both public and private sources) research and development efforts in the domains related to the Digital Patient.

PERSONALIZED MEDICINE

Historically, understanding in detail and with certainty what is going on within the human body has been an elusive quest. Partial glimpses and general understanding are the best we have been able to do with the data we have at our disposal and within the limitations of population-normed theories of what the data mean for the diagnosis and treatment of individuals. In the not-too-distant future, however, that will change as the Digital Patient is developed. The capacity to measure one's personal physiological and social metrics, compare those metrics with the metrics of millions of other humans, personalize needed therapeutic interventions, and measure the resulting changes will realize the vision of personalized medicine. The capacity to aggregate and integrate data from millions of individuals will provide a means to improve health across populations with differing cultures and behaviors.

President Barack Obama stated in the 2015 State of the Union speech that his administration wants to increase the use of personalized genetic information to help treat diseases such as cancer and diabetes. He urged Congress to boost research funding to support new investments in precision medicine. Obama wants "the country that eliminated polio and mapped the human genome to lead a new era of medicine—one that delivers the right treatment at the right time" [2, 3].

He will seek hundreds of millions of dollars for a new initiative to develop medical treatments tailored to genetic and other characteristics of individual patients. "Most medical treatments have been designed for the average patient," said Jo Handelsman, associate director of the White House Office of Science and Technology Policy. "In too many cases, this one-size-fits-all approach is not effective." Dr. Ralph Snyderman, a former chancellor for health affairs at Duke University, often described as the father of personalized medicine, said he was excited by the president's initiative. "Personalized medicine has the potential to transform our healthcare system, which consumes almost $3 trillion a year, 80% of it for preventable diseases," said Dr. Snyderman [3].

THE BEST OUTCOMES

A patient is a person who is receiving healthcare. Healthcare involves surveillance, diagnosis, treatment, monitoring, and quality assessment. The goal of healthcare is, of course, a healthy outcome. Several analytic frameworks for assessing quality have guided initiatives in the public and private sectors to develop measures of the outcomes of healthcare. One of the most influential is the framework put forth by the Institute of Medicine (IOM), which includes the following goals for the healthcare system [4]:

Safety, avoiding harm to patients from the care that is intended to help them.

Effectiveness, providing services based on scientific knowledge to all who could benefit and refraining from providing services to those not likely to benefit (avoiding underuse and misuse, respectively).

Patient-centered, providing care that is respectful of and responsive to individual patient preferences, needs, and values and ensuring that patient values guide all clinical decisions.

Timeliness, reducing waits and sometimes harmful delays for both those who receive and those who give care.

Efficiency, avoiding waste, including waste of equipment, supplies, ideas, and energy.

Equity, providing care that does not vary in quality because of personal characteristics such as gender, ethnicity, geographic location, and socioeconomic status.

Having the goal of improved healthcare outcomes in mind helps to frame the importance of the Digital Patient: *it is among the most powerful technological tools that we can develop and deploy to improve health outcomes*. The Digital Patient is not a panacea; it will become, however, an essential component of the twenty-first-century healthcare toolkit.

THE EMERGENCE OF THE DIGITAL PATIENT

The Digital Patient's origins are recent, tied as they are to computer and imaging technologies developed during past 40 years. Although some of the modeling related to the human physiome dates back to the early 1980s and the emergence of computers as a significant factor in biomedical research, the clearest point of origin for the Digital Patient is the US Library of Medicine's Visible Human Project (VHP).

The Visible Human

The VHP has now celebrated the twentieth anniversary of the completion of the male (1993) and female (1994) image collections [5]. The data has been used broadly and remains a primary resource for research in the areas of human modeling and simulation of structures. The need for the VHP was predicted by the National Library of Medicine's (NLM) 1986 Long-Range Plan to include applications in education, training, modeling, simulation, morphometrics, information interfaces, reference standards, and entertainment [6].

The VHP (described more fully in Chapter 5) has contributed significantly to the education and training of both healthcare professionals and the general public. The data have been used extensively in atlases of both cross-sections and three-dimensional images of the human anatomy. The segmented image data has been the foundation for models used for 3D printing and virtual and augmented reality surgical simulators. Yet, further dynamic tissue modeling enhancements are needed to bring the Visible Human's cadaveric anatomical images to life.

Dead humans, such as the cadavers used in the VHP, are obviously not the same as living humans. They are, however, very useful models of human anatomy, both diseased and healthy. The data derived from analysis of human anatomic structures is an important component of the Digital Patient. That said, the pressing challenge is to build accurate human simulations, comprising many interacting models, capable of representing living humans moving through time.

THE HUMAN PHYSIOME

There are several international collaborative efforts directed toward the analysis of the human physiome. Two of those most inclusive efforts are described here. The International Union of Physiological Scientists (IUPS) began the Physiome Project in the 1990s. Joining the IUPS Physiome effort in 2006, the European Union funded the Europhysiome initiative. The effort ultimately evolved into the DISCIPULUS Project, which had the goals of further developing both the VPH and a Roadmap toward the Digital Patient. The VPH is a methodological and technological framework that will be capable of enabling the collaborative investigation of the human body as a complex system [7, 8]. The framework will make it possible to share resources and observations formed by institutions and organizations creating disparate, but integrated, computer models of the mechanical, physical, and biochemical functions of a living human body. It is thus central to refining the Digital Patient.

The VPH is a framework that aims to be descriptive, integrative, and predictive [9–11]:

Descriptive. The framework should allow observations made in laboratories, hospitals, and the field, at a variety of locations situated anywhere in the world, to be collected, cataloged, organized, shared, and combined in any possible way.

Integrative. The framework should enable experts to analyze these observations collaboratively and develop systemic hypotheses that involve the knowledge of multiple scientific disciplines.

Predictive. The framework should make it possible to interconnect predictive models defined at different scales, with multiple methods and varying levels of detail, into systemic networks that solidify those systemic hypotheses; it should also make it possible to verify their validity by comparison with other clinical or laboratory observations.

The VPH framework is formed by large collections of anatomical, physiological, and pathological data stored in digital format, by predictive models and simulations developed from these collections, and by services intended to support researchers in the creation and maintenance of these models, as well as in the creation of end-user technologies for clinical practice. VPH models aim to integrate physiological processes across different spatial and time scales (multiscale modeling). These models make possible the combination of patient-specific data with population-based representations. The objective is to develop a systemic framework that replaces the reductionist approach to biology and supports the integration of biological systems by dimensional scale (body, organ, tissue, cells, molecules), by scientific discipline (biology, physiology, biophysics, biochemistry, molecular biology, bioengineering), and by anatomical subsystem (cardiovascular, musculoskeletal, gastrointestinal, etc.) [12–14]. The VPH thus represents the human physiological operating system that is a central component of the Digital Patient.

The Digital Patient

Vanessa Díaz-Zuccarini, one of the leading researchers in the DISCIPULUS project, defines the Digital Patient as *a technological framework that, once fully developed, will make it possible to create a computer representation of the health status of each citizen that is descriptive, interpretive, integrative and predictive* [15].

Peter Hunter, one of the early leaders of the IUPS and VPH efforts, identified three major challenges to the development of the Digital Patient in his 2013 article:

> Providing medical professionals and biomedical researchers with advanced user interfaces based on the Digital Patient metaphor that makes it easier to cope with large amounts of information related to different organ systems, different space/time scales, and different diagnostics;
>
> Providing healthcare practitioners with an information and communications technology (ICT) layer capable of recovering and integrating all available health information for each patient into a coherent whole;
>
> Providing biomedical and clinical researchers technology to capture existing knowledge and the digital artifacts in the form of predictive models and to compose digital quanta of knowledge into integrative models of complex system mechanisms [14].

This perspective views the VPH as a comprehensive collection of models and the Digital Patient as the broader infrastructure, providing the technological and logistical platform required to convert those models to an integrated, patient-specific clinical tool as well as to an improved analytic tool addressing health and health outcomes across populations of different sizes and patient characteristics.

Díaz-Zuccarini also provides one example of *a* Digital Patient in Chapter 2:

> a digital representation of a person's "health" and/or "disease" and a sophisticated decision support system, tailored to each one individual. Imagine, she says, a "virtual twin" of sorts, living in digital form, inside a computer. The virtual twin is shaped by the patient's medical history. It keeps a digital record of insulin levels, which are constantly tracked anyway, by a micro-sensor the doctors installed when they did that angioplasty and stented one of the patient's carotids. The virtual twin is a bit sleep-deprived, just like the patient, since he is not sleeping so well due to that back injury when he fell backwards skiing two years ago. It is allergic to that type of antibiotics and just like the patient, has "let itself go" a little bit, after binging on far too many chocolates.

Implicit in this example, and important for future research, are those characteristics of the "twin" that are related to time, behavior, and social context. Also important to note is the distinction between the realization of *a* Digital Patient and *the* Digital Patient platform.

One manifestation of the Digital Patient discussed in the DISCIPULUS project is the Patient Avatar. It is tempting to conflate the Patient Avatar and the Digital Patient. Although the Patient Avatar is *one* possible realization of the Digital Patient, it is only one such representation. The Digital Patient can be represented in an almost infinite variety of configurations—for example, avatars, mathematical models, curated data repositories, and animated graphs [16].

The DISCIPULUS Roadmap defined different "versions" (or levels of maturity) for the Digital Patient. These different "versions" correspond to what could be a short-/mid-/long-term vision for the Digital Patient. It was too difficult for the experts involved in the DISCIPULUS discussions to come up with definite categorizations and timescales, but nevertheless, the recommendations they provided will be relatively easy to position along a time continuum that goes from "I could come up with a small prototype if I work on this for a little while" to "this is achievable in a sensible time period with a lot of work" to "we don't know how to get there yet" [15].

Díaz-Zuccarini also notes that, in addition to patient data, Big Data in healthcare includes data from a myriad of other sources. For example, it includes data on claims and the cost of products and services, pharmaceutical data related to therapeutic mechanisms, side effects and toxicity, and patient behavior and patient activity data (such as from recordings of activity on smartphones or a Nintendo Wii, just to cite two examples). Important privacy issues are also obviously involved in aggregating and integrating the data required for the Digital Patient. One of the formidable challenges of having this diversity in data sources will be the determination of the ownership of the data: Does it belong to patients or to service providers or both, and who can use the data and under what conditions? These questions raise issues that must also be addressed during the continuing evolution of the Digital Patient.

ENABLING THE DIGITAL PATIENT

As the preceding narrative demonstrates, discussion about the subjects of a virtual human, the human physiome, and the Digital Patient highlights the need for integrating a broad spectrum of related topics. The chapters that follow showcase some of that diversity: various academic disciplines, methodologies, hypotheses, purposes, technologies, and practices that collectively contribute to advancing the Digital Patient. The narrative in this chapter simply foreshadows some of those topics: convergence, systems biology, multiscale modeling, standards, and the progress toward personalized medicine.

In January 2011, the Massachusetts Institute of Technology submitted a report to the health sciences research community introducing a new research model that is essential to the continued development of the Digital Patient. The research paradigm they developed is called *convergence*: the merging of distinct technologies, processing disciplines, or devices into a unified whole to create a host of new pathways and opportunities. Convergence implies the technical tools, as well as the disciplined analytic approaches, from design, engineering, and physics, and their adaptation to the life sciences. The strength in this research methodology is that it does not rest on a particular scientific advancement, but on an integrated approach for achieving advancements [17].

Focusing more directly on the type of convergence essential to the Digital Patient are systems biology and its subdiscipline systems physiology. Systems biology addresses interactions in biological systems at different scales of biological organization, from the molecular to the cellular, organ, organism, societal, and ecosystem levels. It is characterized by its integrative nature as compared to the mostly reductionist nature of molecular biology. It is also characterized by quantitative descriptions of biological processes, using a variety of mathematical and computational techniques. Thus, systems biology combines the development and application of predictive mathematical and computational modeling with experimental studies. The modeling techniques incorporate multiple spatial and temporal scales that are consistent with the integrative perspective of systems biology. Just as physiology is a branch of biology, systems physiology, systems medicine, and personalized medicine are subsets of systems biology. These levels of systems and their supporting informatics are shown in Figure 1.1.

Systems physiology focuses on the function of interacting parts of the system at the cell, tissue, organ, and organ system scales, and it is tightly coupled with structural anatomical information. Systems medicine is a subset of systems biology that addresses applications to clinical problems. Examples include the application of the systems biology framework to develop quantitative understandings of disease processes, to drug discovery, and to the design of diagnostic tools. A subset of systems medicine that relies on individual patient data or the data from a specific group of similar patients is the emerging domain of personalized medicine.

The interest in systems biology has been growing steadily during the past decade. As Noble noted, "Systems biology … is about putting together rather than taking apart, integration rather than reduction. It requires that we develop ways of thinking about integration that are as rigorous as our reductionist programs, but different … It means changing our philosophy, in the full sense of the term" [18].

An important question arises from a systems perspective about the construction of the Digital Patient: *What level of detail is necessary to simulate and, more importantly, accurately predict the efficacy of a patient-specific treatment?*

The understanding of human health, disability, and disease, and the rational design of preventive, diagnostic, or therapeutic strategies, depends on the quantitative knowledge of human anatomy and physiology and biological and social systems captured in reliable, validated mathematical models. Every other scientific discipline (from weather forecasting to the manufacture of everything from cell phones to aircraft) uses *a priori* knowledge of the

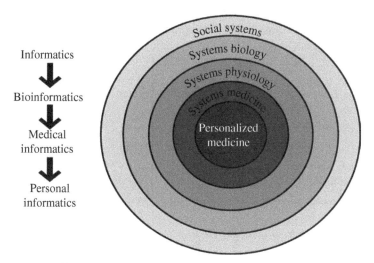

FIGURE 1.1   System of systems and levels of informatics.

physical laws of nature with model-based analysis and design. There is no reason to think that, ultimately, it will not be the same for biology. Indeed, the continued development of the Digital Patient will not be possible without the broad adoption of a system-of-systems analytic approach.

Computational physiology, for example, draws on techniques from numerous disciplines to address anatomical and physiological complexity by solving the mathematical equations that arise when the laws of physics and chemistry are coupled with the measurements of biological material properties. Disease is often a manifestation of the dysfunction of molecular-level processes, but the consequences are seen at scales ranging from the tissue to the organism. Computational physiology must therefore also address the challenges of multiscale physiological processes that operate over a 10^9 range of spatial scale (molecules to organ systems) and 10^{15} range of temporal scale (microseconds of biochemical reactions to the decades of aging processes). As we gain a quantitative understanding of human physiology through multiscale mathematical modeling and begin to adapt these generic models to an individual patient, there is an increasing need to describe disability and disease in terms of model parameters and to incorporate these parameters into electronic health records [19, 20]. The linking of computational models with health information from electronic health records, for example, has the potential to open up new vistas for biomedicine. The vast amount of clinical and wellness data could help validate models and allow for the customization of such models to individual patients and subpopulations [21].

Research and development of applications in the physiome, systems biology, the VPH, and personal health systems share one important challenge: *the need for integration*. That integration is the Digital Patient. To implement the outputs of biomedical research in clinical practice and within the healthcare industry, we need to integrate different data, information, knowledge, and wisdom. There is a need to integrate different types of data for the same patient stored across different systems, across different hospitals, across different countries, and in clinical research databases; patient-specific knowledge; information related to various parts and processes of the human body into a systemic understanding of pathophysiology; knowledge digitally captured via metadata, ontologies and models; and wisdom produced in research laboratories and in clinical practice, which can be formalized in guidelines, standards, and protocols and then used to promote translation of basic science and integrative models into improved healthcare outcomes [14].

One effort to address this required integration is the work of the US Interagency Modeling and Analysis Group (IMAG) and its companion group, the Multiscale Modeling Consortium (MSM). These two groups have several goals:

- to grow the field of multiscale modeling and biomedical biological and behavioral systems;
- to promote multidisciplinary scientific collaboration among multiscale modelers;
- to encourage future generations of multiscale modelers;
- to move the field of biological computational modeling forward in the following disciplines: predictive models of biology, health, disease, bioenergy, and bioremediation;
- to develop accurate methods that cross the interface between multiple spatial temporal scales;
- to promote model sharing in the development of reusable multiscale models; and
- to disseminate the models and insights derived from the models to the larger biomedical biological and behavioral research communities.

The IMAG/MSM efforts focus on the very important point that to realize the Digital Patient, data has to be valid, reliable, and capable of being accessed in many interacting models operating at different scales of time and space [13, 22, 23].

P4 MEDICINE

The convergence of systems approaches to disease, new measurement and visualization technologies, and new computational and mathematical tools can be expected to replace the current, largely reactive mode of medicine, where we wait until the patient is sick before responding with personalized, predictive, preventive, and participatory (P4) medicine that will be cost effective and increasingly focused on wellness.

One of the leaders in this P4 translational effort is Leroy Hood and his colleagues at the Institute for Systems Biology. According to Hood, the benefits of P4 medicine, to the patient and to the system, include new abilities to:

detect disease at an earlier stage, when it is easier and less expensive to treat effectively;

stratify patients into groups that enable the selection of optimal therapy;

reduce adverse drug reactions by more effective early assessment of individual drug responses;

improve the selection of new biochemical targets for drug discovery;

reduce the time, cost, and failure rate of clinical trials for new therapies; and

shift the emphasis in medicine from reaction to prevention and from disease to wellness [24, 25].

P4 medicine promises to sharply reverse the ever-escalating costs of healthcare by introducing personalized diagnosis, less-expensive approaches to drug discovery, a renewed emphasis on preventive medicine and wellness, and numerous cost-decreasing measurement technologies. P4 medicine also promises to improve patient outcomes and to empower both the patient and the physician [26]. Having much more, and more accurate, information to be used by the patient and the physician to make decisions about prevention and treatment is at the heart of aspirations for twenty-first-century medicine.

CONCLUSION

The expansion of the Digital Patient platform and its many possible representations and applications will be possible through careful attention over time to six focus areas: requirements, modeling and simulation, standards, tools and technology, infrastructure, and systems engineering. The focus on requirements highlights the importance of data, system, user, and interoperability requirements in building the Digital Patient out of a collection of simulations. The focus on modeling and simulation highlights the importance of obtaining information about the validity and usability of the many individual simulations that are being merged into the Digital Patient. The focus on standards provides a platform for success by establishing a standard format, language, tool set, and practice for aggregating simulations and forming the Digital Patient. The focus on tools and technology allows for emerging technologies to be integrated into the Digital Patient in the future.

The focus on infrastructure provides an environment through which the users can express their needs and requirements over time. The focus on systems engineering highlights that the Digital Patient needs to have guidelines for how it can be improved upon or updated over time in order to remain useful to the community.

The Digital Patient will not be constructed based solely on new information from all the "omics" studies, from the various efforts to model the human physiome and represent it virtually, from systems analysis, or from Big Data. It will only be realized through the purposeful collaboration of researchers (whether they are patients or scientific, clinical, or policy researchers) on both their research and the framework into which their research will fit. The Digital Patient will continue to depend on the efforts of a wide variety of individual researchers and modelers across many disciplines worldwide. It is inevitably an emergent phenomenon, governable only by sustained cooperation among those with an interest in its development and with guiding principles of openness, flexibility, rigorous validation and reliability processes, and respect for personal privacy.

That takes us back to Rich's observation that "the maps they gave us were out of date by years" and Dickens' statement that "if the courses be departed from, the ends will change." The chapters in this book raise issues and offer suggestions important to the continued realization of the Digital Patient, promising both a more current map and the prospect of a toolkit capable of helping us change the course toward better health.

REFERENCES

1 World Health Organization. Preamble to the Constitution of the World Health Organization as adopted by the International Health Conference, New York, 19–22 June, 1946; signed on July 22, 1946 by the representatives of 61 states (official Records of the World Health Organization, no. 2, p. 100) and entered into force on April 7, 1948.

2 Reuters. (January 20, 2015). Obama Calls for Major New Personalized Medicine Initiative. *The New York Times*. Retrieved January 27, 2015 from http://www.nytimes.com/reuters/2015/01/20/us/politics/20reuters-usa-obama-genomics.html (accessed on July 21, 2015).

3 Pear, R. (January 24, 2015). Obama to Request Research Funding for Treatments Tailored to Patients' DNA. *The New York Times*. Retrieved January 26, 2015 from http://www.nytimes.com/2015/01/25/us/obama-to-request-research-funding-for-treatments-tailored-to-patients-dn (accessed on July 21, 2015).

4 Institute of Medicine (IOM). Crossing the Quality Chasm: A New Health System for the 21st Century. 2001. Washington, DC: National Academy Press.

5 National Library of Medicine (US). The Visible Human Project®. Bethesda, MD: National Library of Medicine (US); 2003 September (updated July 28, 2006). Retrieved April 7, 2015 from http://www.nlm.nih.gov/research/visible/visible_human.html (accessed on July 21, 2015).

6 National Library of Medicine (US). 1986–2006: Two Decades of Progress. In NLM's Long Range Plan 2006–2016. Retrieved April 7, 2015 from http://www.nlm.nih.gov/pubs/plan/lrp06/report/default.html (accessed on July 21, 2015).

7 Clapworthy, G., Kohl, P., Gregerson, H., Thomas, S., Viceconti, M., Hose, D. et al. Digital Human Modelling: A Global Vision and a European Perspective. 2007 Berlin: Springer, 549–58.

8 STEP Research Road Map. Retrieved April 7, 2015 from http://www.digital-patient.net/files/DP-Roadmap_FINAL_N.pdf (accessed on August 12, 2015).

9 Fenner, J.W., Brook, B., Clapworthy, G., Coveney, P.V., Feipel, V., Gregerson, H. et al. (2008). The Europhysiome, STEP and a roadmap for the virtual physiological human. *Philosophical Transactions of the Royal Society A* 366 (1878): 2979–2999.

10 Viceconti, M., Taddei, F., Van Sint Jan, S., Leardini, A., Crisofolini, L., Stea, S. et al. (2008). Multiscale modeling of the skeleton for the prediction of the risk of fracture. *Clinical Biomechanics* 23 (7): 845–852.

11 Clapworthy, G., Viceconti, M., Coveney, P.V., Kohl, P. (2008). The virtual physiological human: Building a framework for computational biomedicine. I. Editorial. *Philosophical Transactions of the Royal Society A* 366 (1878): 2975–2978.

12 Popel, A.S., Hunter, P.J. (2009). Systems biology and physiome projects. *Wiley Interdisciplinary Reviews: Systems Biology and Medicine* 1(2): 153–158.

13 Hester, R.L., Iliescu, R., Summers, R., Coleman, T.G. (2011). Systems biology and integrative physiological modelling. *The Journal of Physiology* 589(5): 1053–1060.

14 Hunter, P., Chapman, T., Covenay, P.V., de Bono, B., Díaz, V., Fenner, J. et al. (2013). A vision and strategy for the virtual physiological human: 2012 update. *Interface Focus* 3: 20130004.

15 "Roadmap for the Digital Patient." (The Digital Patient Community and the DISCIPULUS Consortium). EU Project Discipulus. Vanessa Díaz-Zuccarini, Marco Viceconti, Veli Stroetmann, and Dipak Kalra (editors). 2013.

16 Rosling, H. (February 2006). Hans Rosling: The Best Stats You've Ever Seen (Video). Retrieved April 7, 2015 from http://www.ted.com/talks/hans_rosling_shows_the_best_stats_you_ve_ ever_seen (accessed on July 21, 2015).

17 Massachusetts Institute of Technology. (2011). The Third Revolution: The Convergence of the Life Sciences, Physical Sciences, and Engineering. Washington, DC: MIT Washington Office.

18 Noble, D. (2010). Biophysics and systems biology. *Philosophical Transactions A* 368. Available at: http://rsta.royalsocietypublishing.org/content/368/1914/1125.long (accessed on July 21, 2015).

19 Hunter, P.J., Crampin, E.J., Nielsen, P.M.F. (2008). Bioinformatics, multiscale modeling and the IUPS Physiome Project. *Briefings in Bioinformatics* 9 (4): 333–343.

20 Crampin, E.J., Halstead, M., Hunter, P., Nielsen, P., Noble, D., Smith, N. et al. (2003). Computational physiology and the physiome project. *Experimental Physiology* 89 1: 1–26.

21 Gjuvsland, A.B., Vik, J.O., Beard, D.A., Hunter, P.J., Omholt, S.W. 2013. Bridging the genotype–phenotype gap: What does it take? *The Journal of Physiology* 591: 2055–2066.

22 Interagency Modeling and Analysis Group (IMAG). Futures Meeting Final Report: The Impact of Modeling on Biomedical Research. Bethesda, MD: IMAG; December 15–16.

23 Interagency Modeling and Analysis Group (IMAG). Frequently Asked Questions. Retrieved from http://www.imagwiki.nibib.nih.gov/content/frequently-asked-questions-faq (accessed on March 16, 2015).

24 Hood, L. 2013. Systems biology and P4 (Predictive, Preventive, Participatory and Personalized Health) medicine: Past, present, and future. *Rambam Maimonides Medical Journal* 4(2): e0012.

25 Hood, L., Balling, R., Auffray, C. (2012). Revolutionizing medicine in the 21st century through systems approaches. *Biotechnology Journal* 7: 992–1001.

26 P4 Medicine Institute. The 4Ps: Quantifying Medicine Demystifying Disease. Retrieved from http://p4mi.org/4-ps-quantifying-wellness-and-demystifying-disease (accessed on November 25, 2014).

2

REFLECTING ON DISCIPULUS AND REMAINING CHALLENGES

VANESSA DÍAZ-ZUCCARINI, MONA ALIMOHAMMADI, AND CÉSAR PICHARDO-ALMARZA

Department of Mechanical Engineering, University College London, London, UK

INTRODUCTION

What is a Digital Patient? In loose terms, a Digital Patient (DP) is a digital representation of our "health" and/or "disease" and a sophisticated decision support system, tailored to each one of us. Imagine a "virtual twin" of sorts, living in digital form, inside a computer. Your virtual twin is shaped by your medical history. It keeps inside a digital record of your insulin levels that are constantly tracked anyway by that microsensor the doctors installed when they did that angioplasty and stented one of your carotids. Your virtual twin is a bit sleep deprived, just like you, since you are not sleeping so well due to that back injury when you fell backward skiing 2 years ago. It is allergic to that type of antibiotics and just like you has "let itself go" a little bit, after binging on far too many chocolates.

This description represents a vision of truly personalized medicine, which was at the heart of the project DISCIPULUS (EC funded, FP7/2007-2013, under grant agreement no. 288143) funded by the European Commission. DISCIPULUS was given the task of engaging the EU research community in order to develop a Roadmap toward the *Digital Patient* [1], a key component and conceptual child of the Virtual Physiological Human (VPH) initiative (www.vph-institute.org).

Within the scope of DISCIPULUS, the Digital Patient was defined as "a technological framework that, once fully developed, will make it possible to create a computer

The Digital Patient: Advancing Healthcare, Research, and Education, First Edition.
Edited by C. Donald Combs, John A. Sokolowski, and Catherine M. Banks.
© 2016 John Wiley & Sons, Inc. Published 2016 by John Wiley & Sons, Inc.

representation of the health status of each citizen that is descriptive and interpretive, integrative and predictive" [1].[1]

DISCIPULUS goal was to identify key steps toward realizing the Digital Patient by focusing on the needs of clinical practitioners, healthcare professionals, and biomedical and clinical researchers. In the DISCIPULUS vision, the Digital Patient would be achieved through comprehensive solutions that involve advanced (predictive) modeling and simulation tools, data acquisition, data management, and advanced user interfaces. This vision relies on making the clinical and research data available, creating a positive cycle of effective feedback for building better predictive models. All this would provide sufficient conditions to enable its clinical and industrial translation. One major step in utilizing these advancements would be to incorporate these models in a systematic way into the clinical decision-making process.

Before going into more detail, it is important for us to mention that the main ideas and findings presented in this chapter are the result of the DISCIPULUS Roadmap itself, and a great deal of material within this chapter comes directly from the Roadmap. This is a "digested" version of the discussions that took place. DISCIPULUS was a scientific endeavor that involved the participation and discussion of more than 250 scientists around Europe (and beyond). In this respect, we present the views and ideas of the *Digital Patient* (VPH) community, and do not claim that the information presented here is our own take on the Digital Patient. This is an important point, not only because we would like to give credit where credit is due, but also because it legitimizes the all-encompassing DISCIPULUS vision as the result of wide *consensus*, after much discussion and debate. Many of the definitions and recommendations come straight from the Roadmap since this chapter is supposed to present the DISCIPULUS point of view on the Digital Patient, and this is the primary source for this chapter. For detailed information on each topic, we must refer the reader to the Roadmap itself [1].

A BRIEF CONTEXTUAL BACKGROUND AND A CALL FOR INTEGRATION: PERSONALIZED MEDICINE IS HOLISTIC

Currently, there are numerous efforts underway in the design or development of distinct components of the *Digital Patient*, which is itself (as previously mentioned), part of the VPH initiative. The VPH became the *de facto* EU arm of the *Physiome* project, presented at the meeting of the International Union of Physiological Sciences (IUPS) by its Commission on Bioengineering in Physiology in 1993. The initial setup for the VPH was the outcome of the project "Strategy for the Europhysiome" (STEP, EC funded FP6/2006–2007, grant agreement 027642) and corresponding Roadmap [2]. This continued support from the European Commission has seen the emergence of several,

---

[1] Descriptive—it provides unified access to all information about the patient's health determinants, including those related to life-style, such as physical activity; and interpretative—it helps to gain new understanding.
Integrative—it automatically combines all the available information, so as to provide better decision support based on a large volume of information.
Predictive—the integrated information is used to inform individualized simulations able to predict how specific aspects of subject's health will develop over time, as a function of different interventions.

powerful and innovative projects and initiatives dealing with different aspects of what we could generally call "*in silico* medicine."[2]

Within the vast field of the Digital Patient, there is much fragmentation, partly because the ultimate aim, that is, "personalized medicine" has been used to describe medicine based on "omics" approaches (e.g., genomics, metabolomics, and transcriptomics). However, there is a more encompassing and powerful view emerging—personalized medicine *must* address the challenge of the "whole," by embracing a holistic view. The *Digital Patient* Roadmap follows the blueprint set out by the VPH, in that its approach is better characterized by the term "middle-out," [3] which is based on identifying a level that is relatively well understood in terms of data and processes, and then connecting this to "upper" and "lower" levels of structural and functional integration [4]. This was the fundamental driver behind the Roadmap prepared by DISCIPULUS, and it must be understood in that context. Nevertheless, it is also true that all the work in the "omics" areas not only fits in, but it is an essential constituent. In "Big biology: the 'omes puzzle" [5] the authors point out at the necessity of a "phenome" and even an "integrome"; this clearly signals a road in which information is integrated at the gene scale within a wider context. This is the approach that we have advocated throughout the process of trying to elucidate what the *Digital Patient* is. This "integrative aspect" is highlighted as the fundamental element of systems medicine [6], where molecular data (especially genomic information) is integrated with anatomical, physiological, environmental, and lifestyle data in a predictive model approach, in order to produce "virtual patients." All these approaches can and will contribute to the Digital Patient, and the specifics of these domains have been extensively covered in other roadmaps. DISCIPULUS focused on having integrative modeling and simulation at the core, and in that sense DISCIPULUS' take on this issue made it unique. During the preparation of the DISCIPULUS Roadmap, a number of parallel initiatives were also omitted in order to keep the "problem" of defining what the Digital Patient was somewhat tractable. Some of these initiatives, such as precision medicine, systems medicine, stratified medicine [7], P4 medicine [8], and so on, have been widely reported in the scientific literature and the media. Again, the DP vision represented by DISCIPULUS shares with all these other initiatives the desire for a more integrative approach to healthcare, one where information technology is used as the main instrument to tackle the huge complexity involved.

Finally yet importantly, another term that emerged from the DISCIPULUS discussion is the "Patient Avatar." It is rather tempting to amalgamate the Patient Avatar *and* the Digital Patient as one. However, one of the conclusions of the "Roadmap Toward the Digital Patient" report is that the Patient Avatar *might be a possible realization* of the Digital Patient. Only time will tell if the *Patient Avatar* will become in fact the *Digital Patient*. This "split" will be explained in the following section, albeit succinctly. For more information, the reader is referred to Ref. [1].

---

[2] The VPH vision defined as "a framework of methods and technologies that, once established, will make it possible to investigate the human body as a whole" is a fundamental, multidisciplinary development. When deployed, it will have a profound impact on healthcare and well-being and will present a radical departure from the way medicine is practiced in millions of hospitals across the world. It calls for a total transformation in the way healthcare currently works and is delivered to patients. Underpinning this transformation is substantial technological innovation with a requirement for deeper transdisciplinary research, improved IT infrastructure, better communication, large volumes of high-quality data, and superior tools to those we have now. It also requires a considerable measure of political support; initial developments are likely to be costly, but once the initial deployment costs have been met, overall cost savings are expected to be significant [1].

THE MANY VERSIONS OF THE DIGITAL PATIENT: ON THE ROAD TO MEDICAL AVATARS

As part of the DISCIPULUS initiative, we felt it was necessary to provide a feasible pathway of progression for what the Digital Patient might become. The Digital Patient in our vision was an evolving process directed by a clear need to *make a difference in the clinic*. However, we felt that by reducing the Digital Patient to its ultimate realization (a "Patient Avatar") we would be positioning it as an aspirational goal, almost belonging to the realm of science fiction. Instead, we chose to present it as a metamorphosis: an evolving development able to revolutionize healthcare *from right now*. This is possible, thanks not only to the development of new science and disruptive technologies (which conjures visions of singularities, unique ideas that change a field forever) but also to the "reinvention" of current science, including existing methods and approaches applied in novel ways, incremental scientific advancements in specific areas, and the use and (creative) reuse of current available technologies. Furthermore, we fully acknowledge that although the Patient Avatar as imagined by most of us is too far in the future, there is definitely a space to present the *Digital Patient* (version 1.01) as something that can be achieved in the near future, with current technologies. Our starting point for this reasoning was the fact that given the enormity of the task, the ambition of having a fully functioning Patient Avatar would be perceived as a chimera, which is far from the case if we understand that *the road toward the Digital Patient is a process*. We would rather use the Patient Avatar to signal a direction. In a rather clumsy analogy, when Alexander Graham Bell started working on his "harmonic telegraph" that eventually would become the telephone, he might have dreamed (or not!) of communications without cables in the future. However, the current developments in terms of mobile phones and smartphone technologies are, we are pretty sure, well beyond his wildest dreams. And still, here we are.

With this in mind, we defined different "versions" (or levels of maturity) for the Digital Patient. These different "versions" correspond to what could be a short-/mid-/long-term vision for the Digital Patient. It was rather difficult for the experts involved in the DISCIPULUS discussions to come up with definite categorizations and timescales; but nevertheless, we believe that the recommendations they provided will be, for the trained eye, relatively easy to position along a time continuum that goes from "I could come up with a small prototype if I work on this for a little while," to "this is achievable in a sensible time with some/a lot (of) work" to "we don't know how to get there yet." The "maturity levels" are briefly presented in the following (see also Fig. 2.1):

> *Maturity level 1: Interactive health analytics*—Consider the development of exploratory interfaces that enable a more holistic exploration of the data currently available at multiple points of care for each patient; here the goal is improved fusion of all existing knowledge about each patient (individualized knowledge fusion).
>
> *Maturity level 2: Individualized well-being and healthcare management*—This implies that the available clinical data is not only explored but also truly integrated into simulation-based decision support systems that guide fully individualized treatment decisions.
>
> *Maturity level 3: The Patient Avatar*—This involves a more global integration of data collected at the "point of care" and at the "point of life," as well as a broader range of simulations of pathophysiological processes, not necessarily related to the specific

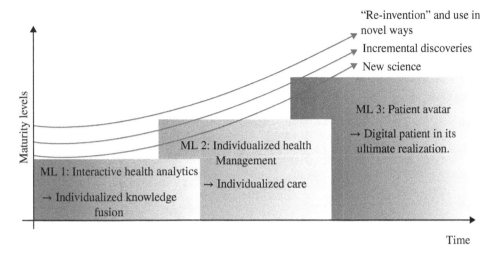

FIGURE 2.1   Different "maturity levels" of the Digital Patient [1].

disease in question. The result is truly integrative medicine, capable of coping with patients with polydiseases, comorbidities, and complex cases more effectively; the goal is the full realization of the Digital Patient vision.

DISCIPULUS: THE DIGITAL PATIENT TECHNOLOGICAL CHALLENGES AND MAIN CONCLUSIONS

The overall concept of the Digital Patient was split into its component parts in order to define the technological challenges, from the initial inputs in terms of data and information to the ultimate goal: translation and adoption. The main areas of technological challenges are illustrated in Figure 2.2.

The different technological challenges reflect areas in which there is still much work to do. These areas are needed in order to achieve the *Digital Patient*, according to the DISCIPULUS vision (Fig. 2.2). These areas are generation of data, biomedical information management, mathematical modeling, clinical user interface, and, last but by no means least, translation and adoption. For each one of these areas, the main outcomes of the Roadmap are described in the section that follows.

Main Outcomes [1]

Area: Generation of Data for Model Construction, Validation, and Application   The generation, standardization, validation, integration, and homologation of data were identified by the wider community to be of the utmost importance. The realization of the Digital Patient vision is heavily dependent on the availability and organization of massive amounts of data for a range of purposes. These purposes can be ascribed to three categories: (i) for building models (i.e., gathering and structuring information to identify interactions and translating them into numeric); (ii) for validating models (i.e., comparing models against some ground truths to falsify/corroborate them); and (iii) for populating models with patient-specific information (i.e., deploying validated models in a clinical context).

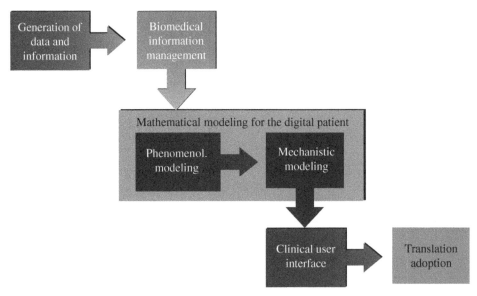

FIGURE 2.2   Different areas needed to achieve the "Digital Patient," according to the DISCIPULUS vision [1].

In order to achieve these goals, we need to considerably focus on facilitating the generation, standardization, certification, and integration of data, targeting the following main application areas: construction and validation of data-driven prediction models, application of data-driven prediction models within primary and secondary healthcare, construction and validation of causal and predictive models, application of causal models within primary/secondary care, and multidimensional phenotypic data analysis, to uncover new important patterns that can serve as inspiration for statistical and causal models.

From the discussions, a few areas emerged as requiring targeted support and significant effort in research and innovation:

1. Exploration of suitable existing and possible new sources of information, development of new acquisition methods, devices, and technological tools, and the use of longitudinal data, both across the disease time course and the life span, including data on comorbidities.

2. Development and adoption of acquisition methods and technology to determine genotype and measure high-level phenotypes—anatomical data obtained from next-generation image modalities such as magnetic resonance imaging (MRI), computerized tomography (CT), and ultrasound (US); new imaging and sensing technologies for the acquisition of data in more physiological conditions such as standing, moving, and exercising; new (wearable, multimodal) sensors and sensor data analysis to obtain functional data, also during daily life (point of life); lab-on-a-chip devices to obtain biomarker and gene expression data; and new phenomics technology.

3. Development and homologation of next-generation acquisition methods (data independent from the acquisition system, the acquisition method, or the acquisition source).

4. Exploitation and initiation of new developments in data formatting and data processing to enable enhanced data provision—advanced ICT solutions to (preferably automatically) collect and format data and provide it to the Digital Patient for use and sharing. This includes denoising and dimensionality reduction of the raw data and of the extracted feature space: data formatted in a predefined standardized and certified way (provided patient consent about the level usage is embedded) for research purposes.

Area: Biomedical Information Management

Whereas the mere acquisition of biomedical data has become relatively trivial and affordable, the management of this data remains a daunting challenge, despite decades of research. Biomedical information management is a complex multifaceted problem, including challenges such as the collection and sharing of data (a paradigm shift within the scientific and broader community such that data are gradually considered a public good), the standardization of data collection, the question of ontology, dimensionality reduction, the question of security and privacy, and the computer and storage infrastructure needed to store enormous amounts of data retrievable rapidly, safely, and from everywhere. These facets are interdependent, which renders biomedical information management extremely demanding. Despite many years of R&D projects and standardization, electronic health record (EHR) systems and diagnostic tools of different modalities often still use different information models and semantics to represent clinical data. This makes it challenging to scale up the corpus of data to support VPH model development and validation, and to ensure that deployed VPH models can safely reason on the holistic information about individual patients. Semantic interoperability remains a major challenge for healthcare and for research. Recommendations are as follows:

1. To develop patient-centered authorization mechanisms that allow automatic requests for secondary use of clinical data after collection and anonymization
2. To develop methods to compute k-anonymity for anonymized secondary use databases of clinical data when combined with any other information available on the Internet
3. To strengthen the efforts to develop dynamic semantic mediation strategies that allow clinical specialists to participate in multicentric data collection with clinical data available in their research warehouses, employing easy-to-use procedures to define the semantic mapping between the local warehouse structure and the collection ontology
4. To develop automatic extraction of quantified phenotypical disease traits, and use these as similarity metrics to retrieve cases comparable to the one at hand from within the warehouse
5. To develop new innovative storage and computing services that enable data-intensive analysis of biomedical big data, preserved economically over long term

Area: Mathematical Modeling for the Digital Patient

The Digital Patient relies on the power of predictive modeling to be able to progress into a "Patient Avatar" as its final realization. This power is intimately linked to models' capacity to transform observational data into knowledge. In fact, it can be argued that modeling is at the core and the most fundamental element of the Digital Patient as it is able to seize observations, data, and explanations to formulate them and/or capture them in a mathematical and numerical form, in order to achieve the goal of explanatory/predictive medicine. It is the extraordinary and compelling power of multiscale predictive models that will help achieving the full potential of the Digital Patient. Within this context, the areas that have been identified as priorities in modeling are as follows:

1. Support the creation of online repositories to house and share disease-specific and patient-specific data and models to enhance collaboration within the VPH community, providing ubiquitous access (in compliance with data protection, privacy, and confidentiality rules)

2. Prioritize the development of relatively simple models that address specific topics in patient studies, for the expansion of diagnostic methods and therapies in the clinic

3. Develop hybrid methods and strategies to automatically and seamlessly combine phenomenological and mechanistic models, exploiting the use of VPH ontologies and annotated online repositories containing well-documented and validated models

4. Develop surrogate modeling methods that make possible to replace computational demanding submodels, typically large PDE models (partial differential equation models), with estimators developed on precomputed solutions, to provide a fast estimate of the model outputs and an upper boundary of the estimation error

5. Develop integrative modeling frameworks that support the abduction cycle that applies inductive reasoning to observations, in order to generate hypotheses on mechanistic relationships, verify these against reference observations, and where predictions are in good agreement with observations, incorporate this new mechanistic understanding into the inductive reasoning, thereby facilitating new discoveries

6. Personalize not only anatomical data but also the physiological/pathological processes taking place (multiscale) by linking model parameters to easily obtainable patient data, leading to an individual patient model rather than a statistical patient model

7. Develop fast numerical restart methods that make it possible to employ user exploration of the information space to rerun the model with different inputs at very low computational cost when compared to the first run

8. Develop a theoretical framework for the analysis of (spatiotemporal) scale separation, and general homogenization and distribution strategies to define space–time relations across scales

9. Develop strategies to formalize and generalize the testing and validation of mathematical models, providing accurate and automatic estimations on the impact that incomplete data has in the personalized models

Area: Clinical User Interface

For citizens or for clinical research? The discussions on this topic dealt with the dichotomy of having potentially two different target groups: clinicians and patients as "users" of the Digital Patient. In line with the vision and strategy for the VPH, the Digital Patient should ultimately be viewed as a tool for citizens, promoting future health and well-being by fostering the maintenance for a healthy lifestyle, by providing early symptom notifications and allowing personal health forecasting.

However, tailoring the Digital Patient framework to accomodate the needs and interests of individual citizens via tools that are sufficiently explained and tested, as well as developed directly for them (and relatively simple), is a long-term vision. By identifying translation and clinical uptake as the primary focuses, the Digital Patient in the Roadmap is intended for clinicians and clinical researchers, and it is in this context that the Roadmap should be understood.

Along these lines, currently working prototypes are available and allow the three-dimensional exploration of large amounts of information on human anatomy, physiology, and pathology, referred to an average subject (generic) in fixed time point (static). Future research should prioritize the following:

1. Support for effective management of individualized data
2. The extension of existing tools to support time-varying, dynamic data, and support multiscale interactive visualization for data defined at different time scales (data defined across different spatial scales)
3. The development of efficient methodologies for the rapid generation of image-based functionalized anatomical models for safety assessment and treatment planning
4. Extensions to support novel human computer interaction and interactive visualization that allow the usage of large-scale data from heterogeneous sources for knowledge discovery
5. Extensions to support effective information retrieval
6. Extensions to support seamless interfacing with the existing healthcare systems under the criteria of clinical adaptability
7. Extensions to support sound evaluations of Digital Patient technologies

Area: Translation and Adoption

Good examples of computational modeling in medicine have been around for 50 years or more, for example, the diagnosis of congenital heart disease [9]. Some methods based on mathematical models have been in routine use for the past 20 years (e.g., in managing CV risk) [10]. What is new are the benefits emerging from current ICT solutions, particularly in terms of speed and data-handling capacity. Mathematical models and techniques have demonstrated, for example, a key role in policy-making, including health economics, emergency planning, and risk assessment, among many others. The area of translation requires the development or the adaptation of formal processes for verification, sensitivity analysis, validation (including clinical trials), risk-benefit and cost-benefit analyses, and, ultimately, leading to product certification. Reference to the pharmaceutical and medical device industries provides guidance on suitable methodological approaches, but further developments will be required.

1. Input is required from regulators to define the full translational path from verification to certification for different types of Digital Patient solutions. This will, by necessity, be a two-way process as regulatory experts will need to be familiarized with the VPH concepts and the DP landscape.
2. Health technology assessment methodologies must be adapted and adopted to compare VPH solutions with current standard of care.

3. It is unlikely that current conceptual prototypes, developed as proof of concept, can be effective for direct clinical translation. It will be necessary to reengineer current prototypes for each specific clinical task, reengineering the user interface to specific prevention, diagnosis, prognosis, treatment planning, and monitoring purposes.

4. Sets of metrics are required, including both objective indicators and subjective indicators that capture the user experience; user cohorts must be stratified to represent realistic and relevant clinical scenarios (e.g., trainees, senior users with low IT exposure, etc.). Clusters of descriptors for patient analyses will have to be revised based upon novel hypotheses generated through VPH/DP technologies.

5. Health economic and business models must be developed to identify and validate the business case of implementing a specific clinical application for each group of relevant stakeholders, placing the Digital Patient within the hospital, clinic, or surgery context, as well as for the health system as a whole.

6. There will be a significant demand for education and training. Training programs will be required to provide technicians with a strong underpinning knowledge base. In early and mid-term stages of translation, training in principles of the respective VPH model/DP solution will be needed for clinical end users.

THE REMAINING CHALLENGES AND BIG DATA

Perhaps and on reflection, the DISCIPULUS Roadmap should have included a more distinct section on "big data." "Big data" challenges were recognized in the Roadmap itself across different technological areas, in particular data, biomedical information management, and mathematical modeling, which is not in itself surprising. As previously explained, the Digital Patient (and VPH for that matter) is firmly rooted on the basis of developing mathematical models capable of accurately predicting what will happen to a biological system. To tackle this huge challenge, multifaceted research is necessary and the challenges of this research are well explained in the *Digital Patient* challenges, described in previous sections. However, the real challenge is the production of multiscale, mechanistic knowledge (defined over space and time) capable of being predictive with sufficient accuracy. Therefore, it follows that recently, especially in the area of personalized healthcare, there is a huge push to use big data technologies as a complementary approach, in order to reduce the complexity that developing a reliable, quantitative mechanistic knowledge involves.

In particular, part of this huge "data explosion" comes from the "omics" fields. As presented in Ref. [11], genomics and postgenomics technologies produce very large amounts of raw data about the complex biochemical processes that regulate each living organism; nowadays, a single deep-sequencing dataset can exceed 1 TB. More recently, we started to see the generation of "deep phenotyping" data, where biochemical, imaging, and sensing technologies are used to quantify complex phenotypical traits and link them to the genetic information. These data are processed with specialized big data analytics techniques, which come from bioinformatics, but recently there is growing interest in building mechanistic models of how the many species present inside a cell interact along complex biochemical pathways. Because of the complexity and the redundancy involved, linking this very large body of mechanistic knowledge to the higher-order cell–cell and cell–tissue interactions remains very difficult, primarily for the data analytics problems it involves. But when this is possible, genomics research results finally link to clinically relevant pathological signs, observed at tissue, organ, and organism scales, opening the door to a true systems medicine.

However, despite the obvious impact of "omics" data in modeling and technologies sequencing huge amounts of data, "big data" aspects permeated all the chapters of the DISCIPULUS Roadmap: from visualization techniques, to the challenge of medical treatment and commercialization (product and service developments). According to the report "Big and Open Data in Europe: A Growth Engine or a Missed Opportunity?" [12], big data has the potential to contribute €206 billion to the European economy by 2020; however, only 5% of this is in the healthcare sector. In particular, the report highlights the healthcare sector as one example where the introduction of ICT is highly valuable, given enormous amounts of data produced ("data produced by monitoring patients and effects of different treatments"), and in light of the current financial and demographic challenges.

As fleetingly mentioned in the Roadmap itself, healthcare is also one of those cases where open data are expected to play an important role by providing additional incentives for management improvements. This might work well in certain countries (e.g., the United States) where the business model for healthcare is more reliant on the private sector. The story is less clear in Europe though, where the healthcare sector, traditionally dominated by public financing, can expect a much smaller return on investments in big and open data projects.

The availability of new data will allow the development of applications to make it easier to share and analyze information, in order to improve healthcare quality and reduce costs. According to Ref. [13], sound use of these applications and data holds the potential to change the landscape of healthcare. To enable such a breakthrough, advanced new computing infrastructure is needed, where storage for big data with offloaded functions plays a key role, as data warehouses are where the data resides most of its lifetime. Such pioneering scalable storage should allow easy sharing and exchange of the data (while maintaining security and confidentiality requirements), support computing close to the data, including powerful analytics, and preserve the data for decades.

Additionally, the need for user-friendly interfaces between the data and users of the data, in particular the clinicians, cannot be underestimated. It is essential that the end user has an unambiguous and clear way to input and extract data, particularly where it may be categorized in various ways. It may be necessary to use alternative categorization from the end-user perspectives, as compared to the data storage, in order to facilitate easy access. Ultimately, the success of the clinical translation of the Digital Patient requires that the clinicians are willing and able to interface with the project on a daily basis [14, 15].

A final consideration is that apart from patient data, big data in healthcare includes also data from a myriad of other sources, for example, from claims and cost of products and services; pharmaceutical data related to therapeutic mechanisms, side effects and toxicity; and patient behavior and patient activity (think about those recording activity on their smartphones or with a Nintendo Wii, just to cite two examples). In addition to the privacy issue, mentioned in the "Biomedical Information Management" section, probably one of the main challenges of having this diversity in the data sources will be to determine the ownership of the data: does it belong to patients or to service providers? This raises all sorts of ethical issues, which need to be addressed alongside the evolution of the Digital Patient.

CONCLUSION

This chapter presented the outcome of the EC-funded project DISCIPULUS and the "Roadmap for the Digital Patient" report. It also presented in a compact way the vision of the Digital Patient by the VPH community, and it discussed some challenges with regard to "big data." The "Roadmap for the Digital Patient" presents a compelling vision in which progressive, evolving technologies might give birth to the Patient (or Medical) Avatar for predictive and personalized medicine.

REFERENCES

1 "Roadmap for the digital patient" (DISCIPULUS Consortium). Vanessa Díaz-Zuccarini, Marco Viceconti, Veli Stroetmann (eds.). 2013. Funded by the European Commission under FP7-ICT, Project reference: 288143. Available at: http://cordis.europa.eu/project/rcn/100758_en.html (accessed on August 27, 2015).

2 Seeding the EuroPhysiome: a roadmap to the virtual physiological human (STEP Consortium). Viceconti M., Clapworthy G. (eds.). 2007.

3 Brenner S., Noble D., Sejnowski T., Fields R. D., Laughlin S., Berridge M., Segel L., Prank K., Dolmetsch R. E. (2001). Understanding complex systems: top-down, bottom-up or middle-out? In Novartis Foundation Symposium: Complexity in Biological Information Processing, Bock G., Goode J. (eds.), Vol. 239, pp. 150–159 Chichester: John Wiley & Sons Ltd. Kaiserin-Freidrich-Haus, Berlin, Germany, July 4–6, 2000.

4 Kohl P., Noble D. Systems biology and the virtual physiological human. *Molecular Systems Biology* 2009; 5: 292.

5 Baker M. Big biology: the 'omes puzzle. *Nature, News Feature* 2013; 494(7438): 416–419.

6 Regierer B., Zazzu V., Sudbrak R., Kühn A., Lehrach H. Future of medicine: models in predictive diagnostics and personalized medicine. *Advances in Biochemical Engineering/Biotechnology* 2013; 133: 15–33.

7 Stratified Medicine Innovation Platform". InnovateUK Technology Strategy Board. Available at: https://connect.innovateuk.org/web/stratified-medicines-innovation-platform/overview (accessed on October 12, 2015).

8 P4 Medicine Institute. Available at: http://p4mi.org/p4medicine (accessed on October 13, 2015).

9 Warner H. R., Toronto A. F., Veasey L. G., Stephenson R. A mathematical approach to medical diagnosis: application to congenital heart disease. *JAMA* 1961; 177: 75–81.

10 Horrocks J. C., McCann A. P., Staniland J. R., Leaper D. J., de Dombal F. T. Computer-aided diagnosis: description of an adaptable system, and operational experience with 2,034 cases. *British Medical Journal* 1972; 2(5804): 5–9.

11 Viceconti M., Hunter P., McCormack K., Henney A., Omholt S. W., Graf N., Morley-Fletcher E., Geris L., Hose R. Big data, big knowledge: big data for personalised healthcare. White paper, published by the Virtual Physiological Human for Integrative Research. Available at: www.vph-institute.org (accessed on August 4, 2015);2014.

12 Buchholtz S., Bukowski M., Śniegocki A. Big and open data in Europe: a growth engine or a missed opportunity? demosEUROPA in cooperation with the Warsaw Institute for Economic Studies (WISE Institute), Warsaw, 2014.

13 Groves P., Kayyali B., Knott D., Van Kuiken S. The 'big data' revolution in healthcare. Accelerating value and innovation. Center for US Health System Reform Business Technology Office. McKinsey & Company, January 2013. Available at: http://mckinsey.com/insights/health_systems_and_services/the_big_data_revolution_in_us_health_care (accessed October 12, 2015).

14 Shah J., Pradhan S., Zaveri A. Electronic data capture for registries and clinical trials in orthopaedic surgery. *Clinical Orthopaedics and Related Research* 2010; 468: 2664–2671.

15 Zheng K., Padman R., Johnson M. P., Diamond H. S. An interface-driven analysis of user interactions with an electronic health records system. *Journal of the American Medical Informatics Association* 2009; 16: 228–237.

3

ADVANCING THE DIGITAL PATIENT

CATHERINE M. BANKS

Virginia Modeling, Analysis and Simulation Center, Old Dominion University, Suffolk, VA, USA

INTRODUCTION

Any preliminary read on the subject of a virtual human … human physiome … digital patient lays bare the need for integrating the wide spectrum of topics and technologies associated with this research and development. Reading through the chapters of this compendium will prove out that diversity—various disciplines, methodologies, hypotheses, purposes, technologies, and practices—contributes to advancing the digital patient. This brief discussion introduces the origins, evolution, and expansion in this field of enquiry. As with all interdisciplinary studies, it will be useful to first layout a common lexicon with the introduction and/or operationalization of phrases and words found in that preliminary read on this subject:

- *Complicated and complex systems*—these systems diverge based on the level of understanding of the system; a physics-based model is complicated because it has numerous parts, but it is not complex in that it is predictable. On the other hand, a complex system like the human body might have fewer parts, but it is complex because it is difficult to ascertain absolutes in the data as humans are organic; one cannot predict the behavior of the human system with any certainty.
- *Computer and computational models*—a computer model refers to the algorithms and equations used to capture the behavior of the system being modeled; while the computational model is a mathematical model that requires extensive computational resources (e.g., computer memory and speed) to study the behavior of a complex system by computer simulation.

- *Interoperability and integration*—the technical term "interoperability" refers to computer systems that can exchange information; integration (of systems) seeks to embed existing and new systems into an existing environment.
- *Live, virtual, constructive simulation*—examples of each in the medical domain are as follows: live—using live actors to mimic illness; virtual—synthetic training environments where people employ simulated equipment like the virtual operating room; constructive—simulated people and simulated equipment augment real-world conditions like the virtual stethoscope.
- *Simulation and simulator*—simulation is a means, a technique, to replace or augment real-world experiences with case studies or guided experiences that represent or replicate substantial aspects of that real-world with an interactive capacity; the simulator is a device that can be used to accomplish this, such as a computerized manikin that can mimic fluid loss.
- *Digital Patient*—an artificial human being to include anatomical, physiological, and behavioral attributes.
- *Anatomical model*—models of the human anatomy ranging in complexity from single cell to organ-to-organ system; single or multiple components (e.g., the femur or the entire skeletal system) with a view to studying form, *what it is*.
- *Physiological model*—models to understand how the anatomy works in totality; how cells, muscles, and organs operate together and interact from the molecular basis to whole integrated behavior of entire body with a view to studying function, *what it does*.
- *Behavioral model*—for purposes of this study, this modeling focuses on representing changes in human behavior the result of a wide range of factors such as information, motivation, ability, and physical change.
- *Individualized and personalized patient care*—moving from treating the individual patient based on the at-large norms for his/her symptoms or disease patterns, then prescribing norm-set treatment options to personalized patient care with specified treatment options that are not norm driven.

THE DIGITAL PATIENT: ITS EARLY START

Numerous efforts have been and currently are underway in the design of and/or distinct components of the digital patient. Some of the earliest work is the concept presented to the International Union of Physiological Sciences (IUPS) by its Commission on Bioengineering in Physiology in 1993. Within 3 years, a workshop on organizing the Physiome Project was underway; by 2001, IUPS designated the human Physiome Project a primary focus of work for the next decade. Heading the research is the Physiome Commission of the IUPS; core to the Commission is the integration of models of components of organisms through the development of databases and models, which would facilitate the understanding of the integrative function of cells, organs, and organisms. The Project's goal is compiling and delivering a central repository of databases, and linking experimental information and computational models from many laboratories into a single, self-consistent framework as a means of promoting a holistic, analytical approach to medicine and physiology. One of the participants in the Physiome Project, the National Simulation Resource at the University of Washington, Department of Bioengineering, provided a number of tools such as data-basing information ranging from functional behavior of molecules, to observations intact cellular systems descriptive models, computational models, and search engines both networked and web-based.

Another group of contributors to the Human Physiome research and development are the scientists at Auckland University (New Zealand). This project is an integrated program aimed at archiving and disseminating quantitative data and models of the functional behavior of human anatomy from molecules to tissues to organism. This project sets apart modeling hierarchies (genes, proteins, biophysical models, constitutive laws, organ models, and whole-body models) and makes them available in various databases. The models are primarily mathematical.[1] The visualization tools are web-based, animated visualizations of computational outputs.

In the United States, the University of Southern California Institute for Creative Technologies (ICT) is home to an extensive effort conducting basic applied research in immersive technologies to advance and maintain state of the art for a human synthetic experience. Many of the participants in the research view the synthetic experience as real. This team is engaging avatars and traditional learning environments to create a mixed-reality setting. The research at ICT is also engaged in behavioral modeling. ICT has developed six research areas: (i) cognitive architecture (integrated digital patients and intelligent robots), (ii) embodiment (nonverbal behavior), (iii) emotion (computational systems that use emotion to communicate and to influence memory), (iv) integrated digital patients (provides a prototype to create your own digital patient), (v) multicomp lab (visual cues), and (vi) natural language processing (digital patients interacting with people).

At Stanford University holograms are used as a means to understand interactions among people in immersive virtual reality and other forms of digital representation in media. The depth of this research begs the question, what does this project present in the way of representing the body's physiological and behavioral systems?

Another significant effort is the LINDSAY Digital Patient, a three-dimensional, multiscale, interactive computer model of male and female anatomy and physiology. The University of Calgary is leading this collaborative project: Departments of Computer Science and Undergraduate Medical Education, and the faculty of medicine—Virtual Medical Education Unit. The goal of the LINDSAY project is to present biological models and computational tools for research and learning of human anatomy and physiology via a component-based computational framework, facilitating the interrogation of the human body in depth, interactively, and in real time. The simulation ranges from the body systems level to organ, tissue, cell, and subcellular structural levels. These agent-based simulations replicate the physiological processes of these ranges. Coupled with the diverse capability is the availability of the product: the LINDSAY Digital Patient is available as e-Learning software, touch table applications, iPad/iPhone apps, 3D anatomy (Presenter), 4D physiology (Composer). Much of the literature produced as part of this effort focuses on the technical development of these tools.

We should not leave this discussion without presenting a key aspect to engaging all components available as parts of the state of the art: measurement and metrics. One such organization focused on performance metrics is the group founded by Johns Hopkins Medicine, MedBiquitous. Operating at the international level, the group is developing and promoting technology standards for the health professions to advance lifelong learning,

---

[1] The mathematical models range five levels: level 1, molecular; level 2, subcellular Markov models; level 3, subcellular ODE (ordinary differential equations) models; level 4, tissue and whole organ continuum models; level 5, whole body system models.

continuous improvement, and better patient outcomes. MedBiquitous is accredited by the American National Standards Institute (ANSI) to develop information technology standards supporting the health professions. The group is focused on creating a technology blueprint for advancing the health professions that will seamlessly support the learner in ways to improve patient outcomes and simplify the administrative work associated with lifelong learning and continuous improvement. Specific to the digital patient, MedBiquitous has engaged a Virtual Patient Working Group to focus on developing XML standards and web services requirements to enable interoperability, accessibility, and reusability of web-based virtual patient learning content.

ENGAGING THE DIGITAL PATIENT

Simply stated, human biology is a science of complexity. The typical approach to studying this complex entity called the human body has been *reductionist biology* in which the scientist looks at specific segments of the body, in essence taking the pieces apart. This has its place in the examination of individual anatomical components, but it falls short when attempting a holistic analysis of the body. Thus, an approach that accommodates an integrated, interoperable, that is, complex and dynamic, examination of human biology coupled with physiological and behavioral components of the individual's experience is ideal. And that is what simulation delivers in the form of the digital patient. Moreover, a digital patient approach to patient care can provide the best personal health system because it encourages, even requires, that the patient be more aware and take an active role in his own health as opposed to depending on hospitals, clinics, and specialists.

1. *Research*—for purposes of this discussion, research encompasses engaging the digital patient to conduct medical studies and in the development of devices and tools. Medical studies serve to eliminate danger to human subjects: such as disease and treatment studies, pharmaceutical development, and biologic medicine. With regard to devices and tools, the US Food and Drug Administration (FDA) is responsible for the oversight of these apparati under its Center for Devices and Radiological Health. The Center regulates via four evaluation models: animal, bench, computational, and human. Simulation supports this evaluation as it is premised on mathematical modeling, thus the soundness of the device; and the virtual (mirroring real-world) application for an analysis of its effectiveness. In 2014, the FDA published a guidance document, "Reporting Computational Modeling Studies in Medical Device Regulatory Submissions," as a means of encouraging simulation in medical research. The FDA is also involved in developing the Virtual Physiological Patient (VPP), a library of computer models of the human body at various levels of disease states. Additionally, there is the partnership among device developers, software providers, and medical professionals known as the Medical Device Innovation Consortium (MDIC) that serves as a center for disease-specific information gathering. Significantly, the goal of the VPP is to serve as a shared point of reference that will improve both understanding the value and limitations of models. For the FDA and its associate partners these applications are distinct parts of what could grow into a whole representation.

2. *Education*—medical training can be either patient-centric or education-centric with each perspective requiring varying levels of model and/or simulation fidelity. A digital patient can support both. (There is much discussion on this topic in Part 4 of this publication.)

3. *Practice*—the future of healthcare, in the United States and globally, is proving to be an overwhelming challenge. Changing practice to provide holistic, personalized care in an expanding (longer-lived and growing population) and demanding (multiple pathologies and needs per individual patient) environment requires optimizing research, technology, and training. Clinicians must exploit new generation capabilities in diagnostic and therapeutic patient care for the burden of patient needs to be met. Medical technology is very near to providing safe and effective personalized patient care through the use of digital patient technology. Gone will be the *normed set of symptoms standard set of treatments* approach.

And importantly, there is … .

4. *Personalized healthcare*—this should be the primary goal for the digital patient—personalized healthcare with the patient actively participating. There are many organizations associated with this facet of the digital patient. Some advocate for proactive healthcare models using technology for broadband infrastructure, interoperability, and care in the home. The ideal situation is to make care-at-home the default location for the patient in contrast to clinics and hospitals with their associated challenges and costs. Sadly, these individual health-teams address the patient as distinct parts of a body, or as a body with individual pathologies and isolated aspects of physiology. The data prove that healthcare should be a coordinated effort; still, it is widely known that the vast majority of medical errors are the result of miscommunication as varying disciplinary units fail to communicate. The digital patient facilitates a self-care approach coupled with a networking capability that will avert communication gaps while fostering care customization.

CONCLUSION

In January 2011, the Massachusetts Institute of Technology submitted a report to the health science research community introducing a new research model from which this compendium draws upon to discuss how and why connecting the research and development surrounding the digital patient is a must. The research paradigm they developed is called *convergence*. Convergence is the merging of distinct technologies, processing disciplines, or devices into a unified whole to create a host of new pathways and opportunities. Convergence can take the technical tools, as well as the disciplined design engineering and physics approach and apply them to the life sciences. The strength in this methodology is that it does not rest on a particular scientific advancement but on a new integrated approach for achieving advancements.

Specific to interdisciplinary research and development, this approach is inclusive, flexible, and forward-thinking. It is a methodology that supports the merging of the life, physical, and engineering sciences and their respective interdisciplinary research areas. As such, this notion of convergence is a good first step in achieving the purpose behind the discussions among the chapters of this book: the integration of completed work and ongoing work, determining gaps in the research and development, and advancing the completion of a digital patient.

4

THE SIGNIFICANCE OF MODELING AND VISUALIZATION

JOHN A. SOKOLOWSKI AND HECTOR M. GARCIA

Virginia Modeling, Analysis and Simulation Center, Old Dominion University, Suffolk, VA, USA

INTRODUCTION

Any preliminary read on the subject of a virtual human, human physiome, digital patient lays bare the need for integrating the wide spectrum of topics and technologies associated with this research and development. Reading through the chapters of this compendium will prove out that diversity—various disciplines, methodologies, hypotheses, purposes, technologies, and practices—contributes to advancing the digital patient. This chapter addresses a significant component of the digital patient: visualization. At the core of modeling and simulation engineering, visualization is the means by which modeling and simulation articulate; that is, typically, visualization serves to interface with the model, and that model is an approximation of the real-world. However, with the digital patient the aim is to secure more than an approximation; the digital patient must be a true replication of the human physiology. Moreover, it is this component of visualization, both analog and digital, that is critical to that replication. Opportunely and constructively, visualization has the capacity to capture what is undoubtedly the most complex system: the human body.

As engineers, we like to think that the development of a digital patient starts within the realms of modeling, simulation, and visualization engineering. A brief review of the common lexicon within this field of study bears this out. Listed down are some of the phrases and words useful for a preliminary read on this subject at-large as well as how they apply or translate to the digital patient:

- *Complicated and complex systems*—these systems diverge based on the level of understanding of the system; a physics-based model is complicated because it has numerous parts, but it is not complex in that it is predictable. On the other hand, a

The Digital Patient: Advancing Healthcare, Research, and Education, First Edition.
Edited by C. Donald Combs, John A. Sokolowski, and Catherine M. Banks.
© 2016 John Wiley & Sons, Inc. Published 2016 by John Wiley & Sons, Inc.

complex system like the human body might have fewer parts, but it is complex because it is difficult to ascertain absolutes in the data as humans are organic; one cannot predict the behavior of the human system with any certainty.

- *Computer and computational models*—a computer model refers to the algorithms and equations used to capture the behavior of the system being modeled; while the computational model is a mathematical model that requires extensive computational resources (e.g., computer memory and speed) to study the behavior of a complex system by computer simulation.
- *Interoperability and integration*—the technical term "interoperability" refers to computer systems that can exchange information; integration (of systems) seeks to embed existing and new systems into an existing environment.
- *Live, virtual, constructive simulation*—examples of each in the medical domain are as follows: live—using live actors to mimic illness; virtual—synthetic training environments where people employ simulated equipment like the virtual operating room; and constructive—simulated people and simulated equipment augment real-world conditions.
- *Simulation and simulator*—simulation is a means, a technique, to replace or augment real-world experiences with case studies or guided experiences that represent or replicate substantial aspects of that real-world with an interactive capacity played out over time; the simulator is a device that can be used to accomplish this, such as a computerized manikin that can mimic fluid loss.
- *Anatomical model*—models of the human anatomy ranging in complexity from single cell to organ-to-organ system; single or multiple components (e.g., the femur or the entire skeletal system) with a view to studying form, *what it is*.
- *Physiological model*—models to understand how the anatomy works in totality; how cells, muscles, and organs operate together and interact from the molecular basis to whole integrated behavior of entire body with a view to studying function, *what it does*.
- *Behavioral model*—for purposes of this study, this modeling focuses on representing changes in human behavior the result of a wide range of factors such as information, motivation, ability, and physical change.

The above lexicon framework facilitates an explanation of the difficulty of modeling the human physiology.

MODELING A COMPLEX SYSTEM: HUMAN PHYSIOLOGY

Engineers expert at modeling and simulation are well aware of the challenges in replicating or characterizing a real-world entity that is dynamic and organic. Entities that experience some sort of continuous movement (dynamic) and/or ongoing change in structure, comportment (organic) often present themselves as complex systems. As defined by Banks in Chapter 3, a complex system is one that presents itself as *difficult to ascertain data* due to those dynamic, organic variables. In the context of a digital patient, the difficulty in modeling arises due to physiological uncertainty or behavioral unpredictability—again it is that dynamic/organic characteristic. The human body is unequivocally a complex system and modeling it is quite the task.

Expert modelers comfortably admit that modeling is not easy: the more complex the system or entity to be represented or characterized, the more difficult the task of modeling it. Added to that is the difficulty of modeling the organic, dynamic nature of the human body. Case in point is the Physiome Project [1]. The Project presents a physiome bioinformatics matrix of six mathematical modeling levels, of which the first five are linked to biology, physiology, and bioengineering. These mathematical models found among the three disciplines are the foundation for human models developed for simulation purposes.

- Level 1 models: Molecular models
- Level 2 models: Subcellular Markov models
- Level 3 models: Subcellular ODE models
- Level 4 models: Tissue and whole organ continuum models
- Level 5 models: Whole body continuum models
- Level 6 models: Whole body system models

This range of modeling speaks to the complexity of the human anatomy and the complex system of the human body. Therein lies the need for visualization as the means to articulate the mathematical models.

The following sections include discussions on modeling, simulation, and visualization at-large, and visualization specific to the digital patient.

MEDICAL MODELING, SIMULATION, AND VISUALIZATION

In modeling and simulation, we look at describing how something behaves (via modeling) to gain some understanding about the system represented by the model. Simulation facilitates changes to the model as a means to observe it over set periods of time or activities. Thus, the term "simulation" is defined as *models that have been implemented in a temporal manner*. Specific to medical implementations, these simulations can take on three forms: *live, virtual, and constructive simulation*. Live simulation is real people using real equipment but employing the equipment outside the context of a real world. Virtual simulation consists of real people employing simulated equipment. Constructive simulation involves simulated people working with simulated systems. (The concept of a constructive simulation may be somewhat hard to grasp because humans do interface with this simulation by providing input to the simulation, but the simulation carries out the action.) These simulation forms are not restricted to exist in isolation. Combining them can produce a simulation environment known as live–virtual–constructive (LVC) simulation, such as a virtual operating room (Fig. 4.1).

Within the realm of modeling and simulation are paradigms that permit representing the object being modeled as a static or dynamic entity. These paradigms are discrete event simulation and continuous simulation. Discrete event simulation relies on the occurrence of specific events to advance a simulation from one state to another, over time; that is, the variation in a model caused by a chronological sequence of events acting on it. The events are instantaneous occurrences that may cause variations or changes in the state of a system, which are in essence the one or more variables that completely describe a system at any given moment in time. Continuous simulation allows that the system represented changes constantly over time. This is typical when models are governed by the laws of physics.

Still, it is the third facet, visualization, which serves as the means by which information is communicated [2]. This information can be the result of a simulation or a representation of a physical object being simulated inside the simulation, such as the body of a jet plane inside a

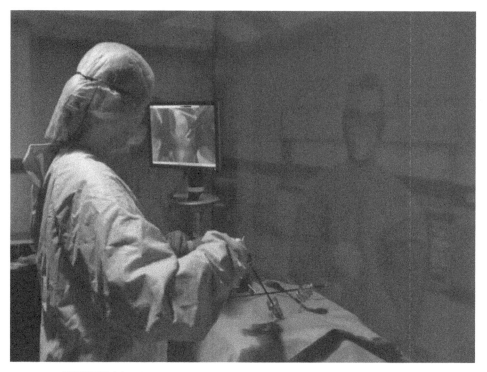

FIGURE 4.1   The virtual operating room at Old Dominion University [38].

virtual wind tunnel or a cardiac pathology discovered via a three-dimensional (3D) image in an ultrasound simulator [3]. Visualization can also include being the model: it can represent the human body or aspects of it. Moreover, to understand how an individual human body functions as a complex system, 3D computer models are patient-tailored as would be in the case of a digital patient [4]. Numerous visualization tools are employed to produce these 3D computer models. These tools are capable of interrogating the parameters of a model, presenting models from the minute molecular level to whole-body level. The visualization tools can also animate computational outputs for analysis, prediction, and prescription [5].

The adage *a picture is worth a thousand words* truly speaks to the fact that complex ideas or information can be more easily represented with an image. In such a sense, the goal of an engaging visualization is to illustrate complex information through an image or a series of images (i.e., videos and interactive visualization). The intent of engaging visualization for a project such as the digital patient is to illustrate complex information. Such images can be either 2D or 3D representation derived from real anatomical or simulated data. By adding a fourth component, 4D medical visualizations can provide additional details about the patient [6]. When the visualization is effective, it enables the understanding of complex relations of large amounts of data with ease [7].

This is why when trying to explain something complex, people often resort to drawing (i.e., sketches, diagrams, mapping directions). The complex nature of the digital patient stresses the need for effective visualization. In effective, successful visualization it is always very important to accomplish two things: (i) show the precise data and (ii) avoid distorting the data [8]. This is done by understanding what to communicate, to whom it is intended, and how it will inform the viewer (Fig. 4.2).

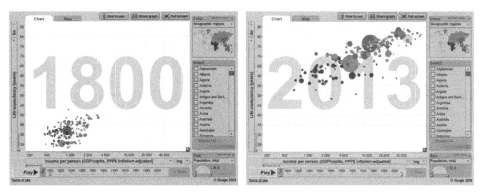

FIGURE 4.2 Bubble graph of the wealth and health of nations over 200 years [39].

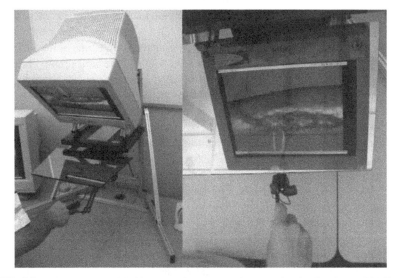

FIGURE 4.3 The wound debridement simulator with haptic feedback at Old Dominion University [40].

Some computer visualizations are presented as a snapshot of a moment in the time of the simulation, and others as a continuous real-time visualization. These options are selected depending on what we are trying to understand; but the focus of the visualization is to stay true to the data so that we can get an accurate illustration from which to make informed decisions. Because of the multidisciplinary aspects of modeling and simulation, visualizations can and often does make use of very distinct delivery platforms. Some simulations use multidisplay systems as in the case of flight simulators, or multiscreen large-scale displays (like the CAVE) [9]. On the other side of the spectrum, visualizations can happen on laptop screens or inside head mounted displays (HMDs) [10]. In addition, the interactions with these systems vary, depending on their purpose. Some use replicas of the physical hardware that interacts with the simulation as in flight simulators [11], others use spatial controllers to manipulate and interact with the data [12]. Still other types of controllers try to simulate a tactile sensation as you interact with the simulation [13] such as those on laparoscopic simulators (Fig. 4.3).

While all of these technologies are available for visualizing data, not all of them are applicable for all uses or are they generalizable. Therefore, while it may be interesting to do a flight-through using Google Earth inside a CAVE display, the use of such display does not gain any additional insight into the data [14].

Visualization vis-à-vis the Digital Patient (Human Anatomy and Physiology) Odd as it might seem, a reference to cartography is a good starting point for this discussion. Centuries ago, cartography was a time-consuming endeavor that ensued for generations. The visualization was a simple, static drawing that nevertheless proved a very important tool. As visualization tools evolved over time, so did the tools for cartography. These visualization tools are now ubiquitous; Google Earth is the perfect example.

Google Earth has mastered the integration of data and placed that data into context. In just one glance, directions, traffic, road networks, and weather are all discernible to the viewer. In essence, this technology facilitates the co-location of separate data sets, illustrating complex relationships between multiple systems. In similar manner, the digital patient makes use of different data sets and simulations that are interdependent and that can be brought together to illustrate multiple functional relationships among the different systems [15, 16]. In some sense, a similarity exists between the cartography that serves as the grounding data for Google Earth and anatomical visualization as the grounding data for visualizations of the human physiology (Fig. 4.4).

Coupled with the art of cartography are the human mappings of the anatomy. The effort to record the human anatomy in the greatest of detail began with Leonardo da Vinci. Through his visualizations of the human anatomy, medical professionals began to gain an understanding of the human body. These early efforts used visualization to present the information gathered, and they were successful because they focused on the substance rather than the methodology. Technologies today also focus on substance: magnetic resonance imaging, X-rays, and computer tomography scans are such tools that have found themselves as integral for medical diagnosis, intervention, and education (Fig. 4.5).

Advancements in computer graphics have greatly enhanced the capabilities for medical visualizations [17]. *Surface rendering* allows for the display of vast amounts of information as surface models, treating the objects visualized as having a surface of a uniform color and in which shading shows the location of light [18]. This is how we get some areas more illuminated than others. Surface rendering keeps all of the detail on the outer surface of

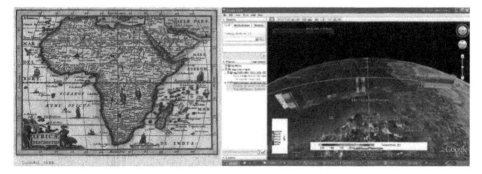

FIGURE 4.4 1683 map of West Africa by the cartographer Cloveris showing Sierra Leone (left) [41]. NASA GES DISC projected and visualized A-Train swath data along with A-train vertical profiles in Google Earth (right) [42].

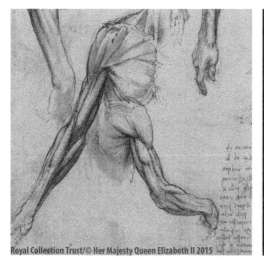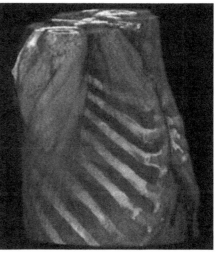

FIGURE 4.5   Da Vinci's sketches of muscles and skeleton (left) [43]. Volume rendering of a native thoracic CT scan (right) [44]. Reproduced with permission of Royal Collection Enterprises.

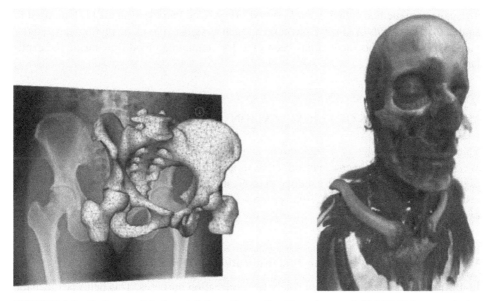

FIGURE 4.6   Surface model of a pelvis bone from a few X-ray images (left) [45]. Volume rendering of CT scan data (right) [46].

the medical data, like a shell, but it can lose the information on the inside. *Volume rendering* allows for the display of the intensity of objects across the entire volume of an object. It is able to represent not only the surface details but also the interior details [19]. Because of the even greater complexity and size of the data used for volume rendering, this technique is used selectively in medical visualization. Still, advancements in graphics processing units or GPUs are making it possible for greater implementation of this technique [20]. For representing anatomical structures, both surface rendering or volume rendering are great visualization methods to use (Fig. 4.6).

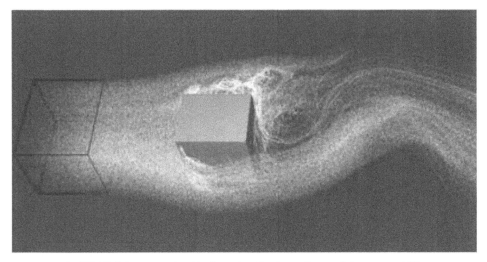

FIGURE 4.7   Interactive 3D flow visualization using particle systems [47].

Specific to simulation and the representing of motion of fluids inside the body, there is a visualization method called *particle systems* (Fig. 4.7). Particle systems [21] are used to simulate certain kinds of "fuzzy" phenomena such as smoke, blood, or anything containing numerous strands. This method has been used for simulating blood flow inside the capillaries and the heart [22].

MODES AND TYPES OF VISUALIZATION

There are many modes of visualization available for representing human physiology. We will discuss two diverse, but effective modes that are supportive to developing the digital patient and each mode's ability to replicate the human anatomy for education and testing. These are classified as visualization as an *explanation tool* and visualization as an *exploratory tool* [23, 24].

Visualization as an Explanation Tool (Education and Practice)

In this mode, visualization is used solely for explanation purposes. This helps advance the use of the digital patient for education and practice (training). When in this mode, it is not necessary for the data to be connected to the original simulation system, but this mode can facilitate presolved simulation data to illustrate a process. The data used for the visualization may be a subsample set of the original data, providing enough detail for practice and education use, but not suitable for research or full simulation purposes. This visualization is performed in real-time and can be interactive. Simulation-based task trainers are an example of this type of mode of visualization. Also included are scientific animations and interactive presentations, such as the Giant Heart project, developed for the Museum of Science and Industry in Chicago [25–27]. Within this visualization mode, virtual guides or visual aids can be added to the underlying data to better help in conveying the message or training outcome (Fig. 4.8).

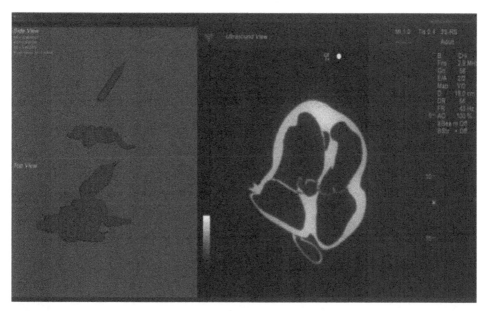

FIGURE 4.8   Ultrasound tool trainer at the Virginia Modeling Analysis and Simulation Center [48].

Visualization as an Exploratory Tool (Research)

In this mode, visualization is used to gain insight of the simulated system, such as the digital representation of the physiology of a patient. The visualization data is connected to the simulation system describing its function, and it contains all of the necessary samples providing enough detail for meaningful simulations. It can be interactive, but the final visualizations must wait for a period of time before the processed result can be presented. It is this aspect that makes this mode primarily suited for research purposes. In this research mode, visualization is the final step of the simulation, and it is used to validate, verify, or gain insight into the model and its results [28]. Once insight or analysis is achieved and verified, the dataset may be subsampled and simplified for use in explanation and/or education purposes, creating a symbiotic relationship between the two modes (Fig. 4.9).

The Usefulness of 3D Computer Graphics   3D computer graphics allow us to visualize information that exists in space [29]. One of the biggest advantages of 3D graphics is the ability to visualize the data from any angle at any moment in time. The data that comprises the 3D model to be visualized is a mathematical model of a 3D object stored in the computer on which calculations can be performed and the results are rendered in a 2D image plane, such as the computer screen and their color represented as a pixel in the resulting raster image.

The data can be either in the form of points, polygons, or voxels. Points and polygons are good at representing simple 3D structures that have a lot of empty or homogeneous filled space as opposed to voxels. These serve best at representing regular grid sampled spaces that are not homogeneously filled [30]. Using a combination of these data models, 3D computer graphics can be used for the visualization and analysis of medical data [31]. Because of the advantages of 3D graphics, most current consumer computer products contain specialty processors for handling a mass amount of 3D models, either in polygon form,

(a)   Four-chamber view and vector graphs volunteer < 30 year

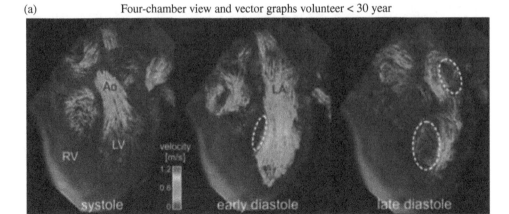

(b)   Four-chamber view and vector graphs volunteer > 50 year

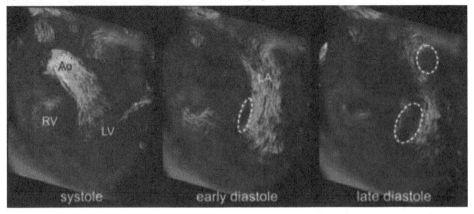

FIGURE 4.9   Vector graph visualization of intracardiac blood flow in a young (a) and an old (b) healthy volunteer. The formation of diastolic vortex flow in the LA and LV is indicated by the dashed circles. Note the reduced diastolic inflow velocities (color coding) and less prominent vortex flow in the older volunteer. Ao, aorta; LA, left atrium; and RV, right ventricle [49].

voxel form, or a combination of both. These products are known as *graphics processing units* (GPUs) [32]. By using this specialty hardware, the visualization of very complex 3D structures is possible, freeing the other computational hardware, such as the CPU, free to do other computations on the model data. This proves significant when working with medical data.

3D Printing, Biomechatronics, and the Digital Patient   Recall the then intriguing 1970s television show, *The Six Million Dollar Man*. The show introduced the notion of a human capable of controlling his robotic/synthetic counterparts to his natural anatomy. The intrigue rested in the fact that this man would use his natural, native biological systems to control and manipulate the robotic. The character in that show was a former astronaut equipped with bionic implants. Fast forward to the twenty-first century: the advancements of 3D printing, electronics, and robotics all combined have resulted in biomechatronic prosthetics that can replace or enhance the human capacity of the host biological system. With respect to a digital patient, consideration needs to be given to the interconnects and communication mechanisms and protocols between the body's physiological systems and their biomechatronic counterparts. Current advances in 3D printing, biomechatronics, and the understanding of how some physiological systems work have made this now a reality.

A quick look at one leading company, BiOM® Personal Bionics™, helps us understand how in the future human physiological systems will be enhanced or repaired using personal bionics. No longer will the digital patient system need to simulate the absence or deterioration of a functioning limb or system; it will now process and manage the symbiotic relationship between the biological and the synthetic. Advancements in these integrating technologies will result in digital patients whose whole health depends on these synthetic augmentations. Moreover, as these technologies are developed, a greater understanding of the *biological counterpart function* is gained.

VISUALIZATION FOR PATIENT-SPECIFIC USEFULNESS

Even when the daunting task of representing and simulating a complex system like the human body is completed, we would still need to present the simulation results to explain and explore it in some manner. We could present the information in its binary format, as a series of 0s and 1s, but the practical utility of such a means for a human would be nonexistent. Another way to present the information is reams of chart-like monitors and spreadsheets with numbers, but for the noninitiated this would be even more confusing. Visualization is unequivocally one of the most important ways of presenting the complex system of the human body as human data. Visualization enables the presentation of complex dynamics and relationships in an easy to understand method, and it facilitates a personalized physiological digital copy of the individual as a means to tell the story of the body: where it has been, where it is, and where it is going.

Because of the advantages integral to 3D graphics, it is now possible to visualize patient-specific data via imaging systems like the CT scan or the MRI. Visualization enables the presentation of complex dynamics and relations in an easy to understand method, but it would also help us achieve some of the more important reasons of having a personalized digital copy of patients. These visualizations can be used to practice a plan of action, a surgical intervention, a drug therapy [33, 34]. Alternatively, visualization can be used to educate a patient about his or her life's choices and behaviors, and how those choices affect individual health and well-being (Fig. 4.10).

CONCLUSION

In this chapter, we discussed what is visualization and how it can help us meet the challenges of the digital patient, how 3D graphics are helping pave the way for engaging visualizations, and how to use two modes of visualization when presenting the data for different purposes, be it research, practice, or education. Visualization is a major component of the digital patient, and we have seen how it can be used to inform and to help gain insights into the data. The digital patient has the potential to be a game changer in the healthcare industry as it will allow for a truly personalized care as well as provide insight to the people with their digital double, at least when it pertains to anatomy, physiology, and behavior. The applications of visualization for the digital patient are wide and varied, and we must always make sure that the visualization stays true to the data and that it focuses on the substance rather than the methodology no matter the application (Fig. 4.11).

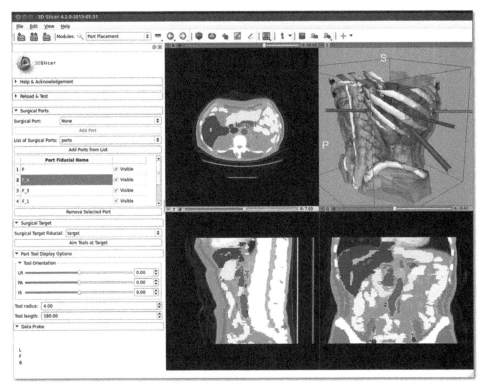

FIGURE 4.10 Laparoscopic surgery port placement visualization module [50].

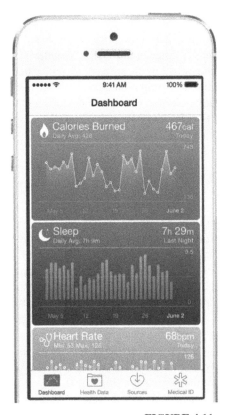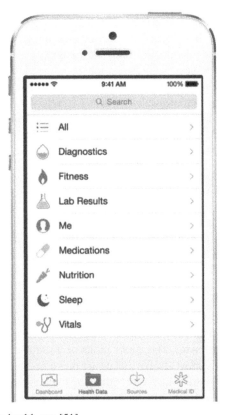

FIGURE 4.11 Apple's health app [51].

The digital patient is the next level of personalized medicine, and it will be brought to the public by the use of visualizations. This is evident in the use of visualization for patient-specific usefulness by the myriad of applications that work on smart phones or specialty health monitoring sensors [35]. These applications use visualization as the main tool to inform the user of their specific condition based on the readings of sensors that monitor heart rate, oxygenation levels, pulse, ways to monitor caloric intake, and caloric output to mention a few. Moreover, by doing so, it can paint a picture of your health based on personal readings and how they can be improved [36]. The digital patient is taking visualization to the next level. It can add simulations of each patient's physiological processes derived from their own medical data, and use those to customize the visualization to help you understand the specifics of how your body works and how you can help maintain and optimize it [37].

REFERENCES

1   Hunter, Peter J. and Borg, Thomas K. "Integration from proteins to organs: The PhysiomeProject." *Nature Reviews. Molecular Cell Biology* 4(3) (2003): 237–243.

2   Pousman, Zachary, Stasko, John T., and Mateas, Michael. "Casual information visualization: Depictions of data in everyday life." *IEEE Transactions on Visualization and Computer Graphics* 13(6) 2007: 1145–1152.

3   Humphrey, William, Dalke, Andrew, and Schulten, Klaus. "VMD—Visual Molecular Dynamics." *Journal of Molecular Graphics* 14(1) 1996: 33–38.

4   Hohne, Karl Heinz, Bomans, Michael, Riemer, Martin, Schubert, Rainer, Tiede, Ulf, and Lierse, Werner. "A 3D anatomical atlas based on a volume model." *IEEE Computer Graphics and Applications* 12(4) 1992: 72–78.

5   Dede, Chris, Salzman, Marilyn C., and Loftin, Richard B. Science space: Virtual realities for learning complex and abstract scientific concepts. In Proceedings of the IEEE Virtual Reality Annual International Symposium, March 30–April 3, 1996, Santa Clara, CA. New York: IEEE Press, pp. 246–253.

6   Tory, Melanie, Röber, Niklas, Möller, Torsten, Celler, Anna, and M. Stella Atkins. 4D space-time techniques: A medical imaging case study. In Proceedings of the Conference on Visualization'01, October 21–26, 2001, San Diego, CA, USA. IEEE Computer Society.

7   Joshi, Alark, Qian, Xiaoning, Dione, Donald P., Bulsara, Ketan R., Breuer, Christopher K., Sinusas, Albert J., and Papademetris, Xenophon. "Effective visualization of complex vascular structures using a non-parametric vessel detection method." *IEEE Transactions on Visualization and Computer Graphics* 14(6) 2008: 1603–1610.

8   Tufte, Edward R. and Graves-Morris, Peter R. 1983. The Visual Display of Quantitative Information, vol. 2, no. 9. Cheshire: Graphics Press.

9   Cruz-Neira, Carolina, Sandin, Daniel J., and DeFanti, Thomas A. 1993, Surround-screen projection-based virtual reality: The design and implementation of the CAVE. In Proceedings of the 20th Annual Conference on Computer Graphics and Interactive Techniques, SIGGRAPH 1993, August 2–6, 1993, Anaheim, CA, USA. New York: Association for Computing Machinery (ACM), 135–142.

10   Birkfellner, Wolfgang, Figl, Michael, Huber, Klaus, Watzinger, Franz, Wanschitz, Felix, Hummel, Johann, Hanel, Rudolf. "A head-mounted operating binocular for augmented reality visualization in medicine-design and initial evaluation." *IEEE Transactions on Medical Imaging* 21(8) (2002): 991–997.

11   Rolfe, John M. and Staples Ken J., eds. 1988. Flight Simulation. 1. Cambridge, NY: Cambridge University Press.

12 Hand, Chris. "A survey of 3D interaction techniques." *Computer Graphics Forum* 16(5) 1997: 269–281.

13 McNeely, William A., Puterbaugh, Kevin D., and Troy, James J. "Six degree-of-freedom haptic rendering using voxel sampling." ACM SIGGRAPH 2005 Courses, Los Angeles Convention CenterLos Angeles, CA, USA, July 31–August 4, 2005. New York: ACM Press/Addison-Wesley Publishing Co, pp. 401–408.

14 Qi, Wen, Taylor, Russell M. II, Healey, Christopher G., and Martens, Jean-Bernard. 2006. A comparison of immersive HMD, fish tank VR and fish tank with haptics displays for volume visualization. In Proceedings of the third Symposium on Applied Perception in Graphics and Visualization. July 28–29, 2006 in Boston, MA, New York: ACM, pp. 51–58.

15 Maes, Frederik, Collignon, Andre, Vandermeulen, Dirk, Marchal, Guy, and Suetens, Paul. "Multimodality image registration by maximization of mutual information." *IEEE Transactions on Medical Imaging* 16(2) (1997): 187–198.

16 Marescaux, Jacques, Clément, Jean-Marie, Tassetti, Vincent, Koehl, Christophe, Cotin, Stéphane, Russier, Yves, Mutter, Didier, Delingette, Hervé, and Ayache, Nicholas "Virtual reality applied to hepatic surgery simulation: The next revolution." *Annals of Surgery* 228(5) 1998: 627–634.

17 Rossler, Friedemann, Botchen, Ralf P., and Ertl, Thomas. "Dynamic shader generation for GPU-based multi-volume ray casting." *IEEE Computer Graphics and Applications* 28(5) (2008): 66–77.

18 Levoy, Marc. "Display of surfaces from volume data." *IEEE Computer Graphics and Applications* 8(3) 1988: 29–37.

19 Drebin, Robert A., Carpenter Loren, and Hanrahan Pat. "Volume rendering." *ACM Siggraph Computer Graphics* 22(4) 1988: 65–74.

20 Zhang, Qi, Eagleson, Roy, and Peters, Terry M. "Dynamic real-time 4D cardiac MDCT image display using GPU-accelerated volume rendering." *Computerized Medical Imaging and Graphics* 33(6) (2009): 461–476.

21 Reeves, William T. "Particle systems—A technique for modeling a class of fuzzy objects." *ACM Transactions on Graphics (TOG)* 2(2) 1983: 91–108.

22 Dzwinel, Witold, Boryczko, Krzysztof, and Yuen David A. "A discrete-particle model of blood dynamics in capillary vessels." *Journal of Colloid and Interface Science* 258(1) 2003: 163–173.

23 Silén, Charlotte, Wirell, Staffan, Kvist, Joanna, Nylander, Eva, and Smedby, Örjan "Advanced 3D visualization in student-centred medical education." *Medical Teacher* 30(5) (2008): e115–e124.

24 Wu, Keqin, Chen, Jian, Pruett, William, and Hester, Robert L. Hummod browser: An exploratory visualization tool for the analysis of whole-body physiology simulation data. 2013 IEEE Symposium on Biological Data Visualization (BioVis), Atlanta, GA, October 13–14, 2013. IEEE, pp. 97–104.

25 Gibson, Sarah, Samosky, Joe, Mor, Andrew, Fyock, Christina, Grimson, Eric, Kanade, Takeo, Kikinis, Ron "Simulating arthroscopic knee surgery using volumetric object representations, real-time volume rendering and haptic feedback." In CVRMed-MRCAS'97, March 19–22, 1997. Springer: Berlin/Heidelberg, 1997, pp. 367–378.

26 McGhee, John. "3-D visualization and animation technologies in anatomical imaging." *Journal of Anatomy* 216(2) 2010: 264–270.

27 Giant heart project. http://bbinet.com/index.php/portfolio/museums/msi-giant-heart/ (accessed on August 1, 2015).

28 Barna, Maria and Niswander Lee. "Visualization of cartilage formation: Insight into cellular properties of skeletal progenitors and chondrodysplasia syndromes." *Developmental Cell* 12(6) 2007: 931–941.

29   Angel, E.. 2012, Interactive Computer Graphics: A TopDown Approach with Shader-Based OpenGL (6th ed.). Boston, MA: Addison-Wesley.

30   Bhaniramka, Praveen and Demange, Yves. OpenGL Volumizer: A toolkit for high quality volume rendering of large data sets. In Proceedings of the 2002 IEEE Symposium on Volume Visualization and Graphics, October 28–29, 2002, Boston, MA, USA. IEEE Press: Piscataway, NJ, pp. 45–54.

31   Diri, Banu and Albayrak, Songul. "Visualization and analysis of classifiers performance in multi-class medical data." *Expert Systems with Applications* 34(1) 2008: 628–634.

32   Fogal, Thomas, Childs, Hank, Shankar, Siddharth, Krüger, Jens, Bergeron, R. Daniel, and Hatcher, Philip. Large data visualization on distributed memory multi-GPU clusters. In Proceedings of the Conference on High Performance Graphics, June 25–27, 2010, Saarbrucken, Germany. Aire-la-Ville: Eurographics Association, pp. 57–66.

33   Gering, David T., Nabavi, Arya, Kikinis, Ron, Hata, Noby, O'Donnell, Lauren J., Grimson, W. Eric L., Jolesz, Ferenc A., Black, Peter M., and Wells, William M. "An integrated visualization system for surgical planning and guidance using image fusion and an open MR." *Journal of Magnetic Resonance Imaging* 13(6) 2001: 967–975.

34   Sloot, Peter, Chen, Fan, and Boucher, Charles. "Cellular automata model of drug therapy for HIV infection." In Cellular Automata. Springer: Berlin/Heidelberg; 2002, pp. 282–293.

35   Gay, Valérie and Leijdekkers, Peter. "A health monitoring system using smart phones and wearable sensors." *International Journal of ARM* 8(2) 2007: 29–35.

36   Tamura, Toshiyo, Togawa, Tatsuo, Ogawa, Mitsuhiro, and Yoda, Mikiko. "Fully automated health monitoring system in the home." *Medical Engineering & Physics* 20(8) 1998: 573–579.

37   Bouwman, Jildau, Vogels, Jack T.W.E., Wopereis, Suzan, Rubingh, Carina M., Bijlsma, Sabina, and van Ommen, Ben "Visualization and identification of health space, based on personalized molecular phenotype and treatment response to relevant underlying biological processes." *BMC Medical Genomics* 5(1) 2012: 1–9.

38   Scerbo, Mark W., Belfore, Lee A., Garcia, Hector M., Weireter, Leonard J., Jackson, Michael W., Nalu, Amber, Baydogan, Emre, Bliss, James P., and Seevinck, Jennifer A virtual operating room for context-relevant training. In Proceedings of the 51st Human Factors and Ergonomics Society Annual Meeting, Vol. 51, no. 6, October 1–5, 2007, Baltimore Marriott Waterfront Hotel, Baltimore, MD. Thousand Oaks, CA: SAGE Publications, pp. 507–511.

39   Rosling, Hans. "Gapminder: World." http://gapminder.org/world (accessed on August 1, 2015), 2008.

40   Seevinck, Jennifer, Scerbo, Mark W., Belfore II, Lee A., Weireter, Jr., Leonard J., Crouch, Jessica R., Shen, Yuzhong, McKenzie, Frederick D., Garcia, Hector M., Girtelschmid, Sylva, Baydogan, Emre and Schmidt, Elizabeth A. "A simulation-based training system for surgical wound debridement." *Studies in Health Technology and Informatics* 119 2005: 491–496.

41   Original 1683 map of West Africa by the cartographer Cloveris showing Sierra Leone. http://www.sierra-leone.org/artifacts-maps.html (accessed on August 1, 2015).

42   NASA GES DISC projected and visualized A-Train swath data along with A-train vertical profiles in Google Earth http://disc.sci.gsfc.nasa.gov/gesNews/google_earth_a_train_swaths (accessed on August 1, 2015).

43   Clayton, Martin and Philo, Ron. 2012, Leonardo da Vinci: Anatomist. London: Royal Collection Publications.

44   Volume rendering of a native thoracic CT scan, retrospectively gated to avoid motion artifacts. https://www.flickr.com/photos/voxel123/4431164722/ (accessed on August 1, 2015).

45   Zachow, Stefan, Zilske, Michael, and Hege, Hans-Christian. 2007. 3D reconstruction of individual anatomy from medical image data: Segmentation and geometry processing. ZIB Report 07-41, Berlin: Zuse Institute.

46   Kroes, Thomas, Post Frits H., and Botha Charl P. "Exposure render: An interactive photo-realistic volume rendering framework." *PloS One* 7(7) 2012: e38586.

47   Kruger, Jens, Kipfer, Peter, Konclratieva, P., and Westermann, Rüdiger "A particle system for interactive visualization of 3D flows." *IEEE Transactions on Visualization and Computer Graphics* 11(6) 2005: 744–756.

48   Sokolowski, John A., Banks, Catherine M., Garcia, Hector M., and Richards, William T. "Developing an Ultrasonography Simulator Training Tool." *International Journal of Privacy and Health Information Management (IJPHIM)* 1(2) 2013: 17–27.

49   Muñoz, Daniel Rodriguez, Markl, Michael, Moya Mur, José Luis, Barker, Alex, Fernández-Golfín, Covadonga, Lancellotti, Patrizio, and Zamorano Gómez, José Luis. "Intracardiac flow visualization: Current status and future directions." *European Heart Journal—Cardiovascular Imaging* 14(11) 2013: 1029–1038.

50   Image from The Port Placement visualization module extension for Slicer 4.2. http://www.kitware.com/source/home/post/124 (accessed on August 1, 2015).

51   Image from Apple's Inc. Health App. https://www.apple.com/ios/whats-new/health/ (accessed on August 1, 2015).

PART 2

STATE OF THE ART: SYSTEMS BIOLOGY, THE PHYSIOME, AND PERSONALIZED HEALTH

5

THE VISIBLE HUMAN: A GRAPHICAL INTERFACE FOR HOLISTIC MODELING AND SIMULATION

VICTOR M. SPITZER

Center for Human Simulation, University of Colorado-Denver, Aurora, CO, USA

INTRODUCTION

The Visible Human Project (VHP) has now celebrated the twentieth anniversary of the completion of the male (1993) and female (1994) image collection. The data has generally been utilized for its anticipated purposes and is still a primary resource for research in the areas of human modeling and simulation of structures in the larger-than-millimeter-resolution range. The value and need for the Visible Human were predicted by the National Library of Medicine's (NLM) 1986 Long-Range Plan to include (i) education, (ii) training, (iii) modeling, (iv) simulation, (v) in situ morphometrics, (vi) information interface, (vii) reference standard, and (viii) entertainment. This chapter will concentrate on utilization of the Visible Human in the areas of education, modeling, simulation, and information interface. The Visible Human as a resource for in situ morphometrics is somewhat of a given by the quantitative nature of the data. As a reference standard, it has not explicitly been designated as such—but numerous laboratories have utilized portions of the data in developing precise and traceable models of the heart [1], liver [2], pancreas [3], and kidneys [4]. Image processing algorithms have been developed and tested on the cross sections [5, 6]—again, not as a reference standard but as an easily accessible collection of complex three-dimensional (3D) imagery. The final category of utilization by the entertainment industry has certainly exceeded expectations with museum exhibits [7–11], movies [12, 13], television [14, 15], literature [16–19], and art [20, 21] all playing their anticipated roles of interest in the beauty and function of the human body.

The term "Visible Human" used in the remainder of this chapter is not limited to the single male and female specimens of the NLM's VHP. It is instead intended to encompass any and all visualization of the entire human body produced via the same or similar

The Digital Patient: Advancing Healthcare, Research, and Education, First Edition.
Edited by C. Donald Combs, John A. Sokolowski, and Catherine M. Banks.
© 2016 John Wiley & Sons, Inc. Published 2016 by John Wiley & Sons, Inc.

methods. That method being, the complete sampling (of visible light emission or reflection) of an entire 3D object, one cross section at a time. Imaging of the VH was completed with 330 mm pixels and 1 mm image spacing [22]. The female specimen was imaged with 333 mm voxels. Using the same process we used in the production of the original VH but with substantially more accurate slice spacing, the University of Colorado Center for Human Simulation (CHS) is now routinely producing 3D image data with 50 μ voxels. The resolution improvement, in 2D space, of the acquisition is demonstrated in Figure 5.1. The same process has been utilized in producing a VH Korean and multiple VH Chinese volumetric image datasets [23]. Image resolution in these specimens range from 1 to 0.1 mm.

A 50μ imaging recently completed at CHS has only utilized regional specimens. Extending this process to the entire body is now possible and upon completion will produce a dataset of more than 35,000 images of 80 MPixels each. A full dataset of nearly 3 TPixels and over 18 TBytes (each color image is captured utilizing 48 bit pixels) will comprise the whole body archive. We have occasionally followed white light imaging with UV illumination, thus doubling the size of the image archive. The time required for sectioning

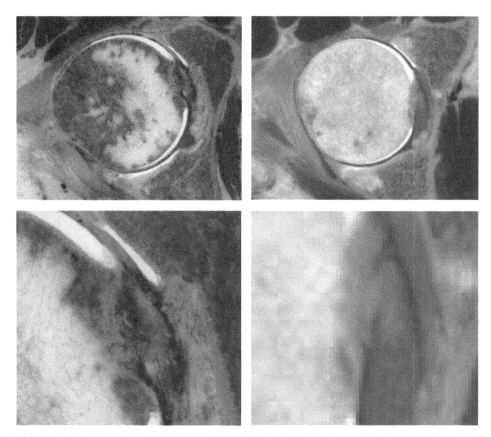

FIGURE 5.1   Visible Human Male images through the right femoral head are on the right. Corresponding images of a specimen sectioned and imaged at 50 μ resolution is on the left. The lower images are magnified views from the region of the foveal ligament and accentuate the nearly two orders of magnitude difference in image resolution. (The VH Male images were acquired with 330 μ pixels while their plane spacing was 1 mm.)

and imaging the Visible Human Female was 1 year (for over 5,000 slices) of 4–6 h days. Currently, we section 24/7 and the cycle time is just under 1 min. Therefore, the anticipated time for the complete sectioning and imaging of an entire body at 50 μ voxel resolution is about 35,000 min or 25 days. This highly automated process for image data acquisition makes the vision of a reference library of VHs a reasonable expectation.

EDUCATION

Two decades of open access to the image data has produced hundreds of education applications including web-based data browsers, [24–27] whole body labeled atlases [28–30], specialty atlases for regions and systems [31–33], physical anatomic models, physiologic and fluid dynamic models, and a journal (VHJOE) [34]. Three Visible Human Conferences (1996, 1998, and 2000) held at the Natcher Conference Center, National Institutes of Health, Bethesda, MD, and a fourth Visible Human Conference held in Keystone, CO in 2002 included a combined total of over 150 scientific papers utilizing VH data in research and education, anatomy, anatomical informatics, modeling, and computer science.

The VH has and will continue to play a major role in assisting healthcare professionals develop and maintain a 3D understanding of the human body in general, and more specifically in their patients. The need for this cross-sectional or 2D understanding of 3D, internal anatomy is exploding as the power of ultrasound imaging is added to the diagnostic tools of primary healthcare providers. VH data provides a unique resource in whole body visualization and a synthesis of cross-sectional and 3D structure. The correlation of 3D objects intersecting 2D cutting planes from the same photorealistic image data reveals the spatial relationships of neighboring structures of interest. The power of the 3D presentation is extended when the user is allowed to control movement of the cutting plane through the data. Figure 5.2 illustrates the effect of revealing the intersection of the 2D and 3D data.

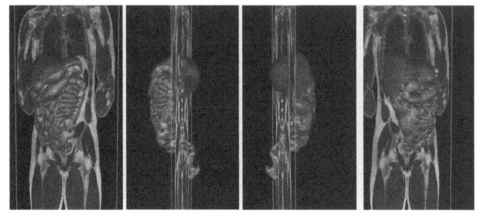

FIGURE 5.2 This sequence from left to right demonstrates the alimentary system three-dimensionally extending both anteriorly and posteriorly from a coronal plane through the esophagus. The left and right images are rotated 40° off an orthogonal view of the coronal plane. The center images are rotated 80° off an orthogonal view of the coronal plane. Image courtesy of Touch of Life Technologies, Inc., from the VH Dissector. Reproduced with permission of Touch of Life Technologies, Inc.

Oblique cutting planes intersecting 3D structures provide a unique atlas with information like that of an unconstrained ultrasound transducer. Real-time ultrasound is currently the driving clinical force for teaching and learning with real time oblique slicing, but many other clinical imaging scenarios—such as patient reorientation and planes through the principal axes of anatomical structures such as the heart or regions of interest such as the pelvis or skull base—benefit from the ability to slice data at any user-defined angle. This feature is demonstrated in Figure 5.3 on a system containing the entire VH Male dataset in fast-access memory. With the advent of ultra high–definition displays, increasing speed and capacity of random access memory and algorithms to compute only displayable data, the opportunity to provide this feature with new datasets an order of magnitude or two larger than the original VHP is possible.

An innovative educational application of the VH image data is shown in Figure 5.4 where the whole body segmented data is projected on the surface of a student's side or back in order to approximate the location of internal organs [35]. The surface projection of these anatomical structures has also been marked on the skin or shirt of a student for visualization throughout the laboratory period. A similar technique has also been used at the WELLS Simulation Center in Aurora, CO to approximate the location of internal organs of mannequins used in simulation scenarios. A further extension of this concept is through augmented reality where the learner wears a head-mounted display to visualize the internal 3D anatomy (in 3D stereo) deep to the plastic skin of the mannequin [36].

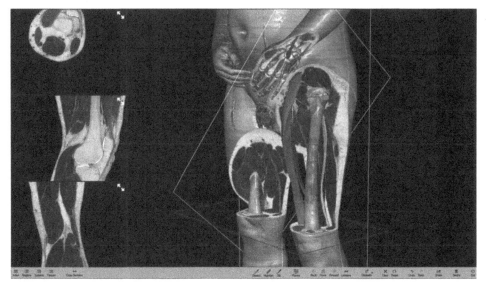

FIGURE 5.3   This screen capture from a VH Dissector Sectra Visualization Table illustrates real-time oblique slicing through the full resolution Visible Human Database. The multitouch interface provides collaborative interaction as students explore and reveal 3D anatomy and its extension from the 2D transverse plane (horizontal plane outline through the distal femurs), 2D coronal plane (vertical plane outline posterior to the femoral shafts), and 2D oblique plane (plane outline through the left hip and just superior to the right knee). Reproduced with permission of Touch of Life Technologies, Inc.

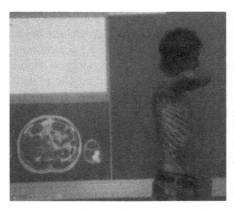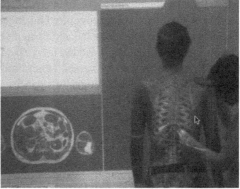

FIGURE 5.4   These images demonstrate an innovative interactive and engaging use of the Visible Human in the VH Dissector by Debra Patten at Durham University, Durham, UK. The projection adds photorealistic internal anatomy on the skin surface of the students. These projections might serve as a template for body painting or marking. Reproduced with permission of Touch of Life Technologies, Inc.

MODELING

Segmentation of VH image data has given rise to new methods and techniques for distinguishing color photographic image data [37, 38]. A novel approach was offered by Senger who employed haptic feedback related to color values to guide the segmentation of structures [39]. Rapid prototyping or 3D printing of segmented VH data has opened a whole new outlet for communicating the structure and function of complex anatomical detail. Models printed from the VH offer extensibility to the whole body [40, 41].

The future for VHP data in research and education is still bright as researchers develop deformable models to simulate the dynamic anatomy of the living human. Dynamic anatomy requires deformable models; and although significant work has been done on deformation of surface models extracted from the volumetric data, there is still much work to be done in order to apply second- and third-order force transfer to adjacent tissues and to calculate and display the resultant tissue deformation [42–46]. The ultimate goal is to reflect surface changes as a result of tissue displacement or volume changes in surrounding tissue. Peristaltic motion, for example, must obey the laws of fluid dynamics, and the plasticity of the surrounding anatomical structures defines the boundary values for the mathematical behavior of the processes. Likewise, the more rapid voiding of the reservoirs for these processes must be defined. Higher frequency tissue deformation and volume change associated with the organs and vessels of respiration and the cardiac cycle must be exhibited in surrounding tissue and surface models in order to accurately display chest motion and distal arterial pulses [47]. The biomechanics of joint motion must display surface model changes for the involved muscles and propagate those changes to the skin and intervening tissue models. On the low-frequency end is modeling the volumetric changes and resultant models of processes of normal and pathologic growth and development. High-frequency dynamic tissue modeling must accommodate the rapid motion of the larynx, auditory ossicles [48], and the extreme deformation caused by impulses from impact or shock waves.

The assignment of acoustical impedance and speed of sound to each segmented tissue makes the generation of simulated ultrasound feasible [49]. An immediate and important application for the modification of deep voxels in response to changes in polygonal surface models is the tissue response required during ultrasound examination. Transducer force on a body surface must produce the anticipated venous compression. Figure 5.5 demonstrates this effect in a simulated ultrasound image from the VH when a virtual transducer is applied to the skin superficial to the vessel. Other modeling applications include the assignment of tissue properties such as electrical impedance and ionizing radiation absorption to segmented image data in order to model processes such as EKGs and radiation dose [50–52].

VIRTUAL REALITY TRAINERS AND SIMULATORS

Anatomically intensive skill trainers have utilized VH data in order to provide a more realistic and complete simulator such as that in Figure 5.6. The trainer shown in Figure 5.7 was originally developed with a generic human form and a single line of text display, to teach triangulation skills for injecting neuromuscular targets for BOTOX™ therapy. The version of the trainer in Figure 5.7 displays the path of the needle in the transverse cross section as well as in the 3D rendering of the torso of the VH Male. The torso was built to the geometry of the VH. The syringe and, therefore, the needle location and orientation is followed with a Polhemus motion tracking system. The VH torso orientation is tracked with the same technology. The needle is shown in real time as it penetrates the skin and each deep structure (not just FDA-approved muscles). At any time, the advancement of the

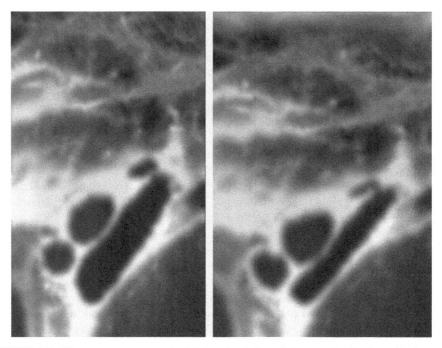

FIGURE 5.5   The screen capture on the left is a simulation of ultrasound reflection with the transducer contacting the surface just enough to visualize the blood vessels. The two circular dark areas are arteries, while the elongated shape is a vein. The second image shows the same area with the transducer pressed with greater force. The arteries are slightly deformed, while the vein is substantially collapsed.

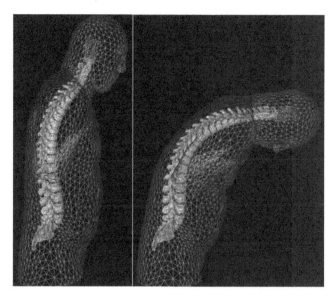

FIGURE 5.6   Flexion of the VH Male neck (left) and further neck flexion accompanied by more extensive spinal flexion (right) is required for optimal patient positioning for needle access to the spinal canal. Some modification to the soft tissues overlying the skeletal components has been applied. Reproduced with permission of Touch of Life Technologies, Inc.

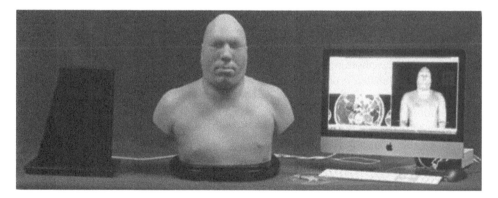

FIGURE 5.7   The rubber bust and skeletal system are built to the geometry of the VH Male. The vertical position of the tip of the "real" needle attached to a "real" syringe (just toward the left of the keyboard) determines which transverse cross section is displayed on the monitor. The syringe and needle are also displayed (updated in real time) on the right-hand side of the monitor. Rotation of the bust rotates the 3D rendering on the monitor. As the user penetrates deep to the skin with the tip of the needle (the entire length of the needle if the syringe and needle are held in a horizontal plane at the correct location of the needle is displayed in the cross section. The needle position can be frozen at any time and the 3D rendering dissected to reveal the entire needle in the 3D VH rendering. An optional display utilizes the orientation of the syringe and needle to control the display of an oblique cross section in place of the transverse cross section. The full length of the needle is always in the oblique cross section.

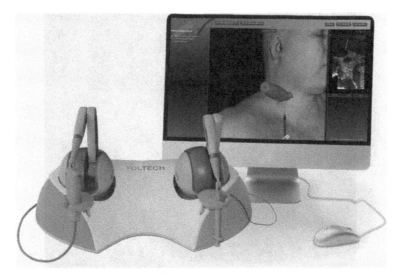

FIGURE 5.8 This virtual reality, partial task trainer is similar to the augmented reality version in Figure 5.7. This trainer includes all the features of the augmented reality version with the addition of ultrasound image guidance training. Haptic response for needle penetration is provided by 3D Systems Omnis. Reproduced with permission of Touch of Life Technologies, Inc.

needle can be suspended and the 3D visualization of the graphical VH can be dissected one structure at a time—to reveal the precise location of the tip of the needle in the 3D anatomy.

The "all virtual patient" analog of the aforementioned trainer has also been developed to add more realistic haptic feedback than just the penetration of a rubber skin. The OPUS Mini simulator in Figure 5.8 also demonstrates the path of the needle in real time, but the user feels penetration of the needle through each tissue interface (if appropriate). This trainer includes ultrasound guidance for the needle targeting where the ultrasound image is simulated from the photographic cross-sectional image data of the VH. This approach provides a fully labeled cross-sectional atlas for the ultrasound guidance training. The simulator provides a graphical indication of needle deviation with the application of any nonaxial force. The haptic devices have a small volume of effective overlap, but the VH can be positioned to present the desired anatomy in that volume.

CONCLUSION

The VH has contributed significantly to the education and training of healthcare professionals and the general public. The image data has been used extensively in atlases of both cross-sectional and 3D images. The segmented image data has been the foundation for models used for 3D printing and virtual and augmented reality surgical simulators and trainers. There is a great need for higher resolution data to visualize and model greater detail of the nervous and distal vascular system as well as fascial planes, tissue folds, and tissue directions. Dynamic tissue modeling still has a long way to go—to bring the VH "back to life."

The real power and advantage of virtual reality is yet to be realized—the power to present a patient mix far more encompassing than is available in the normal clinical environment. Presenting anatomical development and variation, the time evolution of pathology, and a diversity of patient gender, age, race, and habitus all in an interactive but risk-free environment will provide experience efficiency that is clearly superior to that of the apprenticeship model we currently depend on. Extension of the benefits of such a training world to include performance evaluation will increase patient confidence and safety in the healthcare future of our nation and the world.

REFERENCES

1 Trunk, P, Mocnik, J, Trobec, R, and Gersak, B. (2007) 3D heart model for computer simulations in cardiac surgery. *Comput Biol Med* 37(10): 1398–403.

2 Fasel, JH, Gingins, P, Kalra, P, Magnenat-Thalmann, N, Baur, C, Cuttat, JF, Muster, M, and Gailloud, P. (1997) Liver fo the "visible man." *Clin Anat* 10(6): 389–93.

3 Zhou, ZM, Fang, CH, Huang, LW, Zhong, SZ, Wang, BL, and Zhou, WY. (2005) Three dimensional reconstruction of the pancreas based on the virtual Chinese human—female number 1. *Postgrad Med J* 82(968): 392–96.

4 Tonar, Z, Zatura, F, and Grill, R.(2004) Surface morphology of kidney, ureters and urinary bladder models based on data from the visible human male. *Biomed Pap Med Fac Univ Palacky Olomouc Czech Repub* 148(2): 249–51.

5 Tavares, JMRS and Jorge, RMN.Computational Vision and Medical Image Processing: VipImage 2011. CRC Press, Boca Raton (FL), 2011.

6 Yoo, TS, Ackerman, MJ, Lorensen, WE, Schroeder, W, Chalana, V, Aylward, S, Metaxas, D, and Whitaker, R. (2002) Engineering and algorithm design for an image processing Api: A technical report on ITK—the insight toolkit. *Stud Health Technol Inform* 85: 586–92.

7 The Tech Museum of Innovation, *Interactive Immersive Theater*. (2003). Available at: https://www.thetech.org/about-us/media-room/interactive-immersive-theater-opens-tech-museum-june-5 (accessed on September 16, 2015).

8 Maryland Science Center, *Inside Out*. (1997). Available at: http://articles.baltimoresun.com/1997-08-11/news/1997223002_1_maryland-science-visible-human-project-exhibit (accessed on September 16, 2015).

9 National Library of Medicine, *Dream Anatomy*. Available at: http://www.nlm.nih.gov/dream-anatomy/da_visible_vishum.html (accessed on September 16, 2015).

10 National Museum of Health and Medicine, *Visibly Human*. (2010). Available at: http://www.medicalmuseum.mil/index.cfm?p=media.news.article.visibly_human_opens (accessed on September 16, 2015).

11 Ontario Science Centre, *The AstraZeneca Human Edge*. (2013). Available at: https://www.ontariosciencecentre.ca/Tour/TheAstraZenecaHumanEdge/ (accessed on September 16, 2015).

12 *The Fifth Element*, directed by Luc Besson (1997).

13 *Blue End*, directed by Kaspar Kasics (2000, Switzerland), released for TV in the USA as the Virtual Corpse (2003).

14 Law and Order "Desperate" (2003).

15 Crossing Jordan "Cruel and Unusual" (2003).

16 Evans, N.The Horse Whisperer. Delacorte Press, New York 1996.

17 Roach, M. Stiff: The Curious Lives of Human Cadavers. W.W. Norton & co., New York 2004.

18 Waldby, C. The Visible Human Project: Informatic Bodies and Posthuman Medicine. Routledge, London 2000.

19 Naisbitt, J. High Tech High Touch. Broadway Books, New York 1999.

20   Humanescence by Rae Douglass. Available at: http://lightrays.com (accessed on July 4, 2015).

21   Quilling Visible Human Cross-sections y Lisa Nillson. Available at: http://lisanilssonart.com/section/282102_Tissue_Series.html (accessed on July 4, 2015).

22   Spitzer, V, Ackerman, MJ, Scherzinger, AL, and Whitlock, D. (1996) The visible human male: a technical report. *JAMIA*, 3(2): 118–130.

23   Dai, J, Chung, MS, Qu, R, Yuan, L, Liu, S, and Shin, DS. (2012) The visible human projects in Korea and China with improved images and diverse applications. *Surg Radiol Anat* 34: 527–534.

24   Jansma, D and DeRuiter, MC. Visible Human Browsers. Department of Anatomy and Embryology, Leiden University Medical Center, the Netherlands. Available at: http://www.caskanatomy.info/browser/ (accessed on July 4, 2015).

25   Visible Human Server. Computer Science Department, Ecole Polytechnique Fédérale de Lausanne, Switzerland. Available at: http://visiblehuman.epfl.ch (accessed on July 4, 2015).

26   The NPAC Visible Human Viewer. Northeast Parallel Architecture Center, Syracuse University, Syracuse, NY. Available at: http://zatoka.icm.edu.pl/vh/VisibleHuman.html (accessed on July 4, 2015).

27   XX. John McNulty and the Stritch School of Medicine, Loyola University Chicago, Chicago, IL. Available at: http://www.meddean.luc.edu/lumen/meded/grossanatomy/x_sec/ (accessed on July 4, 2015).

28   Spitzer, VM and Whitlock, DG. National Library of Medicine Atlas of The Visible Human Male: Reverse Engineering of The Human Body. Jones & Bartlett Learning, Burlington, MA, 1997.

29   Dean, D and Herbener, TE. Cross-Sectional Human Anatomy. Lippincott Williams & Wilkins, Philadelphia, PA, 2000.

30   McCracken, TO and Walker, R eds. The New Atlas of Human Anatomy. LLC, Miami Beach, FL, 1999.

31   Sanders, I and Mu, L. (2013) A three-dimensional atlas of human tongue muscles. *Anat Rec.* 296: 1102–14.

32   Qatarneh, SM, Kiricuta, IC, Brahme, A, Tiede, U, and Lind, BK. (2006) Three-dimensional atlas of lymph node topography based on the visible human data set. *Anat Rec B New Anat* 289(3): 98–111.

33   Bhutani, MS and Deutsch, JC. EUS Pathology with Digital Anatomy Correlation: Textbook and Atlas. People's Medical Publication House, Shelton, CT, 2010.

34   The Visible Human. *Journal of Endoscopy.* Deutsch, J and McNally, P. Eds. University of Colorado Center for Human Simulation. Available at: http://www.vhjoe.org/index.php/vhjoe (accessed on July 4, 2015).

35   Patten, D. (2007) What lies beneath: The use of three-dimensional projection in living anatomy teaching. *Clin Teach* 4: 10–4.

36   Rolland, JP, Hamza-Lup, FG, Ha, Y, and Martins, R. (2005) Development of head-mounted projection displays for distributed, collaborative, augmented reality applications. *Presence-Teleop Virt* 14(5): 528–49.

37   Vaidyanath, S and Temkin, B. (2006) Registration and segmentation for the high resolution visible human male images. *Stud Health Technol Inform* 119: 556–8.

38   Schiemann, T, Tiede, U, and Hohne, KH. (1997) Segmentation of the visible human for high-quality volume-based visualization. *Med. Image Anal.* 1(4): 263–70.

39   Senger, S. Integrating haptics into an immersive environment for the segmentation and visualization of volumetric data. In WHC '05 Proceedings of the First Joint Eurohaptics Conference and Symposium on Haptic Interfaces for Virtual Environment and Teleoperator Systems. IEEE Computer Society, Washington, DC 2005, pp. 487–90.

40   Kapakin, S. (2011) Stereolithographic biomodelling to create tangible hard copies of the ethmoidal labyrinth air cells based on the Visible Human Project. *Folia Morphol* 70(1): 33–40.

41   The NIH 3D Print Exchange. Displaying models from Bill Lorensen (1st lumbar vertebrae, medulla, cerebral ventricle and hemisphere) and from Dave Chen (the male skull). Available at: http://3dprint.nih.gov/discover/visible-human (accessed on March 16, 2015).

42   Higgins, G, Athey, B, Bassingthwaighte, J, Burgess, J, Champion, H, Cleary, K, Dev, P, Duncan, J, Hopmeier, M, Jenkins, D, Johnson, C, Kelly, H, Leitch, R, Lorensen, W, Metaxas, D, Spitzer, V, Vaidehi, N, Vosburgh, K, and Winslow, R. (2001) Final report of the meeting "modeling & simulation in medicine: towards an integrated framework," July 20–21, 2000, National Library of Medicine, National Institutes of Health, Bethesda, MD, USA. *Comput Aided Surg* 6(1): 32–9.

43   Spitzer, VM and Whitlock, DG. (1998) The visible human dataset: The anatomical platform for human simulation. *Anat Rec (New Anat)* 253: 49–57.

44   Reinig, K, Lee, C, Rubinstein, D, Bagur, M, and Spitzer, V. (2006) The United States military's thigh trauma simulator. *Clin Orthop Relat Res* 442: 45–56.

45   Reinig, KD, Lee, C, Rubinstein, D, Bagur, M, Prince, L, and Spitzer, V. (2006) Using the Visible Human Male for Modeling and Displaying Trauma. SAE 2005 Transactions Journal of Passenger Cars – Electronic and Electrical Systems, pp. 807–17. Available at: http://papers.sae.org/2005-01-2719 (accessed on September 16, 2015).

46   Pan, B, Xia, JJ, Yuan, P, Gateno, J, Ip, HH, He, Q, Lee, PKM, Chow, B, and Zhou, X. (2012) Incremental kernel ridge regression for the prediction of soft tissue deformations. *Med Image Comput Comput Assist Interv* 15(1): 99–106.

47   Mithraratne, K, Ho, H, Hunter, PJ, and Fernandez, JW. (2012) Mechanics of the foot. Part 2: A coupled solid-fluid model to investigate blood transport in the pathologic foot. *Int J Numer Method Biomed Eng* 28(10): 1071–81.

48   Brummund, MK, Sgard, F, Petit, Y, and Laville, F. (2014) Three-dimensional finite element modeling of the human external ear: Simulation study of the bone conduction occlusion effect. *J Acoust Soc Am* 135(3):1433–44.

49   Pinton G. (2012) Three dimensional full-wave nonlinear acoustic simulations of ultrasound imaging and therapy in the entire human body. In Ultrasonics Symposium (IUS), 2012 IEEE International; October 7–10, 2012; Dresden, Germany. Piscataway, NJ: IEEE, Institute of Electrical and Electronics Engineers, pp. 142–5.

50   Jiang, Y, Hong, W, Farina, D, and Dossel, O. (2009) Solving the inverse problem of electrocardiography in a realistic environment using a spatio-temporal LSQR-Tikhonov hybrid regularization method. *IFMBE Proc* 25(11): 817–20.

51   Al Abed, A, Guo, T, Lovell, NH, and Dokos, S. (2013) Optimisation of ionic models to fit tissue action potentials: Application to 3D atrial modelling. *Comput Math Methods Med* 2013(7): 1–16.

52   Xu, XG, Chao, TC , andBozkurt, A. (2000) VIP-MAN: An image based whole-body adult male model constructed from color photographs of the Visible Human Project for multi-particle Monte Carlo calculations. *Health Phys* 78: 476–85.

6

THE QUANTIFIABLE SELF: PETABYTE BY PETABYTE

C. DONALD COMBS AND SCARLETT R. BARHAM

School of Health Professions, Eastern Virginia Medical School, Norfolk, VA, USA

Have you ever considered how information-rich your stool is?

—Larry Smarr

INTRODUCTION

Understanding in detail and with certainty what is going on within one's own body has been an elusive quest. Partial glimpses and general understanding are the best we have been able to do with the data we have at our disposal and with the limitations of population-normed theories of what the data mean for diagnosis and treatment of individuals. In the not-too-distant future, however, that will change as the Digital Patient platform is developed. The capacity to measure one's personal physiological and social metrics, compare those metrics with the metrics of millions of other humans, personalize needed therapeutic interventions, and measure the resulting changes will realize the vision of personalized medicine. Incorporating all of this rich data in simulations will have significant impacts on medical research, education, and healthcare systems around the world, as more interventions are simulated and assessed *in silico* prior to their use in therapy.

Major technological advancements in recent years have paved the way for more systematic approaches to modeling, simulation, and visualization of biological and social processes. Modeling now encompasses high degrees of complexity and holistic methods of data representation. Various levels of simulation capability allow for improved outputs and analysis of discrete and continuous events. Simulation complements both natural language and mathematical and statistical analysis by introducing new ways of thinking. Simulation also provides tools to build understanding and generate insight into complex biological systems and processes [1].

The Digital Patient: Advancing Healthcare, Research, and Education, First Edition.
Edited by C. Donald Combs, John A. Sokolowski, and Catherine M. Banks.
© 2016 John Wiley & Sons, Inc. Published 2016 by John Wiley & Sons, Inc.

There are three distinct modes of modeling and simulation fundamental to the medical and health sciences. These modes include live, constructive, and virtual. The live mode utilizes real people employing real equipment for training purposes. The constructive mode is a means of engaging medical modeling and simulation by developing simulated people and simulated equipment to enhance real-world conditions for training and experimentation purposes. Lastly, the virtual mode comprises real people employing simulated equipment to improve physical skills and decision-making ability [2].

Modeling, simulation, and visualization are widely used in the medical and health sciences, including research, assessment, education, training, and policy-making. One of the fundamental enablers of new medical and health science simulations will be the Digital Patient platform that is described throughout this book. This chapter explores Larry Smarr's research and his study of the quantified self, as an exemplar of the quantified self-movement and as an important prequel to completion of the Digital Patient.

The term "quantified self" appears to have been proposed in San Francisco, CA, by *Wired Magazine* editors Gary Wolf and Kevin Kelly in 2007 as "a collaboration of users and tool makers who share an interest in self-knowledge through self-tracking" [3]. In 2010, Wolf spoke about the quantified self-movement at TED; and, in May 2011, the first international conference was held in Mountain View, California. There are now regular conferences in America and Europe, and the global quantified self-community has over one hundred groups in 34 countries around the world. The largest groups, in San Francisco, New York, London, and Boston, have over 1000 members each [3].

During the past 15 years, Larry Smarr has become a pioneer in the fields of quantified self-research and its medical application, just as he was previously recognized as a thought leader in information infrastructure and supercomputing. Although he is not the only leader in this endeavor (Thomas Goetz and Stephen Wolfram also come to mind), he has created the most robust individual database. Ultimately, the quantified self is an effort to combine human curiosity about our bodies and health with new and innovative research efforts spanning the biomedical and social sciences. This chapter reviews Smarr's discoveries concerning his personal physiology, as well as his research attempting to break down the human microbiome into useful data [4]. Additionally, the chapter describes the vision of the emerging quantified self-movement and reviews critiques of Smarr's research. Finally, the implications of the quantified self-movement for the Digital Patient are discussed.

SMARR'S QUANTIFIED SELF

Quantified self-analysis is an innovative approach to understanding and managing personal health that is becoming available to anyone who wants to participate (with the caveats of having access to the necessary data and analytical tools and the requisite personal persistence). It represents a unique combination of patient autonomy, personal responsibility, and interaction with healthcare providers through the systematic, purposeful gathering, and analysis of personal physiologic and social data. Larry Smarr has undertaken what is now a 15-year investigation to progressively quantify his body. Smarr's journey began with simple quantifications, such as daily weigh-ins. Analysis of one metric, however, led to others, causing him to delve deeper into a broad array of biochemical variables. Through his journey of self-quantification, he discovered four primary factors that are easily quantified and can be analyzed to provide the understanding that can lead to a healthier self. These factors include diet, exercise, sleep, and blood chemistry [2].

At the beginning of Smarr's self-quantification journey, he began researching nutrition, tracking his weight daily, and reading a wide variety of books about weight loss. He gradually discovered that people should alter food intake to accommodate their individual biochemical systems, not merely alter their food intake to achieve weight-loss goals. Understanding and modifying the food intake to accommodate the biochemical systems of the body are critical because it is the subcomponents of food, such as proteins, fats, and carbohydrates, which influence the human digestive and hormonal systems.

Smarr changed his nutrition to what he refers to as the 'Zone' approach. The Zone approach involves caloric restriction, with the goal of lowering cellular inflammation by adhering to a diet consisting of 40% low glycemic carbohydrates, 30% lean proteins, and 30% omega-3-enriched fats [2]. Cellular inflammation results when individuals have too strong of an inflammatory response when fighting off microbial invasions. With too much of an inflammatory response, the body disrupts cellular communication systems, which is the impetus for gaining weight, developing chronic disease, and accelerating the aging process [5].

In an effort to monitor his adherence to the Zone approach to nutrition, Smarr quantified his food intake. For a number of days throughout the year, he measured each ingredient in the food he ate, converting each measurement into calories and grams of protein, fat, carbohydrate, sodium, sugar, and fiber. He averaged the number of days measurements were taken and developed a typical daily intake food profile. Through this profile, he was able to determine which food components he needed to modify in order to match his ideal Zone profile [2].

Smarr's self-quantification journey also identified exercise as a critical component of monitoring and improving overall health. He began with simple changes, such as opting for stairs instead of elevators, turning meetings into "walk and talks," and increasing his involvement with household chores and gardening. These simple changes were also paired with routine elliptical workouts, which he measured using devices that track both activity and caloric expenditure. He used pedometers and the BodyMedia® arm band, which measures various components such as skin temperature, heat fluctuation, galvanic skin response, and acceleration. The BodyMedia armband then uses algorithms to convert the data collected into the number of calories burned per minute. BodyMedia software uploads the data and displays graphs illustrating the physical progression of the day [2].

Smarr then turned to sleep, another critical component of health. Many people do not know how critical good sleep is to health, nor do they know how to determine if they are getting enough deep sleep. The Zeo Personal Sleep Manager (Zeo) is a device that enables individuals to quantify sleep using a headband wirelessly connected to an alarm clock, sampling sleep statistics every 30 s. The periodic sampling measures if the individual is awake, in light sleep, in deep sleep, or in dream rapid eye movement (REM) sleep, as well as the length of sleep. Using this sampling of sleep data, the Zeo ultimately calculates an individual's "ZQ," which is an overall score of the quantity and quality of the individual's sleep each night [2].

The fourth critical health component that Smarr identified through his self-quantification journey was blood chemistry, which can be broken down into three primary blood chemical values: omega-3 and omega-6 fatty acids, cholesterol, and C-reactive protein (CRP). He describes blood as "the window into the well-being of many organs," highlighting its often unacknowledged importance to improving overall health. Smarr had blood tests performed four to eight times per year and kept a spreadsheet of all values across the approximate 60 markers he tracked, allowing trending to be visualized over time. Smarr noted during his

10-year study that he believes tracking his blood samples allowed him to improve his health beyond the results of simply exercising and changing his diet [2].

Omega-3 and omega-6 fatty acids influence the body's inflammation through eicosanoid signaling hormones. Omega-6-enriched foods are generally proinflammatory, and omega-3 foods are generally anti-inflammatory. Smarr used an online service offered by Your Future Health to obtain an omega blood test to measure the inflammation level in his body driven by the ratio of omega-3 to omega-6 fatty acids. He also focused on the ratio of arachidonic acid (AA) to eicosapentaenoic acid (EPA), which directly compares the blood levels of omega-6 to omega-3.

The human body cannot produce fatty acids; therefore, the balance of these fats in diet drastically affects the body's eicosanoid-controlled functions. This is critical because eicosanoid-controlled functions have effects on cardiovascular disease, blood pressure, and arthritis. Additionally, because overconsumption of omega-6 foods increases inflammation, this also increases the risk of obesity and heart disease [2].

Smarr also focused on measuring cholesterol levels, particularly given the association between cholesterol and coronary disease. His cardiologist prescribed him Crestor®, and he began keeping quantitative track of his blood samples to monitor levels of low-density lipoprotein (LDL) and high-density lipoprotein (HDL). He noticed a dramatic decrease in his LDL through quantitatively tracking his blood samples [2].

CRPs are the third key blood marker Smarr tracked, using a high-sensitivity test. CRP is the generic blood marker used to measure inflammation. CRP should be less than 1 mg/L; however, his CRP never dropped below 5 in 3 years, indicating his body was chronically inflamed. After tracking his CRP for 2 years, he noticed it more than doubled in less than 1 year. Chronic inflammation is a cofactor with LDL in forming arterial plaque, meaning even if an individual has low LDL, if the CRP is high, the individual can still have unhealthy levels of plaque formation. Because of this, Smarr quantified the growth rate of plaque thickness in his arteries using an ultrasound analysis of the carotid artery. Due to the large size of the carotid artery, the ultrasound is able to image cross sections of the artery and rate of blood flow, which also directly measures the thickness of plaque on both sides of the artery [2].

Through Smarr's extensive efforts to quantify his health, he discovered he had inflammatory bowel disease (IBD) that had been undiagnosed by his doctors. Because his CRP marker indicated he was chronically inflamed and was experiencing increased plaque thickness, he deduced there was something else driving the inflammatory reaction. Smarr began taking stool samples along with his blood samples and noticed a new set of markers that measured inflammation and immunologic status, particularly lactoferrin. Smarr notes that had he not graphed the digital markers over time, he would never have discovered the IBD because there were no visible symptoms other than rectal bleeding. The combination of lactoferrin markers, a colonoscopy, and biopsies led his doctor to conclude he had late-onset Crohn's disease (CD) [2].

Due to Smarr's discovery, he took his self-quantification journey further by quantifying and analyzing his DNA. He utilized *23andMe, Inc.*, and *Navigenics, Inc.*, genomic services that expose an individual's single nucleotide polymorphism (SNP) sites along the DNA, where single base pair changes occur in approximately 1% of the general population. Individuals can request to search the databases of these services for a specific condition, therefore he searched for CD. He discovered he had a genetic predisposition to colonic inflammation. Anti- and proinflammatory agents usually form an equilibrium; however, if an individual has a proinflammatory SNP, this can overexpress inflammation. He underwent a number of blood tests to determine if food allergies or a colonic microbial imbalance caused the colonic inflammation. The results, which all came back negative, prompted him to quantify his colon's microbial ecology. By tracking human microbiota through periodic stool samples, he was able to reveal the levels of a number of microbial families in his gut. Smarr then began taking probiotics and prebiotics; however, it is unclear if he will be able to return to his original microbial ecological balance prior to taking antibiotics. It is also unclear if the microbial disruption was actually caused by the antibiotics or by the onset of CD inflammation [2].

Fortunately, the continuous decrease in the cost of genome sequencing has revolutionized and transformed the overall scientific understanding of the human microbiome. Quantifying human physiology is a significant and critical component contributing to a substantial move toward predictive, preventive, participatory, and personalized medicine in today's healthcare system. Analysis alone is not enough, however. Building upon this analytic vision of future medicine, Smarr and Harry Gruber recently presented their research on Quantifying Your Superorganism Body Using Big Data Supercomputing. They explain how data from DNA bases are fed into supercomputers, resulting in scalable visualization systems. These systems allow for the examination of patterns, which can then be used to guide and influence clinical analysis [6].

The microbial component of the superorganism Smarr identifies comprises a vast number of species spanning many taxonomic phyla. Microbial ecology and the human immune system are significantly interconnected; therefore, with respect to autoimmune diseases, both the immune system and the microbial ecology are likely to be influential factors in their development.

Smarr's research to quantify the superorganism body utilized trillions of DNA bases of human gut microbial DNA taken from his body, as well as that of hundreds of people sequenced under the National Institutes of Health (NIH) Human Microbiome Project. He used parallel supercomputers to input the data and run bioinformatics software, subsequently managing the data and creating scalable visualization systems. He then used the visualization systems to identify the changes and intricacies of human gut microbial ecology in health and disease [7]. His research also demonstrates how advanced data analytics can be utilized to identify patterns in microbial distribution data that result in ideas for new clinical applications. As he once noted, "This is the gift of the computer age: things once considered too big to count can now be counted" [8].

EXTENDING SMARR'S RESEARCH

Quantified self-research advocates view it as the first step in a process that will eventually lead to the development of "a distributed planetary computer of enormous power" that will allow scientists to create a computational model of individualized bodies [8]. The model will not be a generalized model of the human body, but one that is specific to a unique individual, taking into consideration that particular individual's physiology and genetic makeup. The model generation will likely come from data collected by nanosensors and transmitted through smartphone technology. People will ultimately be able to have personalized genetic codes and medical imaging stored in a cloud database, along with charts of vital signs and detailed nutritional analysis of everything they consume [9]. They can then compare this data with data on millions of other similarly monitored bodies across the world, resulting in a colossal database (now widely referred to as Big Data) mined by software that can utilize the data to provide specific, personalized guidance regarding diet, vitamins, supplements, sleep, exercise, medication, treatments, social interactions, and overall health [8]. That, simply stated, is the overarching goal of the Digital Patient.

Big Data refers to the collection of massive amounts of unstructured and semistructured data [10]. Big Data can be utilized to aggregate the behavior of individuals for a variety of research purposes, including being utilized as a public health surveillance tool [10]. There are an abundance of innovative opportunities for Big Data scientists to develop new models to support quantified self-data collection, integration, and analysis. There is also the significant opportunity (or challenge, depending on one's point of view) to define open-access database resources and privacy standards regarding exactly how personal data is used. A few of these potential quantified self-applications include demonstrating the importance of quantified self-data as it pertains to behavior change, establishing biomedical baseline metrics, applying pattern recognition techniques, as well as aggregating multiple self-tracking data streams from wearable electronics, biosensors, mobile phones, genomic databases, and cloud-based services. A long-term vision of quantified self-activity is the development of a monitoring system that measures an individual's personal information and provides performance optimization suggestions in real time [11].

The research outcomes summarized in Smarr's "Quantifying Your Superorganism Body Using Big Data Supercomputing" also have a number of implications for future research. Despite extensive research, the etiology of CD is unknown, with the potential for its pathogenesis to involve the interplay of host genetics, immune dysfunction, and microbial and environmental influences. Because of the variety of unknown causes, Smarr quantified all three factors. Through this research effort, he was able to effectively demonstrate how advanced data analytics tools are capable of finding patterns in microbial distribution data, which can be used to suggest additional hypotheses for clinical research. The findings from that expanded research will serve as a key factor in the progress toward predictive, personalized, preventive, and participatory medicine [7]. The cost of sequencing a human genome has also fallen drastically in the past 10 years, enabling sequencing of both human and microbial genomes. Ultimately, 99% of DNA genes are in microbe cells; therefore, the inclusion of the microbiome will undoubtedly change the understanding of effective healthcare.

Ultimately, the combination of trending time series analysis of individual biochemical markers paired with population-wide comparisons to people with a variety of different health outcomes will revolutionize biomedical research and healthcare practice. Individuals are becoming increasingly more active in monitoring their own bodies and health, as well as recognizing changes and deviations in trends and are acting more assertively in what they perceive as being in the best interests of their health.

The quantified self-movement will also have a considerable impact on personalized preventive medicine as it relates to addressing public health concerns. The goals of healthcare are increasingly moving toward the idea of personalized disease prevention and health maintenance. Preventive medicine addresses the metrics of the 80% of the life cycle before symptoms become clinically observed. Personalized preventive medicine has great potential in solving ongoing public health challenges, such as increasing healthcare costs, declining outcomes, and emergent problems, such as the diabetes and obesity epidemics [10].

It is important to note that a shift toward preventive healthcare is not simply that of a patient's treatment becoming more personalized, but rather that the individual receiving the treatment becomes the center of empowerment and, therefore, much more influential in the action-taking aspect of his or her healthcare [10].

Moving forward, there is an increasing potential for applying more data to personalized healthcare with additional research regarding the microbiome [4]. Eventually, we will have "personalized doctors with us at all times, instead of two 15-minute visits a year" [4]. Utilizing software and sensors, individuals will have the capability to measure their unique biological variables, contributing to ongoing maintenance and monitoring of overall health, as opposed to simply reacting to acute symptoms as they arise. That is, at least, one of the emerging goals of the emerging quantified self-movement.

Consumer genomics is another result of the quantified self-movement. Current US Food and Drug Administration (FDA) concerns about entities such as *23andMe, Inc.* aside, the likelihood is that, in the near-term, accurate, inexpensive genomic data will become widely available. Direct access to consumer genomic data will be one of the first times individuals have had readily available access to significant amounts of personal health-related data without the mediation of medical professionals. As the quantification movement continues to gain momentum, the healthcare model will transform from an emphasis on the treatment of chronic illness to an emphasis on the maintenance of health and wellness [2].

THE QUANTIFIED SELF-VISION, SIMPLIFIED

Tim Chang articulates the simple vision of the quantified self-movement in his article, "The 'So What' of the Quantified Self":

Using sensors in our smartphones and other wearable devices, we can chart how many calories we burn, our body fat percentage, how many steps we take in a day, how long we sleep, even how many hours a week we spend commuting or sitting at a desk. Soon we'll be able to access the same kind of statistics on our digital selves: Social reach and influence; tastes and preferences; achievements; credibility and reputation; habits; expertise. All that information at your fingertips at all times theoretically allows you to carefully chart a path for improvement, and share your winning strategy and stats with others. On a grand scale, that makes for an interconnected world of healthier, happier people making much more informed decisions [12].

A perusal of the web (definitely not an exhaustive search) identifies more than one hundred types of personal data trackers capable of gathering continuous data on activity, diet, weight, heart and respiration rates, sleep patterns, and blood chemistry. So, simply stated, the vision, as exemplified here by Smarr, is constant monitoring through improved technology, sophisticated analysis, persistence and discipline over time, and improved health through prevention and early personalized treatment.

CRITICISM

There are a number of criticisms surrounding Smarr's research and the self-quantification movement that need to be considered. The main arguments questioning the value of quantified self-monitoring relate to how much information is really necessary for one to understand their personal health status and trends and whether the quantified self-movement and its various applications are scientifically sound.

Critics argue that people do not need to know every detail of their health and genomic makeup and that such an obsession with one's health can prove to be unhealthy. Individuals who consistently monitor themselves closely are almost guaranteed to find something wrong, yet, in many cases, abnormality is actually normal. An obsession with self-quantification and self-monitoring has the potential for individuals to become hypochondriacs or, more likely, hyper anxious [8].

Dr. H. Gilbert Welch, a professor of medicine at the Dartmouth Institute for Health Policy and Clinical Practice, compares the self-quantification movement with the popular trend a few years ago of individuals getting full-body CT scans. Approximately, 80% of individuals who underwent a full-body CT scan found something abnormal about themselves that had not (and may not ever) become symptomatic. Welch believes constant monitoring inevitably leads to everyone being determined to be sick and in need of medical attention. This overuse of healthcare presents further health risks because interventions often involve powerful medical and/or surgical technologies, both of which carry additional risks of their own. Welch explains that doing no harm to the body often requires doing nothing. He notes that the human body has significant capacity to heal itself. Ultimately, tracking and analyzing an overabundance of data "is guaranteed to unleash a lot of intervention on people who are basically healthy" [8].

While the idea of a quantified self has significant potential for individuals with chronic diseases, such as Smarr, the average person may not receive enough benefit to justify the cost of time, money, and psychic peace. Self-quantification through trackers and health-monitoring applications, such as Fitbit, GPS-enabled running watches, and calorie counting phone applications can, of course, guide people in the right direction in terms of their health and fitness. However, much as with diet fads or exercise programs, people also have a tendency to abandon their monitoring programs. For example, according to a report from market research firm Endeavor Partners, approximately one-third of the owners of wearable devices stop using them within 6 months [13].

James Beckerman, a cardiologist from the Providence Heart and Vascular Institute, also poses the problem that those who are in the worst health are also the individuals who are often unsuccessful and feel depressed when attempting to adhere to certain diet and exercise fads or programs. Beckerman argues that those individuals who are successful and who substantiate their effectiveness are often already in good shape. He further explains that the majority of individuals embracing tracking and self-quantification are those who are already making healthy choices about diet, exercise, and sleep and are only interested in self-quantification to reinforce their existing healthy behaviors [13]. This brings into question the applicability of the quantified self as the future of healthcare for the general population, as opposed to those who are already in good shape and good health. Lastly, the scientific soundness of the quantified self-movement has been criticized. In the scientific community, there are ongoing concerns regarding the "utility and interpretive validity" [10] of personal genomic information and physiologic data.

The actual quantification aspect of the quantified self is a considerable obstacle. Having access to an almost unlimited amount of data, ranging from sleep to eating habits, has great potential; however, the likelihood of every individual understanding the data and its utility is questionable. Thomas Goetz notes in his article "The Diabetic's Paradox" that:

> It's easy to let the futuristic allure of technology obscure the fact that people with diabetes have been tracking their own health for 30 years now. *They* are the real early adopters here, and their jaded experience challenges those—like myself—who would argue that self-tracking tools are the salve for so many conditions. In short, the paradox is this: If self-tracking is so great, why do diabetics hate it so much? The fact that

diabetics have been doing this for years, and that *they largely loathe the experience*, not only serves as a caution to the vogue of self-tracking. It also offers an opportunity, serving as an object lesson in what works, and what doesn't work, when people track their health.

In the case of diabetes, the distaste falls into three categories: Self-monitoring for diabetes is an unremitting and unforgiving labor; the tools themselves are awkward and sterile; and the combination of these creates a constant sense of anxiety and failure [14].

The average person is unlikely to spend much time analyzing data and creating data visualizations and calculations using information gained from phone applications or wearable devices. An additional problem is the inconsistency of metrics across different device measurements. For example, different trackers and phone applications may measure "one step" or the number of calories actually burned during any given type of activity differently. The useful quantification of such data will continue to be a challenge until common metrics are adopted across devices [13].

CONCLUSION

President Barack Obama stated in the 2015 State of the Union speech that his administration wants to increase the use of personalized genetic information to help treat diseases, such as cancer and diabetes. He urged Congress to boost research funding to support new investments in precision medicine. Obama wants "the country that eliminated polio and mapped the human genome to lead a new era of medicine—one that delivers the right treatment at the right time" [15, 16].

He will seek hundreds of millions of dollars for a new initiative to develop medical treatments tailored to genetic and other characteristics of individual patients. "Most medical treatments have been designed for the average patient," said Jo Handelsman, associate director of the White House Office of Science and Technology Policy. "In too many cases, this one-size-fits-all approach is not effective" [16]. Dr. Ralph Snyderman, a former chancellor for health affairs at Duke University, often described as the father of personalized medicine, said he was excited by the president's initiative. "Personalized medicine has the potential to transform our healthcare system, which consumes almost $3 trillion a year, 80% of it for preventable diseases," Dr. Snyderman said. Although the new tests and treatments are often expensive, he added, personalized medicine can save money while producing better results. "It focuses therapy on individuals in whom it will work," he said. "You can avoid wasting money on people who won't respond or will have an adverse reaction" [16].

The discussion in this chapter has ranged from the self-analysis of a single scientist, Larry Smarr, through a review of an emerging movement to continuously monitor a wide variety of factors related to health status. At the center of the discussion has been the notion of the quantified self—the constant monitoring of physiological and social status, sophisticated and comparative analysis, personalization of disease prevention, diagnosis, treatment, health maintenance, and real-time implementation. Whether the quantified self-movement involves a larger or smaller percentage of the world's population is less important than the precedent it sets for using Big Data to improve the health of individuals through personalized monitoring and intervention. The quantified self and the Digital Patient are not the same, but the former is an important prerequisite for the development of the latter.

REFERENCES

1 Anderson, JG. A focus on simulation in medical informatics. *Journal of the American Medical Informatics Association*. 2002;9(5):554–556.

2 Smarr, L. Quantified health: a 10-year detective story of digitally enabled genomic medicine. *Sns Next Year's News*. 2011;14(36):1–25. Available at: http://lsmarr.calit2.net/repository/092811_Special_Letter,_Smarr.final.pdf. Accessed November 7, 2014.

3 Quantified self. (n.d.). Retrieved November 11, 2014 from http://en.wikipedia.org/wiki/Quantified_Self. Accessed August 4, 2015.

4 Temple, J. The quantified computer scientist: Larry Smarr on the future of medicine. Recode. Available at: http://recode.net/2014/03/08/the-quantified-computer-scientist-larry-smarr-on-the-future-of-medicine/. Accessed October 25, 2014.

5 What is cellular inflammation? Zone Diagnostics. Available at: http://zonediagnostics.com/cellular-inflammation/. Accessed October 20, 2014.

6 Smarr, L. Quantifying the dynamics of your superorganism body using big data supercomputing. University of Washington. Available at: http://uwtv.org/watch/nauF5BCRQLg/. Accessed October 25, 2014.

7 Smarr, L. Quantifying Your Superorganism Body Using Big Data Supercomputing. ACM International Workshop on Big Data in Life Sciences, Newport Beach, CA, September 20, 2014. Retrieved from http://www.cse.buffalo.edu/~jzola/BigLS/BigLS2014/Smarr-BigLS-2014.pdf. Accessed August 18, 2015.

8 Bowden, M. The measured man. *The Atlantic*. 2012. Available at: http://www.theatlantic.com/magazine/archive/2012/07/the-measured-man/309018/. Accessed October 15, 2014.

9 Smarr, L. An evolution toward a programmable universe. *The New York Times*. 2011. Available at: http://www.nytimes.com/2011/12/06/science/larry-smarr-an-evolution-toward-a-programmable-world.html?_r=0. Accessed November 2, 2014.

10 Swan, M. Health 2050: the realization of personalized medicine through crowdsourcing, the quantified self, and the participatory biocitizen. *Journal of Personalized Medicine*. 2012. Available at: http://www.mdpi.com/2075-4426/2/3/93. Accessed October 26, 2014.

11 Swan, M. The quantified self: fundamental disruption in big data science and biological discovery. *Big Data*. 2013;1(2):85–99.

12 Chang, T. (March 31, 2012). The "so what" of the quantified self. *TechCrunch*. Retrieved November 11, 2014 from http://techcrunch.com/2012/03/31/quantified-self-so-what/. Accessed August 4, 2015.

13 Wagstaff, K. Data overload: is the 'quantified self' really the future? *NBC News*. 2014. Available at: http://scitech.nbcnews.com/_news/2014/08/30/25743259-data-overload-is-the-quantified-self-really-the-future?lite. Accessed October 5, 2014.

14 Goetz, T. (April 1, 2013). The diabetic's paradox. *The Atlantic*. Retrieved January 21, 2015 from http://www.theatlantic.com/health/archive/2013/04/the-diabetics-paradox/274507/. Accessed August 4, 2015.

15 Reuters. (January 20, 2015). Obama calls for major new personalized medicine initiative. *The New York Times*. Retrieved January 27, 2015 from http://www.nytimes.com/reuters/2015/01/20/us/politics/20reuters-usa-obama-genomics.html. Accessed August 4, 2015.

16 Pear, R. (January 24, 2015). Obama to request research funding for treatments tailored to patients' DNA. *The New York Times*. Retrieved January 26, 2015 from http://nytimes.com/2015/01/25/us/obama-to-request-research-funding-for-treatments-tailored-to-patients-dna.html?_r=0. Accessed August 4, 2015.

7

SYSTEMS BIOLOGY AND HEALTH SYSTEMS COMPLEXITY: IMPLICATIONS FOR THE DIGITAL PATIENT

C. Donald Combs[1], Scarlett R. Barham[1], and Peter M. A. Sloot[2]

[1] School of Health Professions, Eastern Virginia Medical School, Norfolk, VA, USA

[2] Department of Computational Science, University of Amsterdam, Amsterdam, the Netherlands

INTRODUCTION

Systems biology addresses interactions in biological systems at different scales of biological organization, from the molecular to the cellular, organ, organism, societal, and ecosystem levels. It is characterized by its integrative nature as compared to the reductionist nature of molecular biology. It is also characterized by quantitative descriptions of biological processes, using a variety of mathematical and computational techniques. Thus, systems biology combines the development and application of predictive mathematical and computational modeling with experimental studies. The modeling techniques that are employed incorporate multiple spatial and temporal scales that are consistent with the integrative perspective of systems biology. Just as physiology is a branch of biology, systems physiology, systems medicine, and personalized medicine are subsets of systems biology. These levels of systems and their supporting informatics are shown in Figure 7.1. The Digital Patient will eventually integrate data and models across scales and time, and thereby enable the realization of truly personalized medicine.

Systems physiology focuses on the function of interacting parts of the system at the cell, tissue, organ, and organ system scales and is tightly coupled with structural anatomical information. Systems medicine is a subset of systems biology that addresses applications to clinical problems. Examples include the application of the systems biology framework to develop quantitative understandings of disease processes, to drug discovery and to the design of diagnostic tools. A subset of systems medicine that relies on individual patient data or the data from a specific group of similar patients is the emerging domain of personalized medicine.

The Digital Patient: Advancing Healthcare, Research, and Education, First Edition.
Edited by C. Donald Combs, John A. Sokolowski, and Catherine M. Banks.
© 2016 John Wiley & Sons, Inc. Published 2016 by John Wiley & Sons, Inc.

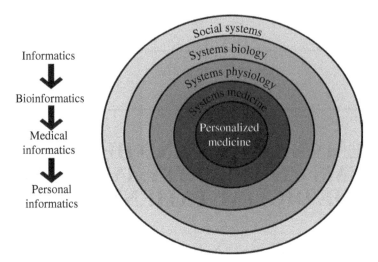

Informatics

↓

Bioinformatics

↓

Medical
informatics

↓

Personal
informatics

FIGURE 7.1   System of systems and levels of informatics.

The interest in systems biology has been growing steadily during the past decade. As Noble noted "Systems biology … is about putting together rather than taking apart, integration rather than reduction. It requires that we develop ways of thinking about integration that are as rigorous as our reductionist programs, but different. … It means changing our philosophy, in the full sense of the term" [1].

Although the framework is being developed, many currently available systems biology studies are not multilevel: they do not integrate physiological responses from the molecular to the cellular, organ, and whole organism levels [2]. The development of an integrated model of human physiology is essential for the understanding of how molecular, cellular, organs, and system levels interact for a total physiological response. Then, of course, the higher levels of biological systems and social systems must ultimately be integrated into the analytic framework.

Biological and physiological systems are highly complex. This complexity results in large measure from the following factors:

Nonlinearities: Many responses have upper and lower boundaries with different levels of sensitivity in between.

Redundancy: Many physiological states are the result of multiple mechanisms pushing and pulling on the observable response. Redundancy makes it difficult to identify important causal mechanisms.

Disparate time constants: The importance of an observation often depends on the timing of the protocol. For instance, the control of arterial blood pressure is a mix of fast-acting neural mechanisms, slow-acting hormonal mechanisms, and long-term effects of body fluid volume and compositions.

Individual variation: Physiological responses are a qualitative and quantitative function of sex, age, body composition, and other individual characteristics.

Emergence: Many high-level, integrative behaviors of the biological system cannot be described solely by aggregating the respective inputs from basic processes.

Biomedical researchers are increasingly using integrative physiological and biological models to better understand fundamental relationships that have been hidden in the complexity [2].

Translational biomedical research has made the integrative analysis of human physiology more relevant to clinical practice. The explosion of data over the past 20 years is providing novel opportunities to develop new clinical treatments. New technologies such as DNA sequencing, imaging, and proteomics provide massive amounts of new information about the human body. The ability to extract useful information from these data is beginning to lead to custom treatments for diseases, such as cancer, infectious diseases, and hematological and metabolic disorders. The existence of these newly available data sources has created a necessity for new methods of analysis. Genetic analysis suggests which genes may be important for clinical outcomes; however, the physiological relevance of changes in genetic makeup is not yet clear. This ambiguity necessitates a systematic approach to the integrative analysis [2].

This chapter expands on the concept of systems biology, explores its implications for individual patients through a description of the work of Dr. Leroy Hood and his colleagues at the Institute for Systems Biology and the broader social implications through a review of the efforts of Dr. Peter M. A. Sloot and his colleagues at the Health Systems Complexity Program in Singapore, and, finally, considers criticisms of the systems approach and the implications for the Digital Patient.

SYSTEMS BIOLOGY

The concept of systems biology centers on the "integration of biology and medicine with information technology and computation." Biomedical systems are multiscale, multiscience systems that link a wide range of temporal and spatial scales [3]. Systems biology focuses on properly assembling a variety of integral moving parts and requires the development of innovative methodologies of thinking about integration.

Systems biology has the potential to provide valuable insights into the physiological workings of the human body. The current goal of systems biology research is to utilize scientific advancements from the past two decades, such as genomics and proteomics, in an effort to develop targeted therapeutic strategies. The effective creation of these strategies, however, can only be realized with an in-depth understanding of the multifaceted etiologies of complex diseases [2].

The highly complex nature of biomedical systems results from several distinct factors previously mentioned. These factors include nonlinearities, redundancy of physiological states as a result of "multiple mechanisms pushing and pulling on the observable response," [2] disparate time constraints, individual variation, as well as the concept that many high-level and integrative behaviors of the biological system cannot be described solely through the sum of inputs from basic processes. Despite the extensive complexities of biomedical systems, researchers are using sophisticated biological and physiological models to better understand fundamental relationships within the biological system [4].

Some scientists predict that understanding the data resulting from the systems biology approach will ultimately lead to the widespread availability of personalized medicine. In order to accomplish this feat, scientists must analyze the data in a manner that recognizes the data as "a highly complex system comprising multiple inputs and feedback mechanisms." Translational medicine, a growing domain within biomedical and population-oriented health research that aims to improve the health of individuals by converting research findings into diagnostic tools and procedures, requires complex functional and conceptual linkages. These linkages include the association of genetics to proteins, proteins to cells, cells to organs, organs to complete systems, as well as systems to the organism itself and to the surrounding social environment [2].

The creation of a comprehensive mathematical model is essential to understand the integration of these systems and to successfully apply a systems biology approach. Such a mathematical model would accurately link the functioning of all organs and systems, providing a useful framework for the development and testing of new hypotheses likely to contribute to improved clinical outcomes [2].

There are currently several intensive efforts under way to develop a human model. A number of centers around the world are in the process of developing specific environments to facilitate the creation of integrative models of human physiology, or "physiomes." The Physiome Project is an effort to develop databases and models with the intent to understand human physiological responses. The International Union of Physiological Sciences (IUPS) Physiome Project focuses on providing a "computational framework for understanding human and other eukaryotic physiology," and comprises databases, markup languages, software for computational models of cell function, as well as software for interacting with organ models. Currently, the primary limitation with the Physiome Project is the lack of integration of the multiple narrow-focus models that could, if successfully integrated, lead to a comprehensive and integrative model of human physiology. Future development and improvement of the human model requires collaboration among scientists worldwide with varying areas of expertise in human biology to develop an accurate and usable human model [2]. One important example of this collaboration is the international effort, based in Europe, to assemble the Virtual Physiological Human (VPH). Chapter 2 written by Dr. Vanessa Díaz-Zucarrini and colleagues earlier in this book describes that effort and its interaction with many of the researchers also involved in the IUPS project. Additionally, Chapter 10 written by Hester and colleagues describes the HumMod, another decades-long integrative, multiscale physiological modeling endeavor.

Many scientists are currently working on various systems biology–driven studies ranging from gene analysis to cellular metabolism and localized blood flow responses. Technological developments during the past few decades have also provided unique opportunities in the development of new clinical treatments. These technologies, such as DNA sequencing, imaging, and proteomics, provide a vast array of new and untapped information about the human body. As scientists are able to extract usable information from the massive amounts of raw data, the research will infiltrate clinical practice in the form of customized treatments for disease in specific individuals. One notable example of this research effort to improve health care at the individual patient level follows.

THE INSTITUTE FOR SYSTEMS BIOLOGY

In Seattle, Washington in 2000, Drs. Leroy Hood, Alan Aderem, and Ruedi Aebersold founded the Institute for Systems Biology (ISB) to address what they saw as the greatest challenge of twenty-first-century science: *the need to understand biological complexity*. The following narrative draws on the extensive information on the ISB website and related articles in Refs. [4–7] to provide an overview of their efforts.

Even the simplest living cell is an incredibly complex molecular machine. It contains long strands of DNA and RNA that encode the information essential to the cell's functioning and reproduction. Large and intricately folded protein molecules catalyze the biochemical reactions of life, including cellular organization and physiology. Smaller molecules shuttle information, energy, and raw materials within and between cells and are chemically transformed during metabolism. Viewed as a whole, a cell is like an immense city filled with people and objects and buzzing with activity.

In the past, biologists sought to understand living things largely by examining their constituent parts. They studied individual genes, proteins, or signaling molecules to learn everything they could about the structure and function of a single and largely isolated biological entity. The scientific strategy pioneered at ISB adds a new dimension to this traditional approach. The researchers there seek to understand both each constituent of a biological network and how all of a network's constituents function together. They use cutting-edge technologies to gather as much information as they can about a biological system. They then use this information to build mathematical and graphical models that account for the behavior of the system. They test these models by gathering additional data, often by perturbing a system through genetic or environmental changes. In this way, they build an understanding of biological systems that can be used, for example, to explore what goes wrong when a biological system becomes diseased and how to treat or prevent that disease [4–6].

The success of some of ISB's research suggests the profound effect that systems biological research will have on medicine, on industry, and on society in the near future. Research at ISB is driving the development of what is known as P4 medicine— a new approach to health care that is predictive, preventive, personalized, and participatory. In the future, physicians will be able to examine the unique biology of each person to assess that individual's probability of developing diseases such as cancer, diabetes, or neurological disorders. They then will be able to prevent or treat that disease using personalized therapeutics. Health care will ultimately shift to a preventive mode in which each individual will have an opportunity from birth to experience optimal health [1, 5].

Systems biology seeks an understanding of how and why complex systems behave as they do, and thus will have far-reaching implications for agriculture, energy production, environmental protection, and many other human activities. As Dr. Hood has noted, biology will be the dominant science of the twenty-first century, just as chemistry was in the nineteenth century and physics was in the twentieth century [5].

Key benefits of P4 medicine [1, 5] to the patient and to the health care system will potentially include being able to:

Detect disease at an earlier stage, when it is easier and less expensive to treat effectively;

Stratify patients into groups that enable the selection of optimal therapy;

Reduce adverse drug reactions by more effective early assessment of individual drug responses;

Improve the selection of new biochemical targets for drug discovery;

Reduce the time, cost, and failure rate of clinical trials for new therapies; and

Shift the emphasis in medicine from reaction to prevention and from disease to wellness.

A coordinated and integrated program is envisioned by ISB to accelerate solving the technical challenges of P4 medicine [1, 4–6]. The program includes the following:

Developing methods for determining individualized genomes and for integrating the findings with diagnostic measurement data.

Developing methods for determining the levels of organ-specific proteins, microRNAs, and other possible biomarkers, including cells, in the blood to assess the health or disease in all major human organ systems and thus enabling the monitoring of the earliest onset of disease.

Digitizing medical records and creating effective, secure databases for individual patient records (new, data intense records with gigabytes of data).

Developing new mathematical and computational methods for extracting maximum information from molecular information on individuals (including their genomes), and from other clinical data and personal history.

Developing new computational techniques for building dynamic and disease-predictive networks from massive amounts of integrated genomic, proteomic, metabolic, and higher-level phenotypic data. (This is the heart of the emerging field of personalized medicine: new methods for interrogating data and understanding the interaction between the environment and the genome of the individual.)

Predicting drug perturbations of biological networks and developing therapeutic perturbations of biological networks (that is, re-engineering of networks in higher organisms with drugs, moving from a diseased state back to normal).

Creating pluripotent cells (stem cells) from normal, differentiated cells, and then differentiating them to specific body cell types. The ability to create stem cells with a given individual's genome will be remarkable, understanding it will be revolutionary.

Developing new *in vivo* molecular imaging methods and analysis methods to follow disease, drug response, drug effectiveness, and drug dosage determinations.

Effectively managing the enormous personalized data sets that will result, which requires the development of broadly accepted policies addressing security, quality control, data mining, privacy protection, and reporting.

Hood and his colleagues view this comprehensive research agenda as technically challenging, requiring significant investment and effort, but nonetheless achievable. Whether that proves to be true is, of course, subject to the same complex factors affecting the research, from the molecular to the societal. That observation leads us to consider an effort to explicitly link the molecular and the societal.

THE COMPLEXITY INSTITUTE

The work of Professor Peter M. A. Sloot and his colleagues is at the forefront of the systems biology and biomedical system movement. Professor Sloot is the codirector of the Complexity Institute at Nanyang Technological University in Singapore. His research interests focus on how nature processes information. He studies this information processing in complex systems through computational modeling and simulation and applies his research efforts to a large variety of disciplines with a focus on biomedicine. Recent work has centered on modeling the virology and epidemiology of infectious diseases, such as HIV, through complex networks, cellular automata, and multiagents. He also attempts to build bridges from biological factors to the sociodynamics of the encompassing societal environment [3].

Sloot's research is based on a complex systems approach to health because as he notes "understanding, preventing and handling diseases requires a holistic approach" [3]. He maintains that there are a number of moving components building upon one another and ultimately developing a connected, hierarchical structure that comprises a complex system. These components include the molecules, genes, transcripts, cell signals, proteins, interactions, and organelles building a cell; the cells, tissues, and organs building an organism; and the organisms ultimately building and affecting society, health care, and health care policies.

Rapidly increasing costs in health services ultimately lead to the recognition of a need for better-informed decisions in the health care decision-making and delivery process. Sloot proposes that this can be accomplished by using an evidence-based, participatory integrative health system that also gives consideration to the findings of the social sciences. When making health care decisions and treating patients, it is critical for health care providers to consider how they can induce patients to pay closer attention to their health, and to assess how the providers can effectively aggregate the information available to them with additional information possessed by individuals to make the best decisions. Further, it is important that more attention be paid to determining how and why social factors become biological factors affecting the health of individuals.

Sloot has developed a Health Systems Complexity Program (see Fig. 7.2) where the overall objective is to develop and maintain an integrative, descriptive, and predictive decision support framework to provide the city-state of Singapore a competitive edge on containing diseases. The primary goals include (i) identifying the interplay between biomedical and social aspects of health, (ii) becoming world leaders in the field, and (iii) to become a Singaporean think tank on health systems. He is convinced that this highly integrative research approach can only be accomplished through a radical transformation concerning the

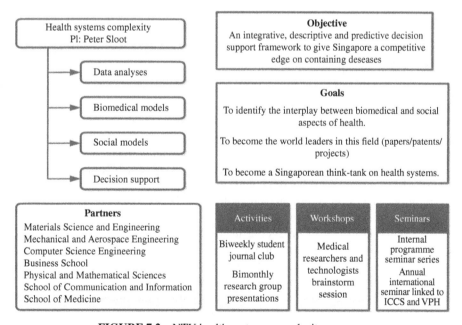

FIGURE 7.2   NTU health systems complexity program.

methods in which biomedical research is conducted [8]. His goals extend beyond those of Hood and his colleagues, in particular through the consideration of the social factors affecting the health of individuals.

Currently, the human body is primarily investigated as if the entity itself is a complex puzzle comprised of a trillion different pieces. Scientists and researchers try to understand the complete picture by assessing one piece, or at the most, a few closely interconnected pieces at a time. Sloot proposes that a societal frame is necessary, although the frame itself is not the entire picture. He further proposes that researchers need to model how the human body works in order to develop patient-tailored computer models capable of being used for diagnosis, prevention, drug treatment, and surgical planning. The overall approach requires integration across temporal and dimensional scales, across complete organ systems, as well as across a variety of disciplines (health care, medicine, bioengineering, and biology) [8].

Specific examples of the research that Sloot and his colleagues are conducting pertains to health systems complexity, biomedical events, multiscale modeling in computational biomedicine, cancer stem cell tumor models, drug–drug interactions, HIV, data management, and infectious disease transmission.

He proposes an approach to research on biomedical events that extracts biomedical events from the literature. There is currently an abundance of biomedical literature, which in turn has attracted significant interest in methodologies that can be used to automatically extract biomedical relationships from the literature. Existing research in this area is primarily focused on extracting binary relations, such as protein–protein interactions and drug–disease interactions. These binary relations, however, are unable to fully and appropriately represent the original biomedical data. Therefore, Sloot identified a need for methods that are able to extract specific and complex relations, referred to as biomedical events. His proposal to extract biomedical events from text has two phases. The first phase involves the mapping of training data into structured representations. This is then used as the basis for the creation of templates that can be used to extract rules automatically. The second phase involves the development of extraction methods to process the obtained rules. With F-scores of 52.34 and 53.34, results from this process are comparable to other state-of-the-art systems, but achieves superior performance in terms of computational efficiency [9].

Sloot expanded on his research on biomedical events in 2014 by proposing a feature-based approach to extract drug–drug interactions from biomedical text. Knowledge of drug–drug interactions is critical for health care professionals to avoid adverse effects when coadministering drugs to patients. Drug–drug interaction is a situation in which one drug increases or decreases the effect of another drug. Text-mining techniques, such as automation relation extraction, have been applied successfully in large-scale experiments to extract a number of relationships efficiently, such as protein–protein interactions. Therefore, he proposes that drug–drug interaction extraction methods can be particularly relevant in obtaining drug–drug interactions from medical records and in corresponding evidence from scientific literature [10].

Sloot's proposal to extract drug–drug interactions from text consists of three steps. These steps involve (i) the application of preprocessing to convert input sentences from a given data set into structured representations, (ii) mapping each candidate drug–drug interaction pair from that dataset into a syntactic structure and generating feature vectors for the candidate drug–drug interaction pairs, and (iii) using the obtained feature vectors to train a support vector machine (SVM) classifier. Results from his research outperformed other state-of-the-art drug–drug interaction systems [10].

Another aspect of Sloot's research addresses multiscale modeling in computational biomedicine. Many multiscale models currently exist or are in the process of development; however, he maintains that a foundational multiscale modeling methodology is missing. His research proposes a multiscale modeling direction that ultimately complements the current dynamic systems approach. To that end, he has conducted two specific case studies pertaining to the transmission of resistance in to the spread of the HIV virus and to in-stent restenosis in coronary artery disease [3].

In these studies, two distinct, mutually dependent scientific activities in computational biology were identified. These activities include knowledge discovery through data and text mining and through modeling and simulation-based analysis. Sloot and his colleagues note that closing the computational gap in systems biology, extracting knowledge on the multi-scale aspects of a biological system, and correlating data on different scales require the construction and integration of a number of models. Web and grid services should be uti-lized to integrate applications and tools for data acquisition, registration, storage, organiza-tion, and analysis, which would ultimately aid in bridging the integration gap. A systems-level approach is also necessary in disseminating processes, data, information, and knowledge across geographic and organizational boundaries within the context of distributed, multidis-ciplinary and multiorganizational collaborative teams [3].

Sloot and colleagues also implemented a systems biology approach in a study that combined epidemiological and genetic networks to address the importance of early treatment in HIV-1 transmission. Current research surrounding the HIV-1 epidemic either uses genetic information of patients' virus to determine past infection events or uses sexual interaction statistics to model a network structure of how the virus is spreading. Methods that take into account both molecular and societal data to create a reliable reconstruction of HIV-1 transmission dynamics are still lacking.

The aim of the early treatment in HIV-1 transmission study was to combine information from both genetic and epidemiological scales in order to adequately characterize and ana-lyze a transmission network of the HIV-1 epidemic in central Italy. Sloot and his col-leagues implemented a filter-reduction method to build a network of HIV-infected patients based on social and treatment information. The social and treatment information was then combined with a genetic network. Their findings revealed noteworthy correlations between high out-degree individuals and longer untreated infection periods by inferring HIV-1 transmission networks using a combined societal and epidemiological approach [11].

The work on systems complexity and its implications for the health of individuals demon-strate the range of systems biology research and serve to illustrate the importance of effective aggregation, analysis, and application of the massive data required to realize the Digital Patient.

THE POTENTIAL OF SYSTEMS BIOLOGY

Systems biology and biomedicine are two fields with profound implications for the biomed-ical sciences, health care, and personal health. These implications include the development of a more effective framework to contain diseases, further advancing the field of computa-tional biomedicine, the continual development of effective integrative physiological models and applications, faster drug discovery, better understanding of drug–drug interactions, and improved, personalized health care just to mention a few.

Understanding of biological phenomena has increased considerably over the past several decades in the scientific community; however, this understanding is not as systematic or integrated as it could be. Advancement of multiscale models and simulations in computational biology will ultimately propel the multiscale models and simulations associated with the IUPS Physiome and VPH projects. For example, the primary concept underlying the multiscale modeling in the Physiome is "the application of continuum field concepts and constitutive laws, whose parameters are derived from separate, finer-scale models." This concept is central to linking molecular systems biology to larger scale systems physiology. The fact that a linked, multiscale model of the heart currently exists and other organ systems multiscale models are in development [8] is proof of the ongoing efforts in this regard.

The implementation of multiscale models, as well as the continued improvement of the effectiveness of such models, will ultimately allow for responses to various stimuli to be predicted, and for results to be displayed using virtual reality technology. In the future, physiome models will have the capability to provide a quantitative description of physiological dynamics and the functional behavior of organisms, while also explaining how all the components of a human body function as part of the integrated whole. A complete VPH, that is, a personalized and four-dimensional model of an individual's unique physiological makeup has the potential to serve as a multifaceted research and testing environment for prevention, diagnosis, and treatment.

Mathematical simulations associated with systems biology and integrative physiological modeling are primarily used in hypothesis testing and experimental design; however, mathematical simulations and integrative models could also be utilized more fully in medical and health professions education. Students, researchers, and clinicians could potentially use these more sophisticated simulations and models to cultivate an understanding of the basic mechanisms necessary to maintain a homeostatic balance in the human body.

The simulations and models could also be used to develop an understanding of alterations that result in pathological states. Mathematical simulations have successfully been used in the past in medical education, lending reasonable hope for the effectiveness of more comprehensive, validated models in the midterm future [2]. There are numerous databases that address anatomical, genome, and proteome data; however, multiscale integrative modeling needs a database of physiological variables that include normal and pathological values [2].

Faster discovery of effective drugs is another implication resulting from the spread of systems biology analytics. Systems biology aims to develop predictive models of human disease, thus influencing drug discovery. Large-scale gene, protein, and metabolite measurements dramatically can accelerate the generation of hypotheses and testing in disease models. Computer simulations will ultimately integrate the understanding of organ and system-level responses, which will help to prioritize drug targets and to design clinical trials [12].

CRITICISM

Although systems biology has a number of innovative and promising implications for research and personal health care, there are currently limitations and criticisms associated with such an approach. Criticisms include a lack of model integration and a general scarcity of systems research, as well as the need for additional scientific breakthroughs before results are valid and applicable in patient care.

Currently there is limited integration among multiple narrow-focus models, for example, in the IUPS Physiome Project. A variety of current models exist, such as the extensive array of models demonstrating various aspects of cardiovascular physiology, but they are not linked together in compelling multiscale physiological models. Integration of these models would allow for a comprehensive, integrative model of human physiology [2]. Additionally, there is scarcity of research on biological multiscale modeling strategies. There are many existing research efforts that present multiscale models; however, there are very few methodological papers or studies on multiscale modeling. One potential solution for this limitation would be the development of a multiscale and multiscience framework for the modeling and simulation of complex systems based on a hierarchical aggregation of single-scale models [3].

Another criticism surrounding systems biology is the notion that the field itself is inherently complex, and because of this complexity requires extensive additional research and scientific breakthroughs. While the field of multiscale modeling in computational biomedicine is emerging and developing, a foundational multiscale modeling methodology is lacking. The field is also lacking in advancements pertaining to experimental devices, advanced software, and software applications, as well as analytical methods. Critics argue these advancements are necessary before the achievements of systems biology can live up to their much-touted potential [13].

CONCLUSION

What this chapter has demonstrated is that biology is an information science. Systems biology is a holistic rather than reductionist approach to addressing biological complexity, using a collaborative, cross-disciplinary approach.

Systems biology integrates many multiscale types of biological information. It supports the development of new experimental approaches to capture temporal and spatial dynamics of biological networks, and it permits the development of predictive and actionable models.

Incorporating the findings of systems biology research into the Digital Patient platform will ultimately lead to the creation of virtual human models and the widespread availability of personalized medicine. It also has the potential to lead to a more participatory, evidence-based approach to health and to better-informed decisions in the health care decision-making and delivery processes.

REFERENCES

1   Noble, D. Biophysics and systems biology. Philosophical Transactions A. February 1, 2010. Available at: http://rsta.royalsocietypublishing.org/content/368/1914/1125.long. Accessed August 5, 2015.

2   Hester, RL, Iliescu, R, Summers, R, Coleman, TG. Systems biology and integrative physiological modelling. *The Journal of Physiology.* 2011;589(5):1053–1060.

3   Sloot, PM, Hoekstra, AG. Multi-scale modelling in computational biomedicine. *Briefings in Bioinformatics.* 2010;11(1):142–152.

4   Hood, L, Balling, R, Auffray, C. Revolutionizing medicine in the 21st century through systems approaches. *Biotechnology Journal.* 2012;7:992–1001.

5   Hood, L. Systems biology and P4 (Predictive, Preventive, Participatory and Personalized Health) medicine: Past, present, and future. *Rambam Maimonides Medical Journal.* 2013;4(2):e0012.

6   Institute for Systems Biology. About systems biology. Available at http://www.systemsbiology.org/about-systems-biology. Accessed November 25, 2014.

7   P4 Medicine Institute. The 4Ps: Quantifying medicine demystifying disease. Available at http://p4mi.org/4-ps-quantifying-wellness-and-demystifying-disease. Accessed November 25, 2014.

8   Sloot, PMA. NITHM: Health Systems Complexity Program. PowerPoint Presentation. Nanyang Technological University, Singapore.

9   Bui, QC, Sloot, PMA. A robust approach to extract biomedical events from literature. *Bioinformatics*. 2012;28(20):2654–2661.

10   Bui, QC, Sloot, PM, van Mulligen, EM, Kors, JA. A novel feature-based approach to extract drug–drug interactions from biomedical text. *Bioinformatics*. 2014;30(23):1–7.

11   Zarrabi, N, Prosperi, M, Belleman, RG, Colafigli, M, Luca, AD, Sloot, PMA.Combining epidemiological and genetic networks signifies the importance of early treatment in HIV-1 transmission. Khudyakov YE, eds. *PLoS One*. 2012;7(9):e46156.

12   Butcher, EC, Berg, EL, Kunkel, EJ. Systems biology in drug discovery. *Nature Biotechnology*. 2004;22(10):1253–1259.

13   Kitano, H. Systems biology: A brief overview. *Science*. 2002;295(5560):1662–1664. Available at: http://www.sciencemag.org/content/295/5560/1662.short. Accessed August 5, 2015.

8

PERSONALIZED COMPUTATIONAL MODELING FOR THE TREATMENT OF CARDIAC ARRHYTHMIAS

Seth H. Weinberg

Virginia Modeling, Analysis and Simulation Center, Old Dominion University, Suffolk, VA, USA

Computational modeling is an excellent tool that facilitates understanding of arrhythmia mechanisms and enables a personalized approach toward treating arrhythmias in individual patients. Emerging computational modeling strategies will enhance the efficiency, efficacy, and safety of invasive arrhythmia therapies.
— Ronald Berger, MD, PhD, Director of Cardiac Electrophysiology
Johns Hopkins Hospital

INTRODUCTION

In 2011, the American Heart Association reported that an estimated 82 million Americans have one or more types of cardiovascular disease, a rate greater than 1 in 3 Americans. Mortality data showed that in one-third of all deaths in the United States (over 800,000), cardiovascular disease was the underlying cause of death. Over 5 million Americans suffer from heart failure, and over 300,000 died from sudden cardiac death that most likely arose from ventricular fibrillation, a highly disorganized, irregular electrical rhythm in the heart [1].

Heart disease is a leading cause of death in North America, and is one of the most common causes of sudden *unexpected* death encountered in medical examiner and coroner's offices.
— Mitchell Weinberg, MD, Assistant Chief Medical Examiner, Edmonton, Alberta

The primary role of the heart is to pump blood through the circulatory system to the lungs and all organs of the body. Cardiac mechanical function is driven by an electrical

The Digital Patient: Advancing Healthcare, Research, and Education, First Edition.
Edited by C. Donald Combs, John A. Sokolowski, and Catherine M. Banks.
© 2016 John Wiley & Sons, Inc. Published 2016 by John Wiley & Sons, Inc.

system that coordinates the appropriate timing for contraction of the atria and ventricles. The regulation of the electrical activity in the heart is complex, with inputs from the parasympathetic nervous system and dependence on hormonal regulation, metabolic levels, and many other physiological signals.

For many decades, computational models have been valuable tools to help understand many physiological and pathological processes. As heart disease is a leading cause of death, in particular unexpected death, *predictive* computational modeling of the heart must be a key component of the Digital Patient. Historically, cardiac models and simulations have provided mechanistic understanding of key aspects of cardiac electrophysiology, including the coupling between electrical and mechanical activity; electrical propagation and failure; the transition from a normal sinus rhythm to an irregular rhythm, or *arrhythmia*; and electrical activity in pathological states such as heart failure. Early computational models were initially developed to reproduce experimental data from animal models; more recently, models of electrical activity in the human heart have been developed [2–4].

In the past few years, advancements in medical imaging and computational processing capabilities have facilitated the development and use of personalized (or patient-specific) cardiac models. In this chapter, we will discuss how such personalized models have great potential to improve the treatment of cardiac arrhythmias. We will provide a window into the previous, current, and future state of cardiac electrophysiology modeling, by way of an overview of relevant cardiac physiology and developments in computational modeling and simulation. We will discuss the development of early models, which focused on electrical signaling within a single cardiac cell, and how such models have been extended to simulate tissue of increasingly larger size and scale, from one-dimensional "cables" up to the entire heart. Our historical overview is by no means exhaustive; the curious reader is encouraged to engage the references provided at the end of the chapter. We will discuss recently published research that is paving the path for personalized treatment of cardiac arrhythmias, present some of the many challenges and opportunities for future work, and significantly, how personalized cardiac models are one piece of the complex system, that is, the Digital Patient.

We begin by asking significant questions: What computational modeling tools can be used to predict cardiac arrhythmias and the efficacy of cardiac therapies or treatments? Can we incorporate pathological conditions and symptoms, for example, genetic mutations, structural or anatomic defects, abnormal neuronal or hormonal regulation, etc., that arise as a consequence of chronic and/or acute stresses or disease into models and simulations? Importantly, what is the Digital Patient in the context of a personalized model for the treatment of cardiac arrhythmias? What patient-specific information is needed to develop and simulate a predictive model?

BASICS OF CARDIAC ELECTROPHYSIOLOGY

Before a discussion of computational modeling, we provide here a brief overview of cardiac electrophysiology. Mechanical contraction of the heart is coordinated by a propagating wave of electrical activity through the myocardium. Under normal conditions, electrical activity originates spontaneously at the sinoatrial (SA) node, also known as the pacemaker. The electrical wave propagates through the left and right atria to the atrioventricular (AV) node, which briefly delays propagation such that the atria can sufficiently contract and blood can flow from the atria to the ventricles. Following the delay, the electrical wave propagates from the AV node through the bundle of His, which splits into two branches, a left bundle branch and a right bundle branch, which activate the left and right ventricles, respectively. Propagation progresses from the bundle branches to Purkinje fibers, consisting of specialized myocytes that facilitate rapid conduction, which in turn activate the ventricular myocardium.

Electrical wave propagation in the heart is a consequence of the generation of an action potential at the cellular level and the subsequent conduction of this electrical signal from cell-to-cell through gap junctions. An action potential is generated by the movement of ions, such as sodium, potassium, and calcium, through ion channels on the myocyte membrane, resulting in a change in the electrical potential across the membrane. During a propagating electrical wave, the flux of current from a neighboring, coupled cell increases, or *depolarizes*, the membrane potential, rapidly activating inward sodium current, which in turn further increases the membrane potential. At this depolarized voltage, inward calcium (which triggers the contraction of the myocyte, as described later in the chapter) and outward potassium currents are activated, while the sodium current is inactivated. Finally, the calcium current is inactivated, and the membrane potential is *repolarized* to resting levels.

From Nobel Origins

Computational modeling of cardiac electrophysiology, and indeed all excitable cell modeling, can trace its origins to the seminal work of Alan Hodgkin and Andrew Huxley, for which they received the 1963 Nobel Prize in Physiology or Medicine. Hodgkin and Huxley developed a mathematical model that describes the electrical activity of neurons using the squid giant axon. In the Hodgkin–Huxley model [5], first published in 1952, the neuron is represented by an electrical circuit: the cell membrane lipid bilayer is represented by a capacitor and ionic currents are represented by resistors, with time- and voltage-dependent conductances (Fig. 8.1).

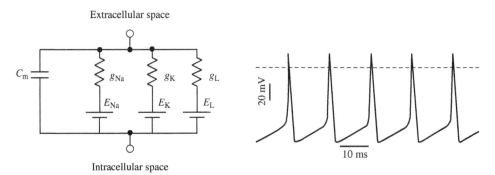

FIGURE 8.1   Hodgkin–Huxley computational model of a neuron. (Left) The circuit diagram represents the electrical properties of the squid giant axon: The cellular membrane is represented by a capacitive element (C_m), and the sodium (Na), potassium (K), and leak (L) ionic currents are represented by resistors with conductances g_{Na}, g_K, and g_L, respectively, each in series with a voltage source, E_{Na}, E_K, and E_L, respectively, which represent the ionic current reversal potential (voltage at which the net current is zero). (Right) A representative simulation reproduces the repetitive firing of the neuron, that is, action potentials, in response to an applied stimulus.

The model includes equations for a capacitive current and three ionic currents: sodium, potassium, and a leak or background current. Using this circuit and Kirchhoff's current law, the equation governing the dynamics of the membrane voltage V, given by

$$C_{\mathrm{m}} \frac{dV}{dt} = -I_{\mathrm{ion}}, \qquad (8.1)$$

where I_{ion} is the sum of the ionic currents and C_{m} is the membrane capacitance, is coupled with equations for additional state variables, called *gating variables*, that govern the ionic current conductance. An additional current term may be added to account for external stimulation. Collectively, these equations constitute a nonlinear system of ordinary differential equations. Significantly, the electrical activity of the neuron can be simulated by integrating this system, illustrating firing of action potentials and the activation and inactivation of individual ionic currents (Fig. 8.1).

Extensions of the Hodgkin–Huxley model of the neuron have been subsequently developed to simulate the dynamics of electrical activity in cardiac myocytes. Denis Nobel developed the first model of a cardiac cell, the Purkinje myocyte, in 1962 [6]. Developments by many groups have produced increasingly detailed models of ventricular, atrial, and

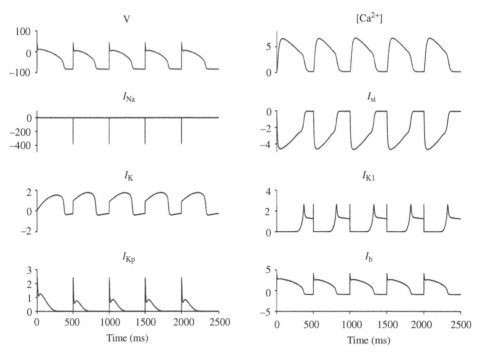

FIGURE 8.2 Luo–Rudy 1991 model of the ventricular myocyte. The myocyte model is stimulated by a brief applied current pulse that elicits an action potential, every 500 ms. The voltage trace is characteristic of the cardiac action potential, with the rapid upstroke, plateau phase, and gradual repolarization. A calcium transient with slow upstroke and recovery follows each action potential. The model contains six currents: sodium (Na), slow inward (typically associated with calcium), three potassium (K) currents, and a background (b) or leak current. The units for voltage, calcium, and ionic currents are millivolts, micromolar, and microamperes/cm², respectively.

sinoatrial node myocytes [7–11]. Several key extensions beyond the Hodgkin–Huxley model include equations to represent additional ionic currents and state variables: calcium currents; several identified potassium currents, ion pumps, and exchangers; ion concentrations; and intracellular stores of calcium. The Luo and Rudy 1991 model is one of the earliest ventricular myocyte models and is still widely used today [7]. A simulation of the model is shown in Figure 8.2.

Model formulations and parameters are continually updated and improved to account for newly available experimental data from a variety of species and cell types, including healthy and pathological human cardiac cells. In the following subsections, we highlight key, but by no means exhaustive, modeling advances and insights that have paved the way toward predictive and personalized models of the heart.

CARDIAC MODELING ADVANCEMENTS

As experimental techniques advanced and enabled the recordings of current from a single ion channel, it became clear that, while Hodgkin–Huxley-type models could well represent ionic current measurements from the entire cell, these models did not reproduce the dynamics (e.g., opening and closing) of individual ion channels. Perhaps most significantly, experiments showed that the timing of ion channel openings and closings is random, a phenomenon that simply cannot be simulated using models governed by deterministic differential equations. Thus, modeling and simulation of myocytes expanded from the realm of nonlinear dynamics to probability and stochastic processes [12]. Studies by many groups demonstrated that ion channel dynamics could be simulated by continuous-time discrete-state Markov chains [10, 13, 14]. Experiments showed that ion channel dynamics are more complicated than transitions between open and closed states; ion channels often exhibit multiple closed states and inactivated states (Fig. 8.3).

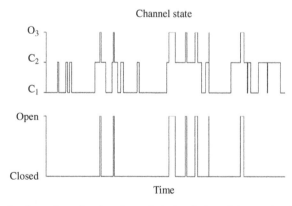

FIGURE 8.3   Stochastic gating of an ion channel. A simulation of the stochastic gating of a three-state ion channel, with a kinetic scheme given by $C_1 \rightleftarrows C_2 \rightleftarrows O_3$, where C_1 and C_2 are two closed states and O_3 is an open state. The simulation shows that the duration of and time between channel openings and closings are random. In the more detailed Markov chain models of ion channel gating, more states may be present, such as inactivated or multiple closed or open states. The transitions between states may depend on voltage, ion concentrations (i.e., calcium), or concentration of a particular ligand or pharmacological agent.

Transitions may depend on voltage, intracellular calcium, or ligand concentrations. Detailed Markov chain models have been developed for several cardiac ion channels from normal myocytes, as well as genetic mutations associated with cardiac diseases such as Long QT and Brugada syndrome [15–17]. Hybrid stochastic-deterministic approaches have been formulated in order to simulate systems of (stochastic) Markov chain ion channel gating and (deterministic) Hodgkin–Huxley-type ionic currents [18].

REGULATION OF INTRACELLULAR CALCIUM

The inclusion of intracellular calcium concentration in cardiac myocyte models was a significant advancement in the modeling of heart disease. In addition to calcium directly triggering the contractile machinery within the cell that leads to muscle contraction, abnormal calcium regulation is associated with a host of genetic diseases, such as catecholaminergic polymorphic ventricular tachycardia (CPVT) [19, 20]. Calcium levels within the cell are highly regulated throughout each cardiac cycle, known collectively as calcium handling or cycling [21] (Fig. 8.4): Intracellular calcium is low at rest. The action potential triggers influx from voltage-dependent calcium channels on the cell membrane. This small calcium influx triggers a large calcium release via calcium-activated channels, called ryanodine receptors (RyRs), from an intracellular calcium store, the sarcoplasmic reticulum (SR). Calcium binds intracellular myofilaments, initiating contraction of the myocyte. Finally, calcium is returned to resting levels via calcium pumps and exchangers. However, this regulation is not one-way; indeed, calcium handling and electrical and mechanical activity are bidirectionally coupled. As a consequence, abnormal calcium signaling can directly lead to life-threatening electrical irregularities or arrhythmias and mechanical dysfunction.

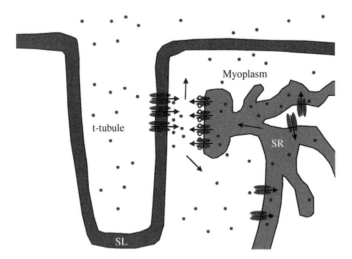

FIGURE 8.4   Calcium signaling in the cardiac myocyte. Illustration of calcium signaling in the cardiac myocyte shows the invagination of the sarcolemma (SL), or cell membrane, known as a t-tubule, and the intracellular store of calcium, the sarcoplasmic reticulum (SR). Voltage-gating calcium channels on the sarcolemma trigger the release of calcium from the SR through channels called "ryanodine receptors." The large efflux of calcium triggers contraction of the myocyte, after which calcium is returned to the SR via ATP-dependent pumps on the SR membrane.

Simulations have shown that accounting for local control of calcium signaling is important [9]: in cardiac cells, the calcium signaling described earlier often occurs in "calcium micro-domains," called dyadic subspaces, in which the calcium-activated channels are regulated by the local calcium concentration, not the concentration of calcium in the myoplasm or "bulk." Systems of ordinary differential equations are often used to account for the calcium concentration in different intracellular "compartments" and the fluxes between these compartments. An example of a simple compartment model representing the calcium concentration in the myoplasm, dyadic subspace, and SR is given by the following system of ordinary differential equations:

$$\frac{d\left[Ca^{2+}_{myo}\right]}{dt} = J_{myo} - J_{pump} \tag{8.2a}$$

$$\frac{d\left[Ca^{2+}_{ds}\right]}{dt} = p_{o,VCC} \cdot J_{VCC} + p_{o,RyR} \cdot J_{RyR} - J_{myo}. \tag{8.2b}$$

$$\frac{d\left[Ca^{2+}_{SR}\right]}{dt} = -p_{(o,RyR)} \cdot J_{RyR} + J_{pump,} \tag{8.2c}$$

where J terms represent fluxes between compartments, and significantly, the flux via the voltage-gated calcium channels (VCC) and RyRs is scaled by an open probability that is time-, voltage-, and calcium-dependent, thus establishing the bidirectional coupling between the voltage and calcium subsystems. These open probabilities may be determined by differential equations or stochastic simulations, as described earlier.

Simulations have recently shown that significant aspects of calcium handling cannot be reproduced by models in which all calcium influx passes through a "common-pool" (as in Eq. 2.2) and neglect "local control" by calcium in the individual dyadic subspaces [22]. Dyadic subspaces are very small in volume (often less than $1\,\mu m^3$), such that at rest only 1–2 calcium ions may be present. As such, calcium diffusion and binding events can produce large fluctuations in the local calcium concentration. Simulations have recently shown that models neglecting these calcium fluctuations may misrepresent important subcellular calcium dynamics that influence the electrical activity of the whole cell and thus potentially the entire heart [23, 24].

FROM CELLS TO CABLES TO SHEETS TO TISSUE TO THE HEART

Extensions of cardiac cell models have proceeded in parallel along many avenues. While single-cell models have extended inward in scope, incorporating increasingly more biophysically detailed representations of ion channels and subcellular signaling, models have also proceeded outward in scope, simulating electrical dynamics of increasingly larger spatial scale, size, and dimension. The electrical circuit analogy of the single cell naturally extends to higher dimensions. The coupling of "single-cell" circuits (Fig. 8.1) via resistors along a single dimension leads to the classical nonlinear cable equation, a mathematical construct often used to study propagation in neuronal axons and dendrites (reviewed in Ref. [25]). In the spatially extended model, the system of ordinary differential equations representing a single cell is replaced with a system of partial differential equations, specifically a reaction–diffusion system in which voltage "diffuses" in the spatial dimensions via cell-to-cell coupling (Eq. 2.3):

$$C_{\mathrm{m}} \frac{dV}{dt} = \nabla \cdot \boldsymbol{D} \nabla V - I_{\mathrm{ion}}, \qquad (8.3)$$

where $\boldsymbol{D}$ is a diffusion tensor. Note that this partial differential equation is identical to the single-cell ordinary differential equation model (Eq. 8.1), augmented by the diffusion term. In higher dimensions, models of two dimensions represent a sheet, while three-dimensional models represent a slab of tissue.

Simulations in 1-, 2-, and 3D have provided significant insights into mechanisms underlying arrhythmia initiation, maintenance, and termination. See Clayton et al., for an excellent review [26]. For example, studies in 1D cable models have demonstrated conditions that lead to electrical propagation failure, which can trigger an arrhythmia [27]. Simulations in two-dimensional (2D) cardiac sheets have shown how rapid electrical waves, known as spiral waves, can become fragmented and chaotic, which is analogous to the transition from a rapid heart rhythm known as a tachycardia to a potentially lethal rhythm fibrillation [28]. Simulations of 3D tissue begin to address the complex issues related to the development of a personalized model of the heart for predictive arrhythmia treatment [29]. Before we discuss these patient-specific models, let us discuss some of the challenges associated with modeling an entire individual heart.

The Heterogeneous Heart

The heart is complex and heterogeneous across many spatial scales. There are regional differences between atrial and ventricular myocytes, such as levels of expression of various ionic currents and calcium handling proteins. Expression levels differ between the left and right ventricle; within the ventricles, there are heterogeneities and gradients from base to apex and transmurally from epicardium to endocardium [30], which influences electrical propagation within the different regions of the heart.

At the tissue level, the myocardium is composed of many cell types. Although myocytes compose the largest component by volume, the much smaller fibroblasts, which play an important supportive role in assembling the extracellular matrix, outnumber myocytes. While the role of fibroblasts in influencing the electrical and mechanical activity of the heart is still an actively investigated area, it is clear that, following myocardial infarction, fibroblasts promote tissue heterogeneity and may couple with myocytes, perturbing electrical activity in and near an infarct region and altering the propensity for arrhythmias [31]. Within the cardiac tissue, expression levels of gap junction proteins vary throughout the ventricular wall and are altered during disease [32, 33].

At the level of individual cells, myocytes can be variable in size and volume, which can further vary in disease. At the subcellular level, ion channels are often localized to particular regions of the cell membrane. The cell membrane topology itself is complex, as deep invaginations of the membrane called transverse tubules (or t-tubules) are present in ventricular myocytes that concentrate membrane calcium channels in the proximity of the SR calcium channels (as described earlier in the chapter).

Beyond these *functional* heterogeneities that occur across many spatial scales, *structural* heterogeneities significantly influence electrical activity within the heart.

Models and simulations using idealized geometries (i.e., cables, sheets, and tissue slabs) can provide insight into electrical activity in the absence of these structural heterogeneities. However, accounting for an individual heart's unique anatomically detailed geometry is an essential step in the development of a personalized model for arrhythmia treatment.

Your Own Personal Heart Model

Returning to Equation 8.3, the partial differential equation for voltage coupled with state variables that collectively describe the electrical activity in cardiac tissue, we are now prepared to ask: How can we formulate a personalized model of the heart? Without trivializing the question too much, we can see that there are essentially two terms we must represent: the ionic currents and the diffusion term. As discussed earlier, ionic current models originated with the Hodgkin–Huxley model of the neuron, followed by development of cardiac models for several animal species and myocyte type (ventricular, atrial, etc.). In 1998, the first human ventricular myocyte model was presented by Priebe and Beuckelmann [34], which notably includes variations for normal physiology and heart failure. Several models of the human ventricular myocyte have subsequently been developed [2–4, 35, 36]. The ten Tusscher model presented in 2004 is a frequently used model in simulation studies and includes variations for myocytes across the transmural gradient (epicardial, endocardial, and midmyocardial cells) [2]. The Iyer–Mazhari–Winslow model, also presented in 2004, notably represents most ionic currents using Markov chain representations [3].

When building the patient-specific model of the heart for the Digital Patient, which model can and should be used? This question gets to the *heart* of one of the most significant challenges associated with personalized models, and indeed large-scale models in general: computational complexity. The Bueno–Orovio human myocyte model consists of four state variables, with representations of three ionic currents, neglecting intracellular calcium handling. In contrast, the Iyer–Mazhari–Winslow model consists of 67 state variables, representing 13 currents and several intracellular calcium compartments. Most other models fall somewhere in between in terms of complexity. From a computational standpoint, using a minimal model enables one to simulate more computationally intensive simulations (e.g., longer duration simulations and more detailed spatial representation), but at the expense of physiological detail at the level of the individual cell. Such minimal cellular-level representations can often still reproduce the same behavior as more detailed models at higher spatial scales. For example, the minimal Bueno–Orovio model reproduces the dynamics of spiral waves in 2D sheets, as observed in the more detailed Priebe–Beuckelmann and ten Tusscher models. However, if a patient has known pathology that includes altered dynamics of a particular ion channel, then ideally a personalized model for this patient should include an explicit representation of that perturbed ion channel. In many cases, this is not always possible, and the influence of the pathology must be accounted for indirectly.

The second key term in the equation governing electrical activity is the diffusion term, which represents the diffusion of voltage throughout the myocardium via gap junctions. While idealized geometries typically assume that cells are regularly spaced on a grid, advancements in medical imaging can be used to determine anatomical geometries based on an individual heart. Early studies used histological sectioning to determine the geometry of small pieces of cardiac tissue. More recently, studies have used computed tomography

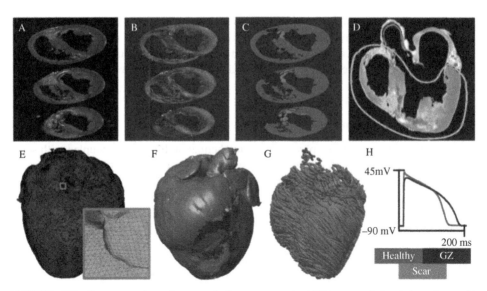

FIGURE 8.5   Reconstruction of anatomical geometry. A. MRI scan of the infarct heart. B. Calculation of myocyte orientation from DTMRI data. C. Segmentation of imaging data into healthy myocardium, periinfarct or gray zone (GZ), and scar tissue. D. Separation of atria from ventricles. E. Finite element mesh. F. Three-dimensional representation of the heart. G. Representation of the DTMRI-reconstructed myocyte orientation. H. Action potentials from the healthy and GZ myocytes. Reproduced from Ref. [42].

(CT) and magnetic resonance imaging (MRI) data to reconstruct individual heart geometries. Diffusion tensor (DT) MRI provides additional detailed information regarding myocyte orientation. Echocardiography, while typically of lower resolution, provides a less invasive and less costly method for anatomical reconstruction. The details of constructing anatomically based geometry are complex and beyond the scope of this chapter. The reader is encouraged to see recent reviews and articles [37–42]. In brief, the process involves segmentation of the imaging data (classification of tissue as normal, infarct, background, and so on), generation of a finite element mesh, and determination of myocyte orientation (see Fig. 8.5).

A Brief Summary of Recent Studies of Personalized Cardiac Models

We briefly summarize a few recent studies of personalized cardiac models. In 2011, Aguado-Sierra and colleagues developed a personalized failing heart model for a patient with a myocardial infarct and left ventricular bundle branch block and simulated electrical activity and hemodynamics, including ventricular pressure throughout the cardiac cycle, which was in close agreement with patient measurements [43]. In 2013, Ashikaga and colleagues performed a retrospective study of catheter ablation targets in patients with scar-related ventricular tachycardia, and their simulations showed close agreement for ablation associated with both success and failure [44]. Their study demonstrates that simulations could be used to predict an optimal ablation site. In 2013, Rantner and colleagues demonstrated that patient-specific simulations could be used to predict optimal placement of implantable cardioverter defibrillators (ICDs) for pediatric and congenital heart defect (CHD) patients to minimize the defibrillation threshold [45].

WHERE CAN WE GO FROM HERE? WHAT IS THE CARDIAC MODEL IN THE DIGITAL PATIENT?

These are difficult questions to answer. Certainly, the Digital Patient should include patient-specific information that is needed to develop a personalized cardiac model. This would need to include anatomical information regarding structure, infarcts, and so on obtained from imaging studies. Beyond this level of information, the answers to these questions are somewhat open-ended. The human myocyte models described earlier were formulated based on average experimental values from many hearts and individual heart cells. Could it one day be feasible to formulate a personalized myocyte model, or many personalized models for different regions of the heart? Such a challenge is daunting and not feasible in a noninvasive manner at present. However, in the short term, human myocyte models can be modified to account for patient-specific information. Such models have already been modified to account for varying degrees of heart failure. As mentioned earlier, ion channels and calcium signaling are altered in patients with certain cardiac diseases, such as CPVT and Long QT syndrome, that are associated with specific genetic mutations. The inclusion of such genetic information in the Digital Patient would enable appropriate *personalized* modifications to a *generic* human myocyte model.

It is worth noting that the aforementioned studies were *retrospective* or focused on *model validation*. While this is a necessary and important step, *prospective* studies and *testing predictions* will ultimately demonstrate the value of personalized models. Many studies, experimental and computational, have shown that accounting for heterogeneity throughout the myocardium across many spatial scales is important to accurately simulate electrical activity, in particular arrhythmias. To what extent and at what spatial scale should a patient-specific model account for heterogeneities? Early patient-specific models have incorporated some detailed heterogeneities, most significantly at the structural and anatomical level, differences in myocytes transmurally, and heart failure modifications. However, accounting for heterogeneities at finer spatial scales and the stochasticity of ion channel openings/closings and calcium signaling may also be important, particularly in the context of calcium-mediated arrhythmias. The Digital Patient should also include information on cardiac-specific interactions with pharmaceutical agents, in particular antiarrhythmic drugs. For example, a recent study of whole heart simulations that included a myocyte model incorporating the binding of two sodium channel blockers into a Markov chain model was able to reproduce the results of the cardiac arrhythmia suppression trial (CAST), in which these drugs paradoxically increased mortality [46].

Importantly, the cardiac model of the Digital Patient should include information regarding inputs from and outputs to the other systems of the body, including the external environment. For example, myocyte models have been developed to simulate the effects of beta-adrenergic stimulation of myocytes [47], modulating contractile strength and heart rate. The integration of a mitochondrial bioenergetics in a myocyte model has been formulated to simulate the influence of increased workload or ischemia [48]. Several studies have coupled whole-heart electrical activity with models of cardiac mechanics, coupling intracellular calcium levels at the single cell with myofilament models, which in turn can predict mechanical deformations using equations from continuum mechanics [49]. Such an electromechanical whole-heart model could in turn be coupled to a personalized model of the cardiovascular network [50] and respiratory system [51]. Simulations could also be used to test novel cardiac therapies in a patient-specific manner [52]. For example, recent simulation studies have tested novel defibrillation approaches, such as high-frequency stimulation [53, 54] and optogenetic therapy [55].

Incorporating all of these levels of detail may be important for predictive modeling but also come at a cost, again touching this important issue of computational complexity. At present, incorporating stochastic ion channel gating into models of the whole heart has not been demonstrated and is likely not feasible with current computational power. Recent advancements in the development of Graphic Processing Units (GPUs) have greatly accelerated and enabled large-scale simulations. Model reduction techniques have been developed that enabled larger-scale simulations that can account for aspects of stochastic phenomenon using deterministic equations [56]. Further research in these areas will enable more computationally intensive simulations.

We conclude with an important question about the construction of the Digital Patient: What level of detail is necessary to simulate, and more importantly, accurately predict the efficacy of a patient-specific cardiac treatment? In the context of personalized cardiac modeling, we would argue that the answer to this question is situation specific. For example, predicting an optimal ablation strategy may not require an ionic model with detailed calcium signaling, whereas predicting the outcome of a treatment for a patient with CPVT likely will. Similarly, predicting the efficacy of a sodium channel drug for the treatment of Long QT syndrome will require a detailed model of the sodium channel but may not require high-resolution imaging data. Of course, great difficulty lies in determining what level of detail is necessary for any particular patient, disease, and therapy. This notion can be summarized by the quote oft-attributed to Albert Einstein:

> Everything should be made as simple as possible, but not simpler.

Just how simple a model should be can often only be answered post hoc. Despite such challenges, personalized cardiac models, individually and as part of the larger Digital Patient, represent a new and powerful tool for clinicians that have great potential to improve, optimize, and revolutionize patient care and treatment.

REFERENCES

1 V. L. Roger, A. S. Go, D. M. Lloyd-Jones, and R. J. Adams, "Heart disease and stroke statistics—2011 update: A report from the American Heart Association," *Circulation*, vol.123, no. 4, pp. e18–e209, February 2011.

2 K. H. W. J. ten Tusscher, D. Noble, P. J. Noble, and A. V. Panfilov, "A model for human ventricular tissue," *Am. J. Physiol. Heart Circ. Physiol.*, vol. 286, no. 4, pp. H1573–H1589, April 2004.

3 V. Iyer, R. Mazhari, and R. L. Winslow, "A computational model of the human left-ventricular epicardial myocyte," *Biophys J*, vol. 87, no. 3, pp. 1507–1525, September 2004.

4 T. O'Hara, L. Virág, A. Varró, and Y. Rudy, "Simulation of the undiseased human cardiac ventricular action potential: Model formulation and experimental validation," *PLoS Comput. Biol.*, vol. 7, no. 5, pp. e1002061, May 2011.

5 A. L. Hodgkin and A. F. Huxley, "A quantitative description of membrane current and its application to conduction and excitation in nerve," *J. Physiol.*, vol. 117, no. 4, pp. 500–544, August 1952.

6 D. Noble, "A modification of the Hodgkin—Huxley equations applicable to Purkinje fibre action and pacemaker potentials," *J. Physiol.*, vol. 160, pp. 317–352, February 1962.

7 C. H. Luo and Y. Rudy, "A model of the ventricular cardiac action potential. Depolarization, repolarization, and their interaction," *Circ. Res.*, vol. 68, no. 6, pp. 1501–1526, June 1991.

8 C. H. Luo and Y. Rudy, "A dynamic model of the cardiac ventricular action potential. II. After depolarizations, triggered activity, and potentiation," *Circ. Res.*, vol. 74, no. 6, pp. 1097–1113, June 1994.

9 J. L. Greenstein and R. L. Winslow, "An integrative model of the cardiac ventricular myocyte incorporating local control of Ca^{2+} release," *Biophys. J.*, vol. 83, no. 6, pp. 2918–2945, December 2002.

10 A. Mahajan, Y. Shiferaw, D. Sato, A. Baher, R. Olcese, L.-H. Xie, M.-J. Yang, P.-S. Chen, J. G. Restrepo, A. Karma, A. Garfinkel, Z. Qu, and J. N. Weiss, "A rabbit ventricular action potential model replicating cardiac dynamics at rapid heart rates," *Biophys. J.*, vol. 94, no. 2, pp. 392–410, January 2008.

11 V. E. Bondarenko and R. L. Rasmusson, "Simulations of propagated mouse ventricular action potentials: effects of molecular heterogeneity," *Am. J. Physiol. Heart Circ. Physiol.*, vol. 293, no. 3, pp. H1816–H1832, June 2007.

12 G. D. Smith, "Modeling the stochastic gating of ion channels," in Computational Cell Biology, 2002, Springer, New York, pp. 1–35.

13 L. A. Irvine, M. S. Jafri, and R. L. Winslow, "Cardiac sdium channel Markov model with temperature dependence and recovery from inactivation," *Biophys. J.*, vol. 76, no. 4, pp. 1868–1885, April 1999.

14 Y. Rudy and J. R. Silva, "Computational biology in the study of cardiac ion channels and cell electrophysiology," *Q. Rev. Biophys.*, vol. 39, no. 1, pp. 57–116, February 2006.

15 C. E. Clancy, and Y. Rudy, "Cellular consequences of HERG mutations in the long QT syndrome: Precursors to sudden cardiac death," *Cardiovasc. Res.*, vol. 50, no. 2, pp. 301–313, May 2001.

16 C. E. Clancy and Y. Rudy, "Na^+ channel mutation that causes both Brugada and long-QT syndrome phenotypes a simulation study of mechanism," *Circulation*, vol. 105, no. 10, pp. 1208–1213, March 2002.

17 Q. Zhou, G. C. L. Bett, and R. L. Rasmusson, "Markov models of use-dependence and reverse use-dependence during the mouse cardiac action potential," *PLoS One*, vol. 7, no. 8, pp. e42295, August 2012.

18 A. Alfonsi, E. Cancès, G. Turinici, B. Di Ventura, and W. Huisinga, "Adaptive simulation of hybrid stochastic and deterministic models for biochemical systems," *ESAIM*, vol. 14, pp. 1–13, September 2005.

19 V. Iyer and A. A. Armoundas, "Unraveling the mechanisms of catecholaminergic polymorphic ventricular tachycardia," *Conf. Proc. IEEE Eng. Med. Biol. Soc.*, Suppl. 6761–6764, 2006.

20 G. M. Faber and Y. Rudy, "Calsequestrin mutation and catecholaminergic polymorphic ventricular tachycardia: A simulation study of cellular mechanism," *Cardiovasc. Res.*, vol. 75, no. 1, pp. 79–88, July 2007.

21 D. M. Bers, "Cardiac excitation–contraction coupling," *Nature*, vol. 415, no. 6868, pp. 198–205, January 2002.

22 M. D. Stern, "Theory of excitation-contraction coupling in cardiac muscle," *Biophys. J.*, vol. 63, no. 2, pp. 497–517, August 1992.

23 S. H. Weinberg and G. D. Smith, "Discrete-state stochastic models of calcium-regulated calcium influx and subspace dynamics are not well-approximated by ODEs that neglect concentration fluctuations," *Comput. Math. Methods Med.*, vol. 2012, no. 12, pp. 1–17, September 2012.

24 S. H. Weinberg and G. D. Smith, "The influence of Ca^{2+} buffers on free $[Ca^{2+}]$ fluctuations and the effective volume of Ca^{2+} microdomains," *Biophys. J.*, vol. 106, no. 12, pp. 2693–2709, June 2014.

25 C. Koch, Biophysics of Computation. Oxford University Press, New York, 2004.

26 R. H. Clayton and A. V. Panfilov, "A guide to modelling cardiac electrical activity in anatomically detailed ventricles," *Prog. Biophys. Mol. Biol.*, vol. 96, no. 1, pp. 19–43, January 2008.

27 A. G. Kléber and Y. Rudy, "Basic mechanisms of cardiac impulse propagation and associated arrhythmias," *Physiol. Rev.*, vol. 84, no. 2, pp. 431–488, April 2004.

28 F. H. Fenton, E. M. Cherry, H. M. Hastings, and S. J. Evans, "Multiple mechanisms of spiral wave breakup in a model of cardiac electrical activity," *Chaos*, vol. 12, no. 3, pp. 852–892, September 2002.

29 F. Fenton and A. Karma, "Vortex dynamics in three-dimensional continuous myocardium with fiber rotation: filament instability and fibrillation," *Chaos*, vol. 8, no. 1, pp. 20–47, March 1998.

30 R. H. Clayton, O. Bernus, E. M. Cherry, H. Dierckx, F. H. Fenton, L. Mirabella, A. V. Panfilov, F. B. Sachse, G. Seemann, and H. Zhang, "Models of cardiac tissue electrophysiology: progress, challenges and open questions," *Prog. Biophys. Mol. Biol.*, vol. 104, no. 1, pp. 22–48, January 2011.

31 K. S. McDowell, H. J. Arevalo, M. M. Maleckar, and N. A. Trayanova, "Susceptibility to arrhythmia in the infarcted heart depends on myofibroblast density," *Biophys. J.*, vol. 101, no. 6, pp. 1307–1315, September 2011.

32 S. Poelzing and D. S. Rosenbaum, "Altered connexin43 expression produces arrhythmia substrate in heart failure," *Am. J. Physiol. Heart Circ. Physiol.*, vol. 287, no. 4, pp. H1762–H1770, October 2004.

33 S. Poelzing, F. G. Akar, E. Baron, and D. S. Rosenbaum, "Heterogeneous connexin43 expression produces electrophysiological heterogeneities across ventricular wall," *Am. J. Physiol. Heart Circ. Physiol.*, vol. 286, no. 5, pp. H2001–H2009, May 2004.

34 L. Priebe and D. J. Beuckelmann, "Simulation study of cellular electric properties in heart failure," *Circ. Res.*, Vol. 82, no. 11, pp. 1206–1223, June 1998.

35 E. Grandi, F. S. Pasqualini, and D. M. Bers, "A novel computational model of the human ventricular action potential and Ca transient," *J. Mol. Cell. Cardiol.*, vol. 48, no. 1, pp. 112–121, January 2010.

36 A. Bueno-Orovio, E. M. Cherry, and F. H. Fenton, "Minimal model for human ventricular action potentials in tissue," *J. Theor. Biol.*, vol. 253, no. 3, pp. 544–560, August 2008.

37 F. Vadakkumpadan, L. J. Rantner, B. Tice, P. Boyle, A. J. Prassl, E. Vigmond, G. Plank, and N. Trayanova, "Image-based models of cardiac structure with applications in arrhythmia and defibrillation studies," *J. Electrocardiol.*, vol. 42, no. 2, pp. 157.e1–157.e10, March 2009.

38 N. A. Trayanova and P. M. Boyle, "Advances in modeling ventricular arrhythmias: From mechanisms to the clinic," *WIREs Syst. Biol. Med.*, vol. 6, no. 2, pp. 209–224, December 2013.

39 N. A. Trayanova and L. J. Rantner, "New insights into defibrillation of the heart from realistic simulation studies," *Europace*, vol. 16, no. 5, pp. 705–713, May 2014.

40 S. Severi, B. Rodriguez, and A. Zaza, "Computational cardiac electrophysiology is moving towards translation medicine," *Europace*, vol. 16, no. 5, pp. 703–704, May 2014.

41 A. Prakosa, P. Malamas, S. Zhang, F. Pashakhanloo, H. Arevalo, D. A. Herzka, A. Lardo, H. Halperin, E. McVeigh, N. Trayanova, and F. Vadakkumpadan, "Methodology for image-based reconstruction of ventricular geometry for patient-specific modeling of cardiac electrophysiology," *Prog. Biophys. Mol. Biol.*, vol. 115, no. 2–3, pp. 226–234, August 2014.

42 H. Arevalo, G. Plank, P. Helm, H. Halperin, and N. Trayanova, "Tachycardia in post-infarction hearts: insights from 3D image-based ventricular models," *PLoS One*, vol. 8, no. 7, pp. e68872, July 2013.

43 J. Aguado-Sierra, A. Krishnamurthy, C. Villongco, J. Chuang, E. Howard, M. J. Gonzales, J. Omens, D. E. Krummen, S. Narayan, R. C. P. Kerckhoffs, and A. D. McCulloch, "Patient-specific modeling of dyssynchronous heart failure: a case study," *Prog. Biophys. Mol. Biol.*, vol. 107, no. 1, pp. 147–155, October 2011.

44   H. Ashikaga, H. Arevalo, F. Vadakkumpadan, R. C. Blake, J. D. Bayer, S. Nazarian, M. M. Zviman, H. Tandri, R. D. Berger, H. Calkins, D. A. Herzka, N. A. Trayanova, and H. R. Halperin, "Feasibility of image-based simulation to estimate ablation target in human ventricular arrhythmia," *Heart Rhythm*, vol. 10, no. 8, pp. 1109–1116, August 2013.

45   L. J. Rantner, F. Vadakkumpadan, P. J. Spevak, J. E. Crosson, and N. A. Trayanova, "Placement of implantable cardioverter-defibrillators in paediatric and congenital heart defect patients: a pipeline for model generation and simulation prediction of optimal configurations," *J. Physiol.*, vol. 591, no. 17, pp. 4321–4334, August 2013.

46   J. D. Moreno, Z. I. Zhu, P.-C. Yang, J. R. Bankston, M.-T. Jeng, C. Kang, L. Wang, J. D. Bayer, D. J. Christini, N. A. Trayanova, C. M. Ripplinger, R. S. Kass, and C. E. Clancy, "A computational model to predict the effects of class I anti-arrhythmic drugs on ventricular rhythms," *Sci. Transl. Med.*, vol. 3, no. 98, pp. 98ra83, August 2011.

47   J. L. Greenstein, A. J. Tanskanen, and R. L. Winslow, "Modeling the actions of beta-adrenergic signaling on excitation—contraction coupling processes," *Ann. N. Y. Acad. Sci.*, vol. 1015, no. 1, pp. 16–27, May 2004.

48   S. Cortassa, M. A. Aon, B. O'Rourke, R. Jacques, H.-J. Tseng, E. Marbán, and R. L. Winslow, "A computational model integrating electrophysiology, contraction, and mitochondrial bioenergetics in the ventricular myocyte," *Biophys. J.*, vol. 91, no. 4, pp. 1564–1589, August 2006.

49   N. A. Trayanova, "Whole-heart modeling: applications to cardiac electrophysiology and electromechanics," *Circ. Res.*, vol. 108, no. 1, pp. 113–128, January 2011.

50   N. Xiao, J. D. Humphrey, and C. A. Figueroa, "Multi-scale computational model of three-dimensional hemodynamics within a deformable full-body arterial network," *J. Comput. Phys.*, vol. 244, pp. 22–40, July 2013.

51   F. Gaudenzi and A. P. Avolio, "Lumped parameter model of cardiovascular-respiratory interaction," *Conf. Proc. IEEE Eng. Med. Biol. Soc.*, vol. 2013, pp. 473–476, 2013.

52   N. A. Trayanova, T. O'Hara, J. D. Bayer, P. M. Boyle, K. S. McDowell, J. Constantino, H. J. Arevalo, Y. Hu, and F. Vadakkumpadan, "Computational cardiology: How computer simulations could be used to develop new therapies and advance existing ones," *Europace*, vol. 14, no. 5, pp. v82–v89, November 2012.

53   H. Tandri, S. H. Weinberg, K. C. Chang, R. Zhu, N. A. Trayanova, L. Tung, and R. D. Berger, "Reversible cardiac conduction block and defibrillation with high-frequency electric field," *Sci. Transl. Med.*, vol. 3, no. 102, pp. 102ra96, September 2011.

54   S. H. Weinberg, K. C. Chang, R. Zhu, H. Tandri, R. D. Berger, N. A. Trayanova, and L. Tung, "Defibrillation success with high frequency electric fields is related to degree and location of conduction block," *Heart Rhythm*, vol. 10, no. 5, pp. 740–748, May 2013.

55   P. M. Boyle, J. C. Williams, C. M. Ambrosi, E. Entcheva, and N. A. Trayanova, "A comprehensive multiscale framework for simulating optogenetics in the heart," *Nat. Commun.*, vol. 4, p. 2370, 2013.

56   G. S. B. Williams, M. A. Huertas, E. A. Sobie, M. S. Jafri, and G. D. Smith, "A probability density approach to modeling local control of calcium-induced calcium release in cardiac myocytes," *Biophys. J.*, vol. 92, no. 7, pp. 2311–2328, April 2007.

9

THE PHYSIOME PROJECT, *open*EHR ARCHETYPES, AND THE DIGITAL PATIENT

DAVID P. NICKERSON, KORAY ATALAG, BERNARD DE BONO, AND PETER J. HUNTER

Bioengineering Institute, University of Auckland, Auckland, New Zealand

INTRODUCTION

Our understanding of human health, disability, and disease, and the rational design of preventative, diagnostic, or therapeutic strategies, will be eventually dependent upon quantitative knowledge of human anatomy and physiology captured in mathematical models. Every other scientific discipline (from weather forecasting to the manufacture of everything from cell phones to aircraft) uses *a priori* knowledge of the physical laws of nature with model-based analysis and design, and there is no reason to think it will not be the same for biology. Computational physiology draws on techniques from these disciplines to deal with anatomical and physiological complexities by solving the mathematical equations that arise when the laws of physics and chemistry are coupled with measurements of biological material properties.

Disease is often a manifestation of the dysfunction of molecular-level processes, but the consequences are seen at the tissue and organ scale. Computational physiology must therefore also address the challenges of multiscale physiological processes that operate over a 10^9 range of spatial scale (molecules to organ systems) and 10^{15} range of temporal scale (microseconds of biochemical reactions to the decades of aging processes). As we gain a quantitative understanding of human physiology through multiscale mathematical modeling and how to adapt these generic models to an individual patient, there is an increasing need to describe disability and disease in terms of model parameters and to link these parameters into electronic health records (EHRs). In this chapter, we discuss the development and use of standards, tools, and software for computational modeling of the

The Digital Patient: Advancing Healthcare, Research, and Education, First Edition.
Edited by C. Donald Combs, John A. Sokolowski, and Catherine M. Banks.
© 2016 John Wiley & Sons, Inc. Published 2016 by John Wiley & Sons, Inc.

human body, including the concept of a physiology circuitboard, and how these could be linked to the encoding of patient data in EHR standards such as *open*EHR.

We discuss the use of *open*EHR Archetypes to help bridge this substantial gap and to illustrate concepts we investigate as an example of a disease arising from a single familial genetic mutation (pseudohypoaldosteronism, associated with mutations of the amiloride-sensitive epithelial sodium channel, ENaC) that yields multiple clinical phenotypes across multiple organ systems.

MULTISCALE PHYSIOLOGICAL PROCESSES

Living organisms are characterized at the molecular level by chaotic thermal energy captured for useful outcomes by dissipative enzyme-controlled processes that are supplied with energy from highly reduced, low-entropy food and oxygen. The primary constituents are carbohydrates, fats, and about 100,000 structurally different proteins (including splice variants) coded by about 20,000 genes whose spatially varying expression is carefully regulated by signaling systems that respond to cues from the local tissue environment as well as the current regulatory state of each cell. The complex interplay between the genome and the environment, now known to include intergenerational epigenetic marking, is described quantitatively by the discipline known as molecular systems biology. The concepts and equations describing behavior at this level include conservation of mass, electrical charge neutrality, the second law of thermodynamics, Gibb's free energy, and the Boltzmann equation. Statistical variation is intrinsic at this level because the underpinning processes are chaotic.

Above the 100 nm scale of proteins and molecular biology, the primary organizational unit is the eukaryote cell (typical dimension 10 m) and mammals have around 300 types—neglecting the much larger number of prokaryotic bacterial cells occupying every possible external epithelial cell-lined niche in our bodies. Physiological function, however, really only emerges at the 100 m scale of primary functional tissue units (pFTUs) that typically embrace five different cell types organized around epithelial conduits (e.g., crypts) or endothelial conduits (capillaries) [1]. Still higher-level secondary FTUs (sFTUs) such as kidney nephrons, liver lobules, cardiac sheets, lung alveoli, bone osteons, colon crypts, etc., are the highly organized tissue structures (each containing multiple pFTUs) that are replicated (often a millionfold) to support the organ-level function of the kidney, liver, heart, lung, musculoskeletal, digestive systems, etc. [1]. Larger animals just include more of these sFTUs in their organs.

Physical processes at the tissue and organ level are described by the equations of mathematical physics: Maxwell's equations for electromagnetic fields, advection–reaction–diffusion transport equations, the Navie–Stokes equations of fluid flow, and the large deformation equations of the finite elasticity theory of solids. These equations capture the laws of the physical universe we live in and, subject to the uncertainty of initial conditions, boundary conditions, and certain constitutive parameters (see later), are predictive. They can be solved on complex mammalian anatomy with numerical methods—predominantly the finite element method but with links to molecular mechanisms [2].

A very important aspect of these equations is that they all contain a black box "constitutive law"—an empirically derived relationship that defines various material properties of the tissue but hides the molecular detail. The viscosity of blood in the Navier–Stokes equations, for example, can be specified empirically as a function of hematocrit, or it can be derived from a detailed analysis of blood constituents. Similarly, the reaction—diffusion equation governing electrical activation in myocardium, for example, contains a current source term that is defined empirically by the measured current–voltage characteristics of each contributing membrane ion channel. The ion channel conductivity and its gating kinetics can be described, if the channel protein structure is known, by molecular dynamic (in fact, atomic-level) equations, but it is often useful to summarize the channel behavior with an empirical relationship that is either directly measured or computed *a priori* from the underlying physics. In all such cases, the ability to derive the constitutive law from the underlying physics is a huge advantage if such an analysis can quantify the influence of disease on the underlying components or processes.

It is abundantly clear that physiological processes, from molecular to tissue scale, are enormously complex and will only be understood quantitatively via biophysically and anatomically based mathematical modeling and numerical computation. The challenge for the Physiome Project (see later) is to establish robust frameworks for computational physiology that ensure reproducibility and reuse of modular model components, and that also enable the use of multiscale modeling in patient-specific (or more realistically subpopulation-specific) drug design and the development of therapeutic strategies. In the following section, we describe the data and modeling standards, databases, and tools that have been developed over the past 20 years to help achieve these goals. The application of this framework to clinical workflows will, however, depend on linking the Physiome standards to medical informatics and EHRs. In subsequent sections, we explore these links and provide an example of how the frameworks can be used to understand diseases associated with mutations of the amiloride-sensitive epithelial sodium channel, ENaC.

PHYSIOME PROJECT STANDARDS, REPOSITORIES, AND TOOLS

Over the past 20 years, a modeling framework for computational physiology has been developed, under the auspices of the Physiome Project [3, 4] and the European VPH project [5, 6]. The overriding goal has been to facilitate reproducibility, modularity, and reuse in computational bioscience: (i) published models and data for biological processes should be available in standardized electronic formats that include annotation of the mathematical components and variables with their biological and biophysical meaning, and allow automated checking of equations for unit consistency; (ii) publications describing these models and data should include an electronic workflow in a standardized format that specifies all information needed to reproduce the results claimed by the publication, including the tables and figures; (iii) the model description framework should facilitate modularity of model construction, for example, using import mechanisms so that complex models can be assembled automatically from simpler components defined as reusable modules.

Modeling Standards

The XML-based standards for the Physiome Project now include CellML [7] for encoding lumped parameter models, FieldML [8] for encoding spatially varying fields, BioSignalML [9] for encoding time-varying signals, and SED-ML [10] for encoding the computational workflow. The molecular systems biology standard (SBML) [11] is also being used as part of the framework. A model repository called "Physiome Model Repository" (PMR) [12] has been developed for CellML-encoded models and now includes about 600 models covering a very wide variety of biological processes. Most of these models are curated (to ensure that

TABLE 9.1   The Data and Modeling Standards in Use in the Physiome Project, and Examples of Repositories and Software Tools Supporting them

Standards	Examples	Repositories	Software
Minimum information standards	MIRIAM MICEE MIASE	MIBBI	
Data encoding standards	BioSignalML RDF, DICOM	Physionet CAPdb	BioSignalML SemSim
Model encoding standards	CellML FieldML SBML	PMR BioModels Database Cardiac Electrophysiology Web Lab	OpenCOR OpenCMISS SBML software
Simulation description standards	SED-ML	PMR BioModels Database Cardiac Electrophysiology Web Lab	SED-ML Showcase

simulations based on the CellML encoding reproduce the outputs reported in the publication) and some are annotated (to provide biological and biophysical meaning to the model components). Various freely available open-source software tools that incorporate Application Programming Interfaces (APIs) for some or all of the CellML, SBML, FieldML, SED-ML, and BiosignalML standards are available. *Open*COR [13], for example, is a general-purpose authoring and simulation environment for CellML models. SBML is designed for molecular systems biology with a focus on encoding biochemical reactions. CellML is designed for any biophysical model, with the syntax (employing MathML for encoding the maths) being agnostic to the application—model components are annotated with biological and biophysical meaning in the RDF-based metadata using appropriate ontologies [14]. Table 9.1 lists some of these standards, data and model repositories, and software tools.

Minimum Information Standards

Minimum Information standards for Biological and Biomedical Investigations (MIBBI) [15] are a set of guidelines for reporting experimental data to ensure that the data can be easily verified, analyzed, and clearly interpreted by the wider scientific community. Each guideline is drawn up by the relevant community of experimentalists. A good example is the Minimum Information about a Cardiac Electrophysiology Experiment (MICEE) [16, 17], which defines a schema that includes information about the tissue preparation, the testing environment, the experimental protocols, the recordings made, and the analysis performed. There are about 40 such standards registered on the MIBBI website, including a minimum information standard for simulation "experiments" called "Minimum Information About a Simulation Experiment" (MIASE) [18].

Physiome Model Repository

The Physiome Model Repository (PMR) [12] is an extensible software system that provides the infrastructure for collaborative development and sharing of models and that supports basic reasoning over the annotations of its component models. The PMR can be trawled to extract a reference to a model, their components and any annotatable object, in particular, model variables. The approximately 600 models in PMR [19] are currently listed under the following categories: *Calcium dynamics, Cardiovascular circulation, Cell cycle, Cell migration, Circadian rhythms, Electrophysiology, Endocrine, Excitation–contraction coupling, Gene regulation, Hepatology, Immunology, Ion transport, Mechanical constitutive laws, Metabolism, Myofilament mechanics, Neurobiology, pH regulation, PKPD, Signal transduction,* and *Synthetic biology* (see Ref. [19]). Each model in this list corresponds to a journal publication and is available as an "exposure," which provides details on the model and the publication from which it is drawn. Various "views" of the model are made available: *Documentation*; *Model metadata*; *Model curation*; *Mathematics* (this displays Presentation MathML generated from Content MathML); *Generated code* (C, C++, Fortran77, Matlab, Python); *Citation information*; *CellML source code*; and, in some instances, a link to launch a software tool to run simulations for that model. Note that RICORDO [20, 21] provides the framework for annotating and adding semantic meaning to the PMR data and models using the resource description framework (RDF).

The next stage of content development for PMR is to provide a list of the modular components of these models each with their own exposure. For example, models for each of the individual ion channels used in the publication-based electrophysiological models will be available as stand-alone models that can then be imported as appropriate into a new composite model. The same is the case for enzymes in metabolic pathways and signaling complexes in signaling pathways. Some examples of these protein modules relevant to the clinical example discussed later are as follows:

Sodium/hydrogen exchanger 3 https://models.physiomeproject.org/e/236/

Thiazide-sensitive Na-Cl cotransporter https://models.physiomeproject.org/e/231/

Sodium/glucose cotransporter 1 https://models.physiomeproject.org/e/232/

Sodium/glucose cotransporter 2 https://models.physiomeproject.org/e/233/

Note that in each case, as well as the CellML-encoded mathematical model, links are provided to the UniProt Knowledgebase for that protein, and to the Foundational Model of Anatomy (FMA) ontology [22, 23] (via the EMBLE-EBI Ontology Lookup Service) for information about tissue regions relevant to the expression of that protein (e.g., *Proximal convoluted tubule, Apical plasma membrane*; *Epithelial cell of proximal tubule*; *Proximal straight tubule*). Similar facilities are available for SBML-encoded biochemical reaction models through the BioModels database [24].

If the data and models based on these XML-encoding standards are to be useful for the Digital Patient, they must be linked to medical informatics. In the next section, we show how the Physiome models are linked into organ systems for studying both physiology and pathophysiology via the ApiNATOMY circuitboard, review the standards for medical informatics, and propose how the two currently rather disparate areas of model encoding standards and medical informatics standards could be brought together.

The Physiology Circuitboard

The modeling standards described earlier deal with the encoding of the model equations in markup languages (CellML, SBML, and FieldML). The variables and parameters of these models are annotated with biological and biophysical meaning via RDF-encoded metadata that provide links to six ontologies maintained by the Open Biomedical Ontologies (OBO) community [25] and adopted by the Virtual Physiological Human community as a standard for resource annotation: ChEBI for chemical IDs [26, 27], GO for cellular components (GO_CC) [28], the CellType ontology (CT) for cellular entities [29, 30], FMA for gross anatomy [22], OPB for biophysics [31], and UniProt for protein citations [32]. Each model represents a module that captures the function (including anatomy if FieldML is used) of some physiological process, and each module could itself have been assembled by integrating multiple modules. As we move up these scales to the more complex processes associated with disease, typically involving multiple tissues, organs, and organ systems, there is a significant challenge in assembling these modules into the larger physiological system picture.

To address this challenge, we have developed the concept of an ApiNATOMY physiological "circuitboard" [33] that contains the entire 50,000 terms of the FMA in an easily accessible form. The term "circuitboard" refers to the formal knowledge we have generated to bridge physiological processes across the body, as well as the circuitboard-style graphics (illustrated in Figure 9.1) used to create a visual depiction of this knowledge. Figure 9.1 shows the circuitboard at the top level (left) and a region where the user has zoomed into a part of the vascular system (right). Note that all epithelial tissue (in contact with the outside world) is depicted on the periphery, adjacent to the organ systems that are in contact with epithelium—the integument (skin), respiratory system, digestive system, genital organs, and various sensory organs.

Modeling molecular transitions, for example, within and between diffusive compartments in tissues entails overcoming two formidable representational challenges of tissue structure and function, namely, how to:

1. apportion tissue space in terms of diffusive parcellations (i.e., a parcel of tissue within which any two points are within diffusion distance of one another) to enable the modeling of transitions in molecular co-location, driven by Brownian motion, across subcellular compartments inside and across nearby cells, as well as,

2. connect these parcellations across distances that are well beyond the diffusion limit (e.g., to describe the transfer of sodium ions from lung tissue to the kidneys) to enable modeling of fluid flow that conveys molecules from one organ to another, or across distant tissue regions within the same organ.

A key goal for the clinical scenario discussed below is the modeling of sodium *a*bsorption, *d*istribution and *e*limination (**ADE**) by multiple tissues. The application of a workflow associated with the physiology circuit board [34] overcomes the earlier two challenges to generate data and models that coherently bridge diffusive and advective processes in support of ADE modeling for sodium. Figure 9.2 illustrates the way in which the use of the FMA ontology allows a FieldML computational model of the vascular system to be overlaid onto relevant tissue types for linking to, for example, CellML pharmacokinetic models.

The physiology circuit board is also a way of linking pFTUs[35] (the pFTU concept described in the first section earlier) in different tissue regions of the body. This is illustrated in Figure 9.3.

Standards for Medical Informatics

Having clinical information in electronic form that is computable has been a grand challenge for biomedical informatics since the dawn of the discipline [36]. Unfortunately, most health information still sits in silos today, and health information exchange for the

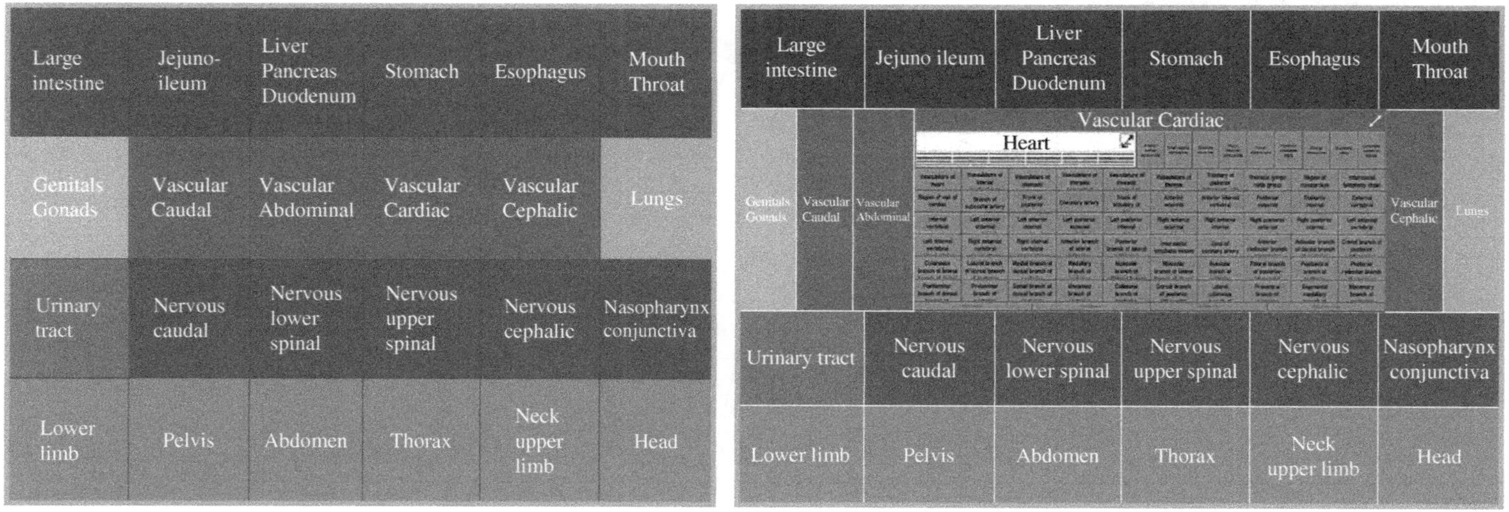

FIGURE 9.1 The physiology circuitboard, showing (left) the major anatomical components of the body and (right) an expanded view of the vascular cardiac system. The terminology is from the Foundation Model of Anatomy (FMA) and all 50,000 anatomical terms of the FMA can be accessed by click/zooming into any region.

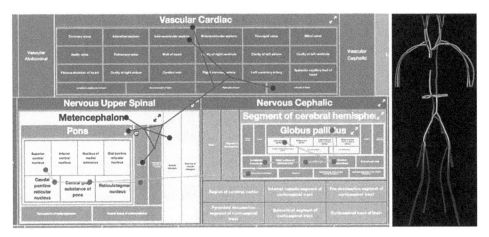

FIGURE 9.2 Overlaying a FieldML model of flow in the cardiovascular system (figure on right) with tissue components of interest in the physiology circuitboard (figure on left). Annotating components of the vascular model with the FMA terms ensures that the 3D computational FieldML model can be projected onto the circuitboard to link with a variety of CellML models operating in different tissue regions. See Ref. [30] for further details.

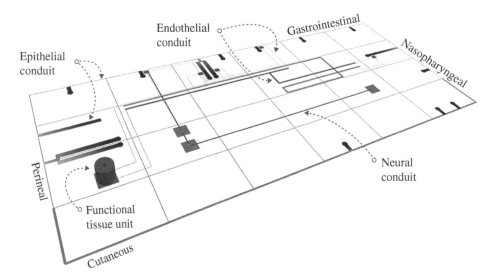

FIGURE 9.3 Mock-up of an ApiNATOMY circuitboard display, showing anatomical layout of a tiled depiction of body regions, edge-based illustration of advective conduits, and a cylindrical pFTU. The histology component of this workflow generates tissue parcellations from 3D histology images, known as primary functional tissue units (pFTUs) [35, 1]—these images are annotated with terms from the FMA and CT. We apply the modeling component of the workflow to link these tissue units to models of long-range fluid flow over the circuit board.

purpose of supporting care between organizations and levels of care (e.g., hospital to primary care) until very recently has been an exception rather than the norm. The size and complexity of the domain and peculiar ethical and medicolegal requirements coupled with the variability of healthcare practice as often encountered render most traditional IT approaches to eHealth unfit, including standardization activities to date. Connecting for

Health Programme in the United Kingdom, for example, is considered one of the largest IT project failures in history [37]. It is fair to say that, to a large extent, health information has been the weakest link in the chain when we consider other related domains like bioinformatics, pharmaceutical, and medical device technology in the quest for integrated biomedicine.

An important rule of thumb in capturing structured and computable clinical data is to obtain them as part of routine clinical practice, as post hoc data collection has been shown to be very expensive, error prone, and at times it is impossible to capture the clinical context in which the data were collected [38]. Data sources can be very diverse and range from operational EHR systems to well-structured longitudinal disease registries and biobanks. The patients' own contribution to health records, increasingly using mobile devices and sensors, is also important and can add valuable insights about environmental and behavioral factors as well (e.g., food, air quality, exercise, and mood).

Being able to make health information linkable and computable requires standardization at various levels (Fig. 9.4). Both data- and terminology-level standards are reasonably mature although there is considerable overlap among certain terminology and ontology systems such as SNOMED CT [39] and LOINC [40]. It is the content standards that have to tackle most of the difficulties arising from breadth, depth, complexity, variability, changeability, and longevity aspects of health information management. Indeed much of the current debate seems to be focussed on such standards, and there are considerable efforts within the discipline to develop fit-for-purpose standards and specifications. Exchange standards (e.g., HL7 v2 messaging [41] or the fast healthcare interoperability resource or FHIR-based API) further tackle the dynamic aspects of health information flow, and ideally they should use the same or a compatible model of information and leverage representational aspects from content standards (e.g., use the same definition for laboratory results or drugs and adverse reactions).

Based on relevance and adoption patterns, we will focus on SNOMED CT as the terminology standard, *open*EHR as the content standard that underpins the Clinical Information Modeling Initiative (CIMI) [42], and ISO/CEN 13606 [43], and HL7 FHIR [44] as the exchange standards.

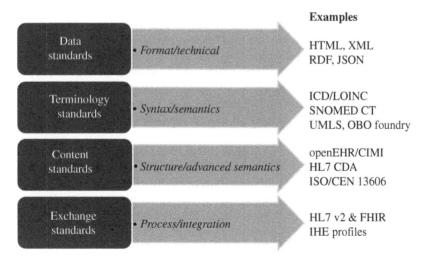

FIGURE 9.4 Different layers of standardization for health information.

SNOMED CT

SNOMED CT is the most comprehensive clinical terminology, encompassing more than 300,000 unique concepts and about 1.4 million relationships with several language translations [39]. Governed strongly by the International Health Terminology Standards Development Organisation (IHTSDO), its scope encompasses the whole healthcare domain for the purpose of encoding the EHR to primarily support care.

Individual concepts are organized into multiple hierarchies (e.g., body structure, clinical finding, pharmaceutical/biologic product, organism, and substance) and linked to natural language descriptors including synonyms and preferred terms. Following ontological principles, SNOMED CT further defines Attributes and Relationships between Concepts. These are mostly "is-a" type relationships that can be used to infer narrower and broader terms, but other types such as "part-of" or "manifestation-of" also exist.

SNOMED CT is underpinned by the powerful Description Logic methodology for formal interpretation of its concepts and relationships and also supports precoordination (e.g., acute gastritis) and postcoordination (gastritis|type: acute) mechanisms to "add more meaning" by combining terms.

There is overlap with the widely used International Classification of Diseases (ICD) [45] terminology in the area of diseases and with Logical Observation Identifiers Names and Codes (LOINC), which is also widely used for ordering and reporting of laboratory tests. There is an ongoing harmonization work between the groups and some mappings are available. A more relevant issue from the point of view of the Digital Patient is that there are also significant overlaps between SNOMED CT and commonly used ontologies in computational physiology such as FMA and ChEBI. While each knowledge resource has been created to serve a particular purpose, mappings between commonly used ontologies in computational physiology and those terminology systems used to encode health information will be critical for any future integration.

*open*EHR

*open*EHR provides open-source specifications and tooling to address the difficulties in representation and handling of health information by means of multilevel modeling. This results in effective separation of concerns (clinical and technical worlds), and also helps tackle the complexity and change. Governed by the *open*EHR Foundation that was founded in 2001 as a not-for-profit organization [46], the approach builds on the EU-funded Good Electronic Health Record (GEHR) project from 1991. Although *open*EHR is not a *de jure* standards development organization, it is increasingly being recognized as a *de facto* standard and being adopted worldwide, especially by the research community. Furthermore, both ISO and CEN have adopted *open*EHR to create a subset standard for the purpose of health information exchange [43].

At the heart of the openEHR formalism is the *Archetype*, which is a computable and reusable discrete model of health information [47]. As opposed to singleton terms usually found in terminological systems such as ICD or SNOMED CT, an Archetype corresponds to a composite and structured but semantically indivisible unit of health information that encapsulates both data and clinical context (e.g., blood pressure measurement). Archetypes formally describe structured health information in a way that can easily be understood and maintained by healthcare professionals. They combine healthcare concepts, clinical context, data elements and their organization, terminology and associated metadata in a technology agnostic way. Practically Archetypes specify labels, data structures and types, valid value ranges, and enumerated values for each information item as well as custom annotations. As an EHR standard, it allows for the data model, user interface, messaging and document exchange, and legacy system integration to be based on the same set of specifications.

A powerful Archetype-based querying language is also part of the specifications: Archetype Query Language (AQL) [48, 49]. As opposed to using table and field references in a relational database or class and property references, AQL queries resemble clinical discourse by leveraging the concept definitions, unique paths, and terminology bindings in Archetypes. Also, it is very fast as the search algorithms can be implemented in a way that uses Archetypes as a map into the data store rather than brute-force searches.

The *open*EHR methodology is commonly known as two-/dual-level or multilevel modeling: The first level is the reference model (RM) comprising fairly stable technical building blocks that depict generic characteristics of health information (e.g., record organization, data structures and types). RM provides the means to define clinical context to meet ethical, medicolegal, and provenance requirements. For example, most generic data types coming out of programming languages or common libraries fall short of representing medication timing in a correct and computable way in a prescription, which is crucial for secondary use. RM is represented using the Unified Modeling Language (UML).

The second level consists of clinical concepts that are constructed by pulling together and constraining the technical building blocks defined in the RM (e.g., by defining optionality, repeatability, sort order, providing default and assumed values) using visual tools. A domain-specific language, the Archetype Definition Language (ADL), is used to express Archetypes. One key distinction of ADL is that one is able to define *Object*-level constraints (e.g., at data instance level) easily as opposed to *Class*-level constraints as offered by other information modeling formalisms such as UML or OWL.

Additional levels exist at the level of *open*EHR Templates (which brings together Archetypes and further constraints for local use) and also at terminology/ontology levels. This effectively reduces the dependency between healthcare and technical professionals by separating the business and technical aspects. A good analogy to understanding how RM, Archetypes, and terminologies relate to each other is by using a limited set of standard LEGO® blocks to assemble many different structures as shown in Figure 9.5.

The blood pressure measurement archetype is a good example. It consists of both the data part that holds the actual measurement data (e.g., systolic and diastolic blood pressure) and also the necessary contextual information required for the correct interpretation by a different system (or a clinician), such as cuff size (e.g., adult and child) and patient position (e.g., lying and sitting). Its mind map representation is given in Figure 9.6.

Archetypes can also import (called slotting) other archetypes so that more comprehensive clinical models can be created. For example, in Figure 9.6 specific archetypes defining the sphygmomanometer used during measurements (e.g., Medical Device) and another for defining a structured model for the patient's exertion status could be slotted into [Device] and [Exertion] slots.

Archetypes contain all possible data elements for a given concept, hence they are *Maximal Datasets*. In practice, only a fraction of data elements defined in an Archetype will be used by any one system; however all data will be interoperable. *open*EHR models can be serialized into other formats, including human readable (e.g., mind maps), computable (e.g., UML, XML, XSD, and OWL), HL7 messages or Clinical Document Architecture (CDA), or FHIRs or profiles. Therefore while the content is managed consistently, downstream technical development can continue without much disruption.

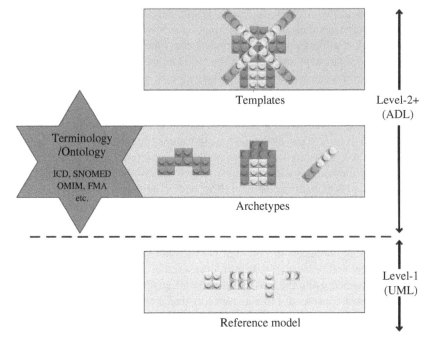

FIGURE 9.5   Schematic representation of the *open*EHR multilevel modeling approach.

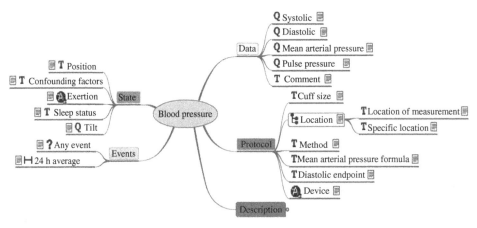

FIGURE 9.6   The openEHR CKM blood pressure measurement archetype mindmap.

ARCHETYPE SPECIALIZATION

Archetypes can be modified safely without breaking original semantics and data-level compatibility by a formal method called "Archetype specialization." New data elements or values can be added, and existing constraints can be made tighter (e.g., making optional data items mandatory or changing free text to coded text). Archetype Specialization is a very powerful, yet simple, mechanism. It ensures backward data compatibility and alignment of datasets with different granularities, and also the ability to run generalized queries against highly granular specialist repositories.

ARCHETYPE DEFINITION LANGUAGE

ADL is a declarative domain-specific language that makes use of existing formalisms such as the Object Constraint Language (OCL) and First-Order Predicate Logic (FOPL). Object Data Instance Notation (ODIN) is an *open*EHR-specific human-readable and computable data representation syntax. It should be noted that the language itself is independent of RM and indeed can be used in domains other than healthcare. The normative ADL version 1 is due to be superseded by ADL version 2, which is reasonably mature and driven by high-profile initiatives like the CIMI as well as various national eHealth programs.

Using ADL constraints for types, values, cardinality, existence, and occurrences can be specified. It is also possible to define local value sets for data items within an Archetype. Every data item defined in an Archetype has a unique path and an internal identifier, thus together with the Archetype identifier they can be referenced from elsewhere. Archetypes can reference other Archetypes, either as a whole (e.g., chaining) or certain items or paths. For the interests of modelin, the Digital Patient the terminology and annotation features will be quite important. The anatomy of an archetype is shown in Figure 9.7.

It should be noted that an Archetype defines how a particular clinical concept can be represented (e.g., data items, structures, value sets, links to external terminologies, annotations, and translations) based on domain knowledge (most archetypes are developed using expert consensus). These constraints would apply to each and every data instance that conform that a particular archetype. On the one hand, Archetypes, as models alone, can be

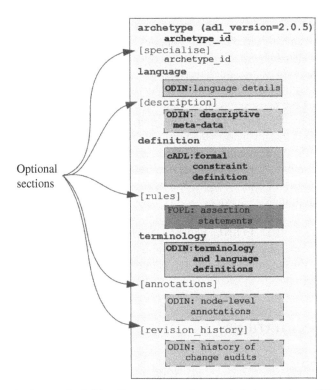

FIGURE 9.7 Archetype Definition Language sections and their notations (ODIN, OCL and FOPL).

used as a source of domain knowledge for the Digital Patient and complement physiological models by providing the definitions for clinical manifestations or parameters.

On the other hand, it is the actual Archetype-based data instances that contain patient-specific information that may provide far more value as these data could be fed into computational models so as to validate them or to generate personalized results. In addition, it is also possible to define instance-level metadata (as opposed to metadata defined at Archetype level). For example, for text type data items it is possible to use the Term Mappings feature to store RDF-like subject- (unique Archetype path), predicate- (with a defined URI), and object- (terminology query or resource with a defined URI) style annotations. In this case, Archetypes can serve as a patient-specific knowledge source by allowing access to instance data.

LINKING ARCHETYPES TO EXTERNAL KNOWLEDGE SOURCES (TERMINOLOGY AND BIOMEDICAL ONTOLOGIES)

Linking Archetypes to related knowledge sources (called "terminology binding") happens in the terminology section. Terminology is used as a broad term referring to various coding, classification and nomenclature systems, controlled vocabularies, and also to biomedical ontologies. *open*EHR defines information in terms of items and their organization for the purpose of *representation*, but their *real-world meaning* and relationships are registered in such resources. Every item, including locally defined value sets, can be linked to one or more terminological resources for the purpose of nonambiguously defining its meaning. Terminology binding allows for expressing much richer semantics and opens up the way for data federation and advanced decision support.

In addition to manual binding, it is also possible to define value sets for certain items by means of semantic terminology queries. Suppose we want to provide list of terms for an Archetype item that defines viral kidney infections. Hence, a query could be written to include "is-a: virus and body-site: kidney" referencing to SNOMED CT. This insulates the clinical model from the complexity and internal workings of complex terminologies. Another advantage is that changes to the terminology can be made without breaking existing applications. HSSP, a joint initiative of HL7 and Object Management Group (OMG), is working on the Common Terminology Service Release 2 (CTS II) standard, which specifies generic properties of terminologies and common operations as well as standard API for accessing the terminology service.

While the current usage of the terminology section is focussed on clinical terminology systems (e.g., ICD, LOINC, and SNOMED), semantic queries relevant to integrating computational physiology data and model resources (DMRs) and clinical data could be formed for modeling the Digital Patient (e.g., FMA, OMIM, UniProt, OBO Foundry, and others).

ARCHETYPE ANNOTATIONS

Annotations are used to provide item-level metadata and specified by (unique) archetype paths and any number of key/value pairs. Where the terminology bindings are found to have shortcomings for the purpose of Digital Patient modeling, it is quite possible to exploit the annotations feature to achieve the desired capabilities. For example, an RDF-based annotation scheme can be implemented, which is compatible with current tooling (e.g., PMR2, RICORDO etc.). These annotations can then be extracted and stored in an existing metadata repository (e.g., in a triple-store as defined in the RICORDO framework) [46]. It is important to note that these are not instance-level annotations.

*Open*EHR MODEL REPOSITORY AND GOVERNANCE

The Clinical Knowledge Manager (CKM) is a web-based clinical models repository and a distributed authoring and governance tool. The *open*EHR Foundation maintains the international CKM instance [50] where registration is free for all. Few other CKM instances exist to meet local or national needs. CKM works like any distributed version control system and supports an editorial process resembling scientific journal peer review. Archetype editors identify a group of domain experts and invite them to a round of CKM review with a due date. Through the web interface each reviewer can then comment on all the individual items of the particular Archetype with a final recommendation as to whether to accept (after minor or major revision) or reject them. There can be as many rounds as necessary, and when the Archetype is considered mature enough it is published. All previous versions and discussions are saved and can be retrieved through the CKM interface. CKM supports a set of APIs to search and access the content, so presumably metadata required for Digital Patient modeling could be extracted with ease.

FAST HEALTHCARE INTEROPERABILITY RESOURCES

FHIR is the latest health information exchange standard from HL7 building on their rather unsuccessful v3 suite of standards and also influenced by other organizations such as *open*EHR, Integrating the Healthcare Enterprise (IHE) [51], and modern web technologies. It is freely available from http://hl7.org/fhir. At the heart of FHIR is the concept of Resources, which are very similar to Archetypes, as the basic unit of interoperability such as a Patient, Adverse Reaction, or Questionnaire. It should be noted, however, that the purpose of FHIR is health information exchange and does not cover the whole of EHR. Therefore, there are marked differences in the design of FHIRs versus *open*EHR Archetypes. First of all, FHIR does not concern creating a maximal dataset for a particular concept. Instead, FHIR strongly advocates the 80/20 rule, in that only items found in 80% of current systems are included in the core specification. The rest can be handled by Extensions, which is a formal mechanism that allows implementers to add new items in a safe and discoverable way.

All Resources have globally unique identifiers and are represented in both XML and JSON. Each Resource embodies a human readable component that summarizes the data in the Resource. Resources can be exchanged in various ways, such as a REST service, inside a Message or a Document.

Like *open*EHR Templates, FHIR Resources can be profiled and bundled to suit certain needs. The significance of FHIR for Digital Patient modeling is manyfold. First, although it is currently not a normative standard, its simplicity for implementation and adherence to modern web standards and technologies have already made it extraordinarily popular in the eHealth domain and almost every serious vendor has already invested in the technology. Second, there is strong drive from many national programs and particularly the US government for the adoption of FHIR [52]. It is therefore almost certain that FHIR will be the actual interface to real-world clinical data in the near future.

It is evident that core *open*EHR Archetypes and FHIRs should be aligned for seamless interoperability. One way to establish this without reinventing concepts for the HL7 community would be to jointly develop further resources and use *open*EHR tooling to create profiles and terminology bindings.

Most vendor systems use proprietary data models and very few have *open*EHR-compliant data repositories. Therefore, FHIR may be the logical pathway to normalize this proprietary data and make it available for secondary use or advanced decision support (possibly based on *open*EHR).

A DISEASE SCENARIO

In this section, we draw upon an example from a clinical scenario to illustrate the application of Physiome modeling approaches and *open*EHR Archetypes to studying pathology mechanisms relevant to a disease condition. We also show how we can draw benefit from the application of ontology- and vocabulary-based standards to provide access to data in support of modeling objectives.

The Pathophysiology of ENaC

The amiloride-sensitive epithelial sodium channel, ENaC, regulates sodium reabsorption over a number of epithelial sites, such as colon, nephron, salivary gland, lungs, and sweat gland [53].

Mutations in the gene for this channel may have two, opposite, effects on sodium physiology:

1. Pseudohypoaldosteronism (PHA): a **reduced** function of the channel may lead to hypovolemia, acidosis, and hyperkalemia [54], as well as a cystic fibrosis-like impact on the lung, giving rise to a predisposition to recurrent chest infection [55].
2. Pseudoaldosteronism (PA): a **hyperactive** function of the same channel may lead to alkalosis, hypokalemia, and an excessive accumulation of sodium in the extracellular fluid, giving rise to hypertension.

The time course for the complications caused by the genetic dysfunction of ENaC can also vary considerably between different mutations—some conditions may resolve through physiological compensation within the first few years of life [56], and others may be fatal unless properly diagnosed and may require life-long monitoring [57].

Challenges to Modeling

The study of the spectrum of the physiological effects of ENaC mutation, therefore, gives rise to the formidable challenge of modeling these effects by taking into account the range of:

1. **Size scales**: For example, representing the impact of altering rates of sodium absorption at cellular level on the pressure of blood at the level of the heart and aorta;

2. **Time scales**: For example, representing the temporal link between the excessive accumulation of sodium in the lung leading to thickening in the consistency of alveolar fluid, and eventual bronchiolar atelectasis, and bacterial overgrowth in the airways;

3. **Interacting sites**: For example, (i) although the same mutated gene is being expressed across the range of tissues described earlier, the simulation of tissue-specific activity of this channel will require parameterization to reflect the effect of the electrochemical environments predominant in those organs. (ii) Modeling the influence that different tissue sites exert on each other (i.e., both within the same organ and between organs) is essential, as in the case of chest infection in PHA that leads further worsening of hyponatremia due to the inappropriate section of ADH by the brain [58, 59].

Applying the Knowledge Representation

The flow modeling strategy to describe the multiscale processes for the handling of sodium ions by ENaC is to link (i) FMA-annotated advective segments conveying blood and other fluid types to (ii) the central advective channel of FMA- and CT-annotated pFTUs generated from the parcellation analysis of the colon, salivary gland, lung, sweat glands, and kidney. This linkage is assembled and visualized via the ApiNATOMY graphical user interface (GUI) described earlier.

Advective flow is modeled through the advective network using OpenCMISS [60]. Time-varying solutions for pressure, flow, and sodium concentration are computed from the relevant models and exported to ApiNATOMY for display on the semantic graphs corresponding to the relevant anatomical region. Once the pressure and flows have been computed throughout the advective systems, an advection–diffusion equation is solved in order to compute the concentration of the sodium ion along these systems. The result of this computation is then a time-varying concentration of the ion in every tissue of the body. This computed transient tissue ion concentration provides an input to combinations of cell models encoded in CellML that share annotations with pFTU-based models. The PMR contains many examples of tissue processes for electrolyte regulation.

Simulations for the effect of tissue expression of ENaC on sodium concentration are carried out on a GET model server (GMS documentation and code available at Refs. [61, 62]), a standalone server that provides web-services for interacting with CellML models. The services relevant here are those related to the model simulation service. The steps linking the execution of the simulation of CellML models using GMS to the ApiNATOMY GUI are illustrated in Figure 9.8.

The ApiNATOMY component contains a central timing module to control and synchronize dynamic model content, such as certain simulations and animations. The timer can run in real time, or be manually controlled through a slider-bar.

By interfacing with the GMS, ApiNATOMY allows direct interaction with CellML models synchronized through the timing module. The semantic metadata repository associated with the PMR allows ApiNATOMY to discover the various variables of a CellML model, and display their traces in a line-chart, or set of line-charts. These charts can also show "alternate timeline" traces for comparison purposes, and will show exact values on mouse-over of glyphs, representing these variables in the correct anatomical context. Mouse-over on graph depictions of blood vessels, also gives rise to displays of location-specific pressure, flow, and ion concentration data.

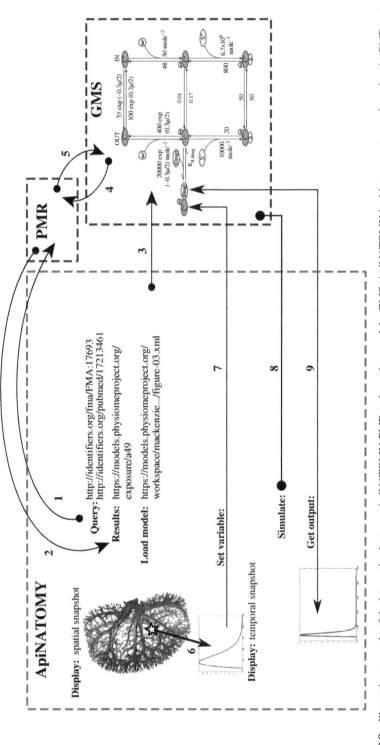

FIGURE 9.8 Illustrative example of the interaction between ApiNATOMY, PMR web services, and the GMS. ApiNATOMY is able to execute queries using the PMR metadata repository (arrow 1, in bold). In the example shown, ApiNATOMY is querying for a given FMA term (for the renal proximal tubule) and a specific paper identified via a PubMed ID. PMR responds to the query providing all matching PMR exposures (arrow 2), from which the ApiNATOMY user selects the appropriate PMR workspace (identified by the URL shown in the diagram). From the selected workspace, the ApiNATOMY user selects a specific CellML model (or the tool infers the required CellML model from information obtained from the exposure definition in PMR) and the GMS is instructed to load that CellML model (arrow 3). Upon receiving this instruction, the GMS will request the model from PMR [12] and instantiate that model into an internal executable form. ApiNATOMY is able to sample spatial fields to extract temporal snapshots for a specific spatial location. Using services provided by the GMS, ApiNATOMY is able to select a particular variable in the instantiated CellML model and instruct the GMS to use the temporal snapshot to define that variable. This service requires the transfer of the temporal snapshot from ApiNATOMY to the GMS using a standard JavaScript array encoded as a JSON string. Once a particular simulation is fully defined, ApiNATOMY instructs the GMS to execute the simulation, over the time interval specified by the central timing module. Following the execution of the simulation, ApiNATOMY requests the simulated variable transient(s) for the desired model variables and presents the results to the user. Once again, this data is transferred as JavaScript arrays encoded in the JSON format.

A Clinical Model

The objective of modeling for this clinical example is twofold: (i) to create a blueprint to represent common clinical features of PHA based on general medical knowledge and population-level data to supplement the computational models and (ii) to create patient or subpopulation-specific models that can be instantiated with real clinical data (possibly aggregated from disparate sources) so as to make possible personalized simulations and visualize temporal disease patterns in the longitudinal health record. It is important to recap the fact that Archetypes define data instance-level constraints on generic RM objects, so building a PHA Digital Patient model with default values and reference ranges taken from generic knowledge or population-level data will serve (i), and using this model to represent actual data (either by *open*EHR-based GUI applications or external data normalized using the model) will serve (ii). In effect, when the model itself and instance data are annotated using clinical terminology and ontologies interoperable with those used by the computational physiology community, a key functionality can be added to ApiNATOMY and other relevant tools to link to real and computable clinical information relevant for that context (e.g., renal disease prognosis when hovering over genitourinary system tile).

As indicated earlier, pseudohypoaldosteronism (PHA) comprises a heterogeneous group of disorders of electrolyte metabolism characterized by an apparent state of renal tubular unresponsiveness or resistance to the action of aldosterone. Clinical characteristics include hyperkalaemia, metabolic acidosis, and a normal glomerular filtration rate. Affected individuals may also present with hypervolemia, renal salt wasting or retention, hypotension or hypertension, and elevated, normal, or low levels of renin and aldosterone based on various underpinning mechanisms.

SNOMED CT has the following entry for PHA:

Pseudohypoaldosteronism (disorder) [77098009]
Pseudohypoadrenocorticalism (synonym)

There are four subtypes:

1. Pseudohypoaldosteronism, type 1, dominant form (disorder) [85880000]
2. Pseudohypoaldosteronism, type 1, recessive form (disorder) [91180009]
3. Pseudohypoaldosteronism, type 2 (disorder) [15689008]
4. Pseudohypoaldosteronism, type 2A (disorder) [703254001]
   (synonym: Gordon hyperkalemia–hypertension syndrome)

Using relationships and hierarchies, we can also infer from SNOMED CT that PHA is a metabolic disorder of transport (disorder) [111394006]. Subtypes of PHA, such as the type 1 recessive form, have additional information indicating that it is a hereditary disorder of the endocrine system and are associated with the adrenal cortex as the body site.

SNOMED CT also includes related entries that may be associated with PHA, for example, Hyperkalemia [14140009], Hyperkalemic acidosis [237847005], Hypercalciuria [71938000], and Renal calculus [95570007]. Figure 9.9 illustrates how these SNOMED CT terms can be bound to the openEHR Problem/Diagnosis Archetype.

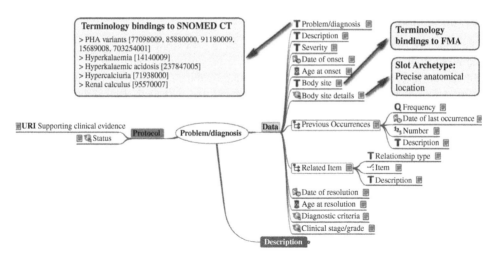

FIGURE 9.9   Problem/diagnosis archetype from *open*EHR CKM with example SNOMED CT bindings.

In order to capture the essential clinical features of PHA, the following Archetypes could be used in the proposed way from *open*EHR CKM:

1. Problem/Diagnosis Archetype (URL: http://openehr.org/ckm/#showArchetype_ 1013.1.169) This archetype is used ubiquitously to record health problems, mostly diagnoses, as recorded by healthcare professionals together with rich clinical context. Archetype item [Problem/Diagnosis] is usually bound to SNOMED CT and hence most EHR systems offer selection of terms from a predetermined list. This Archetype will serve for expressing the clinical condition of PHA together with other associated data and clinical context (Fig. 9.9). At instance level (e.g., in a clinical data repository using Archetyped data), it could be used to identify patients with PHA as well as associated clinical findings (e.g., recurrent chest infection or renal calculus) using the terminology bindings given earlier. Archetype item [Age at Onset] and [Age at Resolution] will provide useful information about the onset and course of the condition and can be used to differentiate the different variants of PHA.

2. Family History Archetype (URL: http://openehr.org/ckm/#showArchetype_ 1013.1.1633) This archetype is used to capture the problems and diagnoses found in genetic relatives and can be configured to denote the various PHA inheritance patterns at model level. Again it can be used at instance level to access real clinical data.

3. Symptom Archetype (URL: http://openehr.org/ckm/#showArchetype_1013.1.195) This generic archetype can be used to define various symptoms related to PHA and also used to retrieve this information from patient records.

4. Pathology Test Result Archetype (URL: http://openehr.org/ckm/#showArchetype_ 1013.1.1401) This archetype and further specializations (e.g., urine protein) can be used to express and retrieve all test result–related information about PHA. In most cases, LOINC will be the choice of clinical terminology for coding of laboratory tests in today's EHR systems.

5. Precise Anatomical Location (URL: http://openehr.org/ckm/#showArchetype_ 1013.1.356) This generic archetype can be used to depict the exact anatomical

location for different types of clinical information required for the PHA patient model, such as [Body Site Details] in the Problem/Diagnosis Archetype or microscopic findings or any kind of medical imaging results. It will have an important role in linking clinical data spatially to multiscale models. [Name of location] for example, can be bound to FMA.

SUMMARY AND CONCLUSIONS

The goal of this chapter has been to summarize the infrastructure being developed for multiscale computational physiological modeling by the Physiome Project and the infrastructure being developed for medical informatics, and to explore ways in which these two fields could be linked through the Archetype data model of *open*EHR. We have used a particular disease model (pseudohypoaldosteronism) to illustrate concepts.

*open*EHR-based models of the Digital Patient can provide key knowledge about clinical concepts and their relationships, which can link to relevant computational models. When real clinical data are available conforming to this model, personalization of computational models becomes possible, and this can pave the way for a whole new raft of advanced clinical decision support tools. Even if source data may not be available in Archetyped format, this Digital Patient model can be used as a canonical health record architecture to normalize disparate data sources, which can then be queried consistently [63]. For example, an AQL query can be formulated to evaluate prognosis of subjects having early-onset PHA with autosomal recessive inheritance and with multiple organ involvement using above Archetypes.

This normalization step can be critical, for example, date/time primitive data types used by the majority of current systems to represent the timing of clinical phenomena (e.g., medication timing) may fall short of meeting the semantic precision required for multiscale temporal representations for computational physiology. It is evident that an important step in any workflow should involve researchers to identify what kind of clinical concepts would be relevant to a particular modeling context (e.g., PHA, cardiovascular disease, or a rare disease) and decide on particular terminology bindings that would facilitate the linkage of multiscale models. Tools working with real clinical data should also incorporate the functionality to annotate Archetyped data instances using preferred open biomedical ontologies.

We can discuss about both model- and data-based inferencing over rich collections of clinical data sources integrated with the computational models. A probable example would be a biobank expressing all its clinical data using the openEHR-based Digital Patient model, which have Archetype terminology bindings not only to clinical terminology but also to other biomedical ontologies like CheBI, UniProt, Gene Ontology, and OMIM as well as instance-level annotations. These metadata can be extracted as semantic annotations for *every* instance and stored in the same metadata repository such as the CellML models, thus offering a one-stop-shop querying capability for researchers to find related data and model resources (DMRs).

Linking computational models with health information has the potential to open up new vistas for biomedicine. The vast amount of clinical and wellness data could help validate such models and allow for customization of such models to individual patients or certain subpopulations (i.e., personalized medicine). Ultimately, this could lead to a new generation of hybrid model and data-driven decision support tools with better predictive power and precision at patient and population levels as well as paving the way for new breakthroughs in our ability to understand biological systems and develop new technology (see, e.g., [64]). The clinical application of the Physiome and *open*EHR standards and software frameworks discussed in this chapter will benefit greatly from the creation of appropriate clinical workflow environments such as the recently completed VPH-Share project [65].

REFERENCES

1 Hunter PJ and de Bono B. Biophysical constraints on the evolution of tissue structure and function. *J. Physiol.*, 592 (11): 2389–2401, 2014.

2 Hunter PJ, Pullan AJ, and Smaill BH. Modeling total heart function. *Annu. Rev. Biomed. Eng.*, 5: 147–177, 2003.

3 Hunter PJ and Borg TK. Integration from proteins to organs: The Physiome Project. *Nat. Rev. Mol. Cell Biol.*, 4 (3): 237–243, 2003.

4 Hunter PJ. The IUPS Physiome Project: A framework for computational physiology. *Prog. Biophys. Mol. Biol.*, 85 (2–3): 551–569, 2004.

5 Hunter PJ, Coveney PV, de Bono B, Diaz V, Fenner J, Frangi AF, et al. A vision and strategy for the virtual physiological human in 2010 and beyond. *Phil. Trans. A Math. Phys. Eng. Sci.*, 368 (1920): 2595–2614, 2010.

6 Hunter PJ, Chapman T, Coveney PV, de Bono B, Diaz V, Fenner J, et al. A vision and strategy for the virtual physiological human: 2012 update. *Interface Focus*, 3 (2), 2013:20130004.

7 Cuellar AA, Lloyd CM, Nielsen PF, Bullivant DP, Nickerson DP and Hunter PJ. An overview of CellML 1.1: A biological model description language. *Simulation*, 79: 740–747, 2003.

8 Christie GR, Nielsen PMF, Blackett SA, Bradley CP, and Hunter PJ. FieldML: Concepts and implementation. *Phil. Trans. A Math. Phys. Eng. Sci.*, 367: 1869–1884, 2009.

9 Brooks DJ, Hunter PJ, Smaill BH, and Titchener MR. BioSignalML—A meta-model for biosignals. *Conf. Proc. IEEE Eng. Med. Biol. Soc.*, 2011: 5670–5673, 2011.

10 Waltemath D, Adams R, Bergmann FT, Hucka M, Kolpakov F, Miller AK et al. Reproducible computational biology experiments with SED-ML—The simulation experiment description markup language. *BMC Syst. Biol.*, 5: 198, 2011.

11 Hucka M, Finney A, Sauro HM, Bolouri H, Doyle JC, Kitano H, et al. The systems biology markup language (SBML): A medium for representation and exchange of biochemical network models. *Bioinformatics*, 19: 524–531, 2003.

12 Yu T, Lloyd CM, Nickerson DP, Cooling MT, Miller AK, Garny A, Terkildsen JR, Lawson J, Britten RD, Hunter PJ and Nielsen PM. The physiome model repository 2. *Bioinformatics*, 27 (5): 743–744, 2011.

13 Garny A and Hunter PJ. OpenCOR: A modular and interoperable approach to computational biology. *Front. Physiol.*, 6: 26, 2015.

14 Beard DA, Britten R, Cooling MT, Garny A, Halstead MDB, Hunter PJ, et al. CellML metadata standards, associated tools and repositories. *Phil. Trans. A Math. Phys. Eng. Sci.*, 367: 1845–1867, 2009.

15 MIBBI—Minimum Information for Biological and Biomedical Investigations. Available from: http://www.dcc.ac.uk/resources/metadata-standards/mibbi-minimum-information-biological-and-biomedical-investigations (accessed on August 6, 2015).

16 Quinn TA, Granite S, Allessie MA, Antzelevitch C, Bollensdorff C, Bub G, Burton RA, et al. Minimum information about a cardiac electrophysiology experiment (MICEE): Standardised reporting for model reproducibility, interoperability, and data sharing. *Prog. Biophys. Mol. Biol.*, 107 (1): 4–10, 2011.

17 Minimum Information about a Cardiac Electrophysiology Experiment. Available from: https://www.micee.org/ (accessed on August 6, 2015).

18 Waltemath D, Adams R, Bergmann FT, Hucka M, Kolpakov F, Miller AK et al. Minimum information about a simulation experiment (MIASE). *PLoS Comput. Biol.*, 7 (4): e1001122, 2011.

19 Physiome Model Repository. Available from: https://models.physiomeproject.org/cellml (accessed on August 6, 2015).

20 De Bono B, Hoehndorf R, Wimalaratne S, Gkoutos G and Grenon P. The RICORDO approach to semantic interoperability for biomedical data and models: Strategy, standards and solutions. *BMC Res. Notes*, 4 (1): 313, 2011.

21 The RICORDO Project. Available from: http://www.ricordo.eu/ (accessed on August 6, 2015).

22 Rosse C and Mejino JLV. A reference ontology for biomedical informatics: The foundational model of anatomy. *J. Biomed. Inform.*, 36 (6): 478–500, 2003.

23 Foundational Model of Anatomy. Available from: http://sig.biostr.washington.edu/projects/fm/ (accessed on August 6, 2015).

24 BioModels Database. Available from: http://www.ebi.ac.uk/biomodels-main (accessed on August 6, 2015).

25 Smith B, Ashburner M, Rosse C, Bard J, Bug W, Ceusters W, et al. The OBO Foundry: Coordinated evolution of ontologies to support biomedical data integration. *Nat. Biotechnol.*, 25 (11): 1251–1255, 2007.

26 Degtyarenko K, de Matos P, Ennis M, Hastings J, Zbinden M, McNaught A, et al. ChEBI: A database and ontology for chemical entities of biological interest. *Nucleic Acids Res.*, 36: D344–D350, 2008.

27 Chemical Entities of Biological Interest (ChEBI). Available from: http://www.ebi.ac.uk/chebi/ (accessed on August 6, 2015).

28 Gene Ontology Cellular Component Organization. Available from: http://www.ebi.ac.uk/QuickGO/GTerm?id=GO:0016043 (accessed on August 6, 2015).

29 Bard J, Rhee SY, Ashburner M. An ontology for cell types. *Genome Biol.*, 6 (2):R21, 2005.

30 CL Ontology Browser. Available from: http://www.ebi.ac.uk/ontology-lookup/browse.do?ontName=CL (accessed on August 6, 2015).

31 The Ontology of Physics for Biology (OPB). Available from: http://sbp.bhi.washington.edu/projects/the-ontology-of-physics-for-biology-opb (accessed on August 6, 2015).

32 The UniProt Consortium. UniProt: A hub for protein information. *Nucleic Acids Res.*, 43: D204–D212, 2015.

33 De Bono B, Grenon P and Sammut SJ. ApiNATOMY: A novel toolkit for visualizing multiscale anatomy schematics with phenotype-related information. *Hum. Mutat.*, 33 (5): 837–848, 2012.

34 de Bono B, Safaei S, Grenon P, Nickerson DP, Alexander S, Helvensteijn M, et al. The open physiology workflow: Modeling processes over physiology circuitboards of interoperable tissue units. *Front. Physiol.*, 6: 24, 2015.

35 de Bono B, Grenon P, Baldock R and Hunter P. Functional tissue units and their primary tissue motifs in multi-scale physiology. *J. Biomed. Semant.*, 8;4 (1): 22, 2013.

36 Haux R. Health information systems—Past, present, future. *Int. J Med. Inform.*, 75(3–4): 268–81, 2006.

37 Campion-Awwad O, Hayton A, Smith L and Vuaran M. The National Programme for IT in the NHS. Cambridge, UK: University of Cambridge; 2014 [cited February 28, 2015]. Available from: http://www.cl.cam.ac.uk/~rja14/Papers/npfit-mpp-2014-case-history.pdf (accessed on August 6, 2015).

38 Institute of Medicine (US) Committee on Quality of Health Care in America. Crossing the Quality Chasm: A New Health System for the 21st Century. Washington, DC: National Academies Press; 2001 [cited February 28, 2015]. Available from: http://www.nap.edu/catalog/10027/crossing-the-quality-chasm-a-new-health-system-for-the (accessed on August 6, 2015).

39 Systematised Nomenclature of Medicine Clinical Terms (SNOMED CT) [cited February 28, 2015]. Available from: http://www.ihtsdo.org/snomed-ct/ (accessed on August 6, 2015).

40 Logical Observation Identifiers Names and Codes (LOINC®)—LOINC [cited February 28, 2015]. Available from: http://loinc.org/ (accessed on August 6, 2015).

41 Health Level Seven International [cited July 30, 2012]. Available from: http://www.hl7.org/ (accessed on August 6, 2015).

42 Clinical Information Modeling Initiative (CIMI) [cited February 28, 2015]. Available from: http://www.opencimi.org/ (accessed on August 6, 2015).

43 ISO Technical Committee 215: Health Informatics, Working Group 1: Health Records and Modelling Coordination. ISO 13606 – Health Informatics-Electronic Health Record Communication. Report No.: ISO 13606. ISO, Geneva.

44 Fast Healthcare Interoperability Resources (FHIR) [cited February 28, 2015]. Available from: http://hl7.org/implement/standards/fhir/ (accessed on August 6, 2015).

45 WHO|International Classification of Diseases (ICD) [cited February 28, 2015]. Available from: http://www.who.int/classifications/icd/en/ (accessed on August 6, 2015).

46 Kalra D, Beale T, and Heard S. The *open*EHR foundation. *Stud. Health Technol. Inform.*, 115:153–73, 2005.

47 Beale T. Archetypes: Constraint-based domain models for future-proof information systems. Eleventh OOPSLA Workshop on Behavioral Semantics: Serving the Customer. Seattle, WA, USA. Boston, MA: Northeastern University; 2002. p. 16–32.

48 Archetype Query Language Description—Specifications—*open*EHR wiki [cited February 28, 2015]. Available from: https://openehr.atlassian.net/wiki/display/spec/Archetype+Query+Language+Description (accessed on August 6, 2015).

49 Ma C, Frankel H, Beale T and Heard S. EHR query language (EQL)—A query language for archetype-based health records. *Stud. Health Technol. Inform.*, 129 (Pt 1): 397–401, 2007.

50 openEHR Clinical Knowledge Manager. Available from: http://openehr.org/ckm (accessed on August 6, 2015).

51 Integrating the Healthcare Enterprise (IHE) [cited February 28, 2015]. Available from: http://www.ihe.net/ (accessed on August 6, 2015).

52 Health Level Seven International (HL7). HL7 Launches Joint Argonaut Project to Advance FHIR. 2014. Available from: http://www.hl7.org/documentcenter/public_temp_1EBAE4D9-1C23-BA17-0CEBCC686D004E0F/pressreleases/HL7_PRESS_20141204.pdf (accessed on August 6, 2015).

53 Chang SS, Grunder S, Hanukoglu A, Rösler A, Mathew PM, Hanukoglu I, et al. Mutations in subunits of the epithelial sodium channel cause salt wasting with hyperkalaemic acidosis, pseudohypoaldosteronism type 1. *Nat. Genet.*, 12 (3): 248–53, 1996.

54 Geller DS, Zhang J, Zennaro M-C, Vallo-Boado A, Rodriguez-Soriano J, Furu L, et al. Autosomal dominant pseudohypoaldosteronism type 1: Mechanisms, evidence for neonatal lethality, and phenotypic expression in adults. *J Am. Soc. Nephrol.*, 17 (5): 1429–36, 2006.

55 Sheridan MB, Fong P, Groman JD, Conrad C, Flume P, Diaz R, et al. Mutations in the beta-subunit of the epithelial Na+ channel in patients with a cystic fibrosis-like syndrome. *Hum. Mol. Genet.*, 14 (22): 3493–8, 2005.

56 Pseudohypoaldosteronism. April 30, 2014 [cited February 19, 2015]. Available from: http://emedicine.medscape.com/article/924100-overview#a0101 (accessed on August 6, 2015).

57 Hogg RJ, Marks JF, Marver D, and Frolich JC. Long term observations in a patient with pseudohypoaldosteronism. *Pediatr. Nephrol. Berl. Ger.*, 5 (2): 205–10, 1991.

58 Babar SM. SIADH associated with ciprofloxacin. *Ann. Pharmacother.*, 47 (10): 1359–63, 2013.

59   Syndrome of Inappropriate Antidiuretic Hormone Secretion. April 29, 2014 [cited February 19, 2015]. Available from: http://emedicine.medscape.com/article/246650-overview (accessed on August 6, 2015).

60   Bradley C, Bowery A, Britten R, Budelmann V, Camara O, Christie R, et al. OpenCMISS: A multi-physics & multi-scale computational infrastructure for the VPH/Physiome project. *Prog. Biophys. Mol. Biol.*, 107 (1): 32–47, 2011.

61   Get – Bitbucket [cited October 30, 2014]. Available from: https://bitbucket.org/get (accessed on August 6, 2015).

62   GET Documentation – GET 0.1 Documentation [cited October 30, 2014]. Available from: http://get-documentation.readthedocs.org/en/latest/ (accessed on August 6, 2015).

63   Atalag K. Using a single content model for eHealth interoperability and secondary use. *Stud. Health Technol. Inform.*, 193: 282–96, 2013.

64   Gjuvsland AB, Vik JO, Beard DA, Hunter PJ, and Omholt SW. Bridging the genotype-phenotype gap: What does it take? *J. Physiol.*, 591 (Pt 8): 2055–2066, 2013.

65   VPH-Share Project. Available from: http://www.vph-share.eu (accessed on August 6, 2015).

10

PHYSICS-BASED MODELING FOR THE PHYSIOME

WILLIAM A. PRUETT AND ROBERT L. HESTER

Department of Physiology and Biophysics, University of Mississippi, Jackson, MS, USA

INTRODUCTION

Until 50 years ago, knowledge acquisition in the biological sciences was a matter of obtaining data and drawing conclusions from observations. Research has shown that the human mind is capable of focusing on a limited number of constructs simultaneously [1]. Biological models consist of nonlinear dynamical systems, and understanding their behavior requires accounting for multiple thresholds and sensitivities simultaneously. Together, these facts imply that the present method of progress in biology is eventually self-defeating: there will come a point where too many factors must be accounted for to understand any system completely. Mathematical modeling represents a method of integrating experiments into a coherent whole, allowing knowledge to be synthesized, rather than attained. In this way, mathematical models make future progress in biology possible.

As a case in point, consider the circulatory model of Guyton, Granger, and Coleman in 1972 [2]. At that point, a great debate was occurring over the causes of hypertension in the physiological human. Guyton used his early research into the concepts of unstressed fluid volume and natriuresis [3–7], Starling's observations on the behavior of the heart at different inflow pressures [8], and observations of the secretory profiles of renin, aldosterone, and vasopressin to create an integrated model of human volume homeostasis. With a focus on quantitative analysis of the feedback mechanisms involved, Guyton's effort was the first model of quantitative integrative physiology; the paradigm that first incorporated physics-based modeling into the biological world, and inspired the *in silico* human. The model synthesized previous observations to create a tool in which hypotheses were testable. Furthermore, because the tool was physics-based, composed of relationships demonstrated in the laboratory, and drawn together with simple physics, its results were readily interpretable and easily acceptable. With the model, Guyton showed that hypertension could not be

The Digital Patient: Advancing Healthcare, Research, and Education, First Edition.
Edited by C. Donald Combs, John A. Sokolowski, and Catherine M. Banks.
© 2016 John Wiley & Sons, Inc. Published 2016 by John Wiley & Sons, Inc.

a cardiac disease, or a vascular disease, but was a disease of the kidney as described by the renal function curve describing urinary output as a function of arterial blood pressure. This model serves as an exemplar of knowledge synthesis, despite anyone's opinion on the conclusions drawn.

Guyton's model offered several lessons concerning the importance of the systems approach. The first was psychological: understanding mechanisms can lead to overestimating the influence of those mechanisms on system-wide behavior. The case in point was the ability of the heart to increase blood pressure by increasing cardiac output. Second, multiple mechanisms may vie for control of a single pathway; understanding the individual mechanisms separately does not guarantee that the pathway will be similarly understood. The importance of feedback, redundant systems, and the nonlinearity of the submodels combined to yield counterintuitive and scientifically unpopular conclusions, which experiments have confirmed over the next decade. What Guyton's model did not do was adapt, in general, to different chronic states. The importance of this lack is apparent: 40 years later and physiologist still cannot explain the origins of hypertension in a majority of cases. The modern view of quantitative systems biology accounts for this lack of adaptation with its insistence on multiscale modeling. Guyton's model was an early example in biology and physiology of a physics-based model (PBM). PBMs use the laws of physics and chemistry to produce results. They are mechanism based and time dynamic, allowing pathology to develop naturally. At the lowest level, models of specific mechanisms are PBMs. At this level, models are representations of the conclusions of basic scientists: they express quantified relationships between physiologically significant entities. Examples include agonist-receptor models [9, 10], second messenger signal models [11–14], finite element models of failure modes in trabecular bone [15–18], model metabolic networks [19–22], or models of blood flow through large arteries or microcirculatory networks [23]. PBMs span the spectrum of physics because human physiology comprises a complex mixture of interacting systems, all predicated on physics and chemistry.

Thinking of such models as atoms, one can see how atoms may be fit together to create a compound structure allowing more subtle analysis to be performed. As such, they provide an ideal framework to extend the work of basic science by integrating conclusions into more complex structures suitable for testing complicated hypotheses. The ability to extend and focus on mechanisms is the principle strengths of PBMs, as they allow straightforward generalization and interpretation. However, carefully maintaining modeling standards is critical to retain these attributes and to represent accurately the evidential value associated with a complex model.

MODELING SCHEMES

Technological advancements have paved the way for new approaches to modeling, simulation, and visualization. Modeling now encompasses high degrees of complexity and holistic methods of data representation. Various levels of simulation capability allow for improved outputs and analysis of discrete and continuous events, and state-of-the-art visualization allows for graphics that can represent details within a single shaft of hair [24].

The human body is an amazing machine comprising multiple organs, tissues that interact to maintain a homeostasis. Pathology is due to alterations in one or more tissues or systems: due to the integrative aspects of the human body, alterations in one system may induce changes in the physiology in other systems.

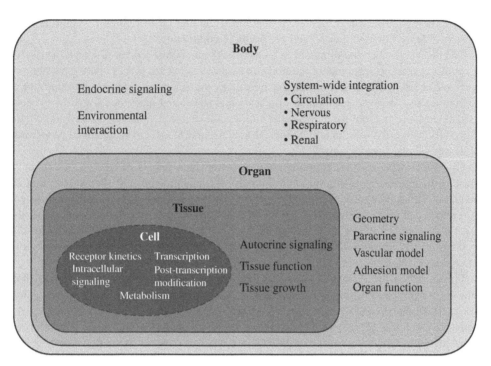

FIGURE 10.1   The hierarchy of model types and levels. The hierarchy of models stretches from the most reductionist intracellular model, developed from data obtained in tightly controlled conditions, through the classical multiscale integration of cellular processes into tissue and organ process, up to the top-down models of macroscopic interactions between organ systems. The digital patient will require full integration through all levels.

Modeling has experienced a philosophical shift, with the advent of genetics, proteomics, and metabolomics. The ability to understand humans at the most fundamental level of biologic detail has encouraged the idea that medicine itself can be personalized. Realizing this goal requires the ability to make accurate predictions about how a patient will react to a treatment (or to no treatment); however, the reductionist approach to science and modeling cannot satisfy that need. Instead, the systems approach to biological modeling has begun to grow in importance as a translational tool. As the perception of the necessity of modeling to understand complex systems and to predict outcomes has increased, systems biology has had to adopt a more mature goal. Now systems biology is engaged in modeling and understanding mechanisms and interactions in a qualitative manner over multiple timescales, creating truly multiscale models and a philosophy of "quantitative systems biology" or "quantitative integrative biology" (Fig. 10.1). The applications of this philosophy in individual disciplines have been reviewed [25–27]. This philosophy acknowledges the importance of the interplay between systems in producing responses in cells, tissues, and individuals.

Several pieces must be in place to realize this interplay in a single mathematical model. These pieces include reductionist modeling at a variety of special and temporal scales, the development of an ontology allowing models to communicate with one another, and finally the creation of a top-level model that allows reductionist models to be "plugged in," creating an integrated model framework that allows testing and generation of hypotheses. Different groups have developed distinct philosophies for approaching these problems, but none has solved the problem completely.

The most common type of model in biology is a reductionist model, in which the scientist looks at specific segments of the body, in essence taking the pieces apart. This philosophy has a strong following because it reinforces the scientific method. By controlling everything else, a single component of a system is tested and understood. PBM has been used extensively as a tool for reductionist biology, for example, in models of cell signaling, especially with cross-talk, pharmacological models, and models of mechanical properties of tissues such as bone or muscle.

Given a collection of reductionist models that cover a system of interest, the models must communicate with one another. Numerous challenges present themselves at this point, including problems of temporal differences between submodels, scaling between different submodels, and differences in the assumptions that underlie the different submodels. These challenges have been approached in a variety of ways, including model translators that provide protocols allowing disparate models to communicate [28] to utilizing strict model languages that require translation of submodels [29, 30].

Finally, a "top-level" model must tie all designated models together in a framework that allows for hypothesis testing and generation. This step has been the most challenging, and has again attracted a variety of solutions. These solutions reflect most acutely the philosophy and intentions of their developers. One such viewpoint is the minimum model philosophy, in which a model is constructed that is minimal with respect to the hypotheses being tested. This philosophy has been common in the clinical and research activities discussed later in the chapter. At the other end of the spectrum is the "whole human" philosophy, which seeks to realize all aspects of man and woman in model form. A diverse collection of consortia that we discuss in the following represents this philosophy.

Modeling Consortia

The approach to creating digital patients has been to create numerous models with the eventual goal of sewing them together to create an integrative model. For this purpose, different groups have adopted language standards to facilitate eventual integration. The groups have specific requirements for model curation and upkeep, guaranteeing a consistent product with clear evidential support.

The IUPS Physiome Project comprises multiple institutions focusing on specific strengths of each research team. This work is found at http://physiomeproject.org/. The Auckland Bioengineering Institute has provided tools, markup languages, and modeling environments as a basis for the project. This site provides individual models developed in CellML, a standard markup language developed by the Physiome Project. The models include an extensive group of models including *Calcium Dynamics, Cardiovascular Circulation, Electrophysiology, Ion Transport, Metabolism, pH Regulation* and *PKPD*.

The Virtual Physiological Human project, based in the European Union, http://www.vph-institute.org/ has the mission "to ensure that the Virtual Physiological Human is fully realized, universally adopted, and effectively used both in research and clinic." The group has developed a three-prong strategy toward realizing digital patients. The first focuses on developing systems that allow clinical and laboratory observations to be cataloged and shared. Currently, data representing anatomy, physiology, and pathology are available. The second focus is on using multiple experts to analyze their data and collaboratively generate hypotheses that integrate different scientific viewpoints. The VPH provides >1000 curated and noncurated computational models of biological processes. Early work has resulted in an ontological system for development. The final focus is on connecting disparate models over multiple timescales and systems to create predictive mathematical models for testing systems spanning hypotheses.

The University of Washington Physiome Project, http://www.physiome.org/ has developed the JSim software, which is used to solve biological models written in Mathematical Modeling Language (MML). Like VPH, the NSR Physiome Project uses a strategy combining data repositories, a knowledge integration step consisting of mathematical modeling at multiple special and temporal scales, and open-source machinery for searching and using the stored data and models. Almost 400 models are available for users.

The NMS Physiome Project was intended to develop simulations of the neuromuscular skeleton systems http://www.nmsphysiome.eu/. The project concluded in 2013 with the release of two model-building software modules. The first module, NMSBuilder, was a toolkit for modeling muscle movement from patient specific data. The second was a probability-based module, which interfaces with models developed in NMSBuilder to extend the range of motion to more realistic levels. The innovation in this project was its focus on using patient-specific biomedical data for its musculoskeletal simulations.

The Ministry of Education, Culture, Sports, Science and Technology in Japan fund the HD-Physiology Project (http://hd-physiology.jp). There are currently three areas of focus: Research and Development of Software Platform for Integrative Multi-Level Systems Biology, Multi-Level Systems Biology of Cardiac Electrophysiological Activity, and Multi-Level Systems Biology of Small Molecular Dynamics in Circulation. At the current time, 2014, this group does not appear to have developed simulation projects that are available to other investigators.

HumMod

All of the consortia discussed thus far began their work with reductionist models and the development of an ontology to allow them to be integrated into a whole model. Guyton took the opposite approach with his model. It incorporated empirical and mechanistic aspects, allowing a framework to be built, to which models that are more detailed could be added. The project was limited by several factors, including the particular questions Guyton and his students asked and the computational tools available to the group.

Over the subsequent years, Dr. Guyton continued to develop his model in FORTRAN, and this model has been used by other investigators [31–34]. Dr. Thomas Coleman continued to modeling effort with "Human" a DOS based simulation written in basic, then QCP, a Windows-based program written in C++. To be able to easily modify the physiology in a modeling environment, Coleman, Hester, Summers, and Pruett developed HumMod, composed of a solver module and physiological content in an XML format [35]. It is a unique top-down model of human physiology. A version of HumMod can be downloaded at http://hummod.org.

The problem with top-down models in general and HumMod in particular is that parts of the model are not mechanism based, but instead are desired responses based on observations. In other words, a blood vessel dilates some amount in response to exposure to a certain stimulus because the code specifies the expected dilation specific to that stimulus, not because intracellular factors combine to alter vessel wall mechanics according to biochemical/physical laws. In other words, the integrative model needs a multitude of reductionist components to mechanistically model real responses. Conversely, reductionist models need a top-down model so that the importance of particular mechanisms in causing responses in systems or organisms can be assessed. This underscores the significance of both types of PBMs, and the extreme importance of linking efforts to create models that accurately reflect real patients in the digital setting.

Population Modeling with PBM

When discussing the digital patient together with PBMs, one needs to consider the factors that make a real patient so complicated. PBMs are by their nature either deterministic or use probability to generate behavior in networks of agents to calculate a systemic response [36]. There are a large number of deterministic simulations of biological pathways. The deterministic design results in simulations that provide consistent results. However, individual human responses are not consistent; patients are different, with different susceptibilities, immunities, and responses. Developing the digital patient then requires a new paradigm.

At the most fundamental level, differences arise because of differences in individual genomes, whether due to inheritance, parental stresses, or environmental factors. This genetic variation manifests as differences in expression levels of proteins or structural factors, or alterations in metabolic capacity, or any number of other subtle or pronounced deviations from some perceived "normal state." As these differences propagate through the nonlinearities in the system, different responses to a given stimulus might appear. The rules that describe how expression levels are decided, and the particular collection of metabolic pathways available to an individual, and all of the other subtle features that make one individual distinct from another, these are the physiome, the informational content of an individual's physiology.

Considering the physiome as the relationships between systemic and environmental factors, any model can be tailored to individuals by refitting its independent variables. In this way, the response to a stimulus and, in a sufficiently advanced model, the adaptation to stimuli in the model is identified with the same response in the individual, and the model becomes a representation of the individual. From the modeling perspective, a digital patient is one sample from all possible physiomes, and ideally, one that matches a particular individual. This observation has applications to personalized medicine in two very distinct ways. First, it suggests an approach allowing the modeler to convert information about a response to information about the individual (the *descriptive problem*). Given a response, one can search for physiomes that match that response. Conversely, given information about an individual's physiome, one can predict the range of responses to a new challenge (the *predictive problem*). In the extreme, this case involves matching an individual to his or her physiome. This is an intractable problem for now, but there are techniques for extracting partial solutions to both problems.

The first step to modeling the physiome is to understand how changes in independent model variables (parameters) affect the model response to perturbations. In essence, this is a sensitivity analysis pointed not at understanding the robustness of the model, but at understanding the physiome through the lens of the model. Thomas's group used a version of Guyton's model and performed a sensitivity analysis when modifying parameters used in the calculations [34]. Restricting their analysis to 96 parameters and 276 variables, they created a population of 384,000 patients. Their focus was on blood pressure regulation, and they found a distribution of blood pressures with a mean pressure of 106 mmHg, with 2/3 of the population having a mean arterial pressure (MAP) greater than 106 (Fig. 10.2). This

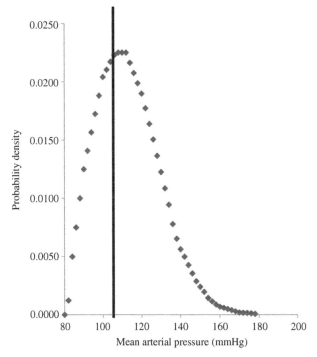

FIGURE 10.2 Population modeling of blood pressure. Thomas's group used one-at-a-time methodology to perform a sensitivity analysis on an extended form of Guyton's model [4]. Calculating mean pressure from diastolic and systolic pressure, almost 2/3 of sampled individuals were hypertensive. (Adapted from Moss et al. [34].)

work provided an excellent sensitivity analysis of those parameters and variables in Guyton's model that were responsible for the increase in blood pressure. This provides possible targets for pharmacologic or lifestyle interventions, with the limitation that all effects were considered singly.

The key development toward solving the descriptive and predictive problems in physics based modeling in physiology has been the appearance of population models. Rather than concentrating on a model that matches the typical human reaction to a stimulus, Monte Carlo sampling of model parameters yields collections of individuals that behave differently to fixed stimulus.

Typically, modelers use Monte Carlo sampling to understand parameter sensitivities or model robustness, or to estimate the model uncertainty with respect to the parameter choices. This approach is common in weather prediction, where parameter variations determine the paths a storm might take, or the range of temperatures a physical location might see in a day. This technique originated in game theory, but moved quickly to biological systems analysis [37].

In the PBM context, populations sampled via Monte Carlo methodology can be calibrated to match the population response. A variety of techniques exist to perform this calibration. Starting from a random sample, bootstrapping methods or Metropolis–Hastings [38] algorithms are viable choices. The human population is identified with the model and its independent variables, and the resulting calibrated object can be used for solving either the predictive or the descriptive problems. Pruett used this technique in a reduced form of

Guyton's model to predict multiple factors that would combine to predict individual response to hemorrhage [39]. This technique has the added benefit that simultaneously sampling a group of model parameters allows the mixed effects to be calculated.

In standard PBM, a model is describing a unique system in which only one outcome may occur, and uncertainty is concentrated in the inputs. In biological PBM, both the input data and the model relationships themselves are subject to uncertainty. In models with a broader basis in physics and lesser emphasis on empirical relationships, parameter (independent variable) uncertainty and measurement uncertainty become the dominant factors. It is critical that we develop techniques for separating and quantifying these effects.

PBM in Education

Simulation for training has been used extensively since the 1930s when Edwin Link developed the flight simulator. Over the next century, training simulators such as for pilots, astronauts, and the military have become extremely realistic and have proven to be valuable in training. Medical simulators started in 1960 with Resusci Annie, but these simulators had minimal physiology. Over the next 50 years, there has been a dramatic improvement in the development of medical simulation tools, from mannequins to task trainers to avatars. However, with all of these systems there is minimal description of the physics-based physiology used to provide medical scenarios. The following provides a brief description of PBM of human physiology used for educational purposes. There are two excellent review of the history of medical simulation [40, 41].

Desktop computer and mannequin PBMs of human physiology have been used in education from the mid-1980s. These packages can simulate acute and chronic medical conditions. Desktop trainers emphasize teaching the mechanisms that underlie patient responses. The majority of the desktop computer-based models have mainly focused on anesthesiology training. Smith's group developed an analog model to understand the uptake and distribution of various anesthetic gases [42, 43]. Over the years, this was expanded and became the "Body" simulation package which the current HumanSim project by Applied Research Associates is based on (http://www.humansim.com/solutions/technologies [29]). Hardman's group created the Nottingham Physiology Simulator [44] (http://www.hardman01.plus.com/index_files/nps.htm [45]). However, at the time this site was accessed (November 2014), the most recent version of the software was not available. Schwid and O'Donnell developed a desktop simulation for anesthesiology [46] which has expanded into a series of healthcare simulations, now marketed by Anesoft (http://anesoft.com/). Dr. Thomas Coleman expanded his work with Dr. Guyton from the 1970s into the development of Human, a Dos-based integrative physiological simulation [47]. Human was converted to the Windows-based Quantitative Circulatory Physiology (QCP) [48] which is the basis for HumMod [35] (both available at http://hummod.org). A list of computer-based simulations can be found at http://www.pennstatehershey.org/web/simulation/home/available/cbs (October 2014).

Unlike desktop simulators, mannequins are used to train the medical professional how to respond to a specific situation. We will consider only high-fidelity hybrid mannequins, which combine the physical mannequin with physiological software and user interfaces to allow scenario programming. Mannequins have been developed for training the treatment of acute scenarios such as hemorrhage, airway maintenance, and drug responses. Because trainees, by altering the timing of interventions and specific dosages and rates in those interventions, have access to an unlimited number of actions, the best mannequins utilize a PBM. However, in most cases the description of the underlying physiology is not disclosed. For example, most mannequin manufacturers state, "vital signs respond to hemorrhage and therapy." However, published experiments in humans suggest that patients respond differently to hemorrhage [28]. Therefore, it is unclear whether the "appropriate" response by the mannequin is consistent with what would be observed in humans.

A recent paper compared the simulation results of the METI HPS during oxygen administration and apnea with human studies [49]. The authors found that oxygen saturation on the METI decreased much later during apnea than observed in clinical situations. The lack of a fall in saturation occurred whether preoxygenation was performed or not. The authors recommend that "The debriefing after simulation of critical situations or the use of the METI simulation to test a new equipment must consider these results" [49]. Although the METI simulator had the most realistic airway of four surveyed mannequins [50], anatomical differences were cited as contributing to the problems in performance. This illustrates one of the challenges facing mannequin producers: matching anatomic reality to allow lifelike behavior in the mannequin complicates interfacing the simulation software with the outside world.

Pettitt, Norfleet, and Descheneaux suggested that the physiological fidelity of the software or mannequin can be adjusted based on the healthcare provider being trained [51]. The two concerns with this proposal are that (i) the simulator outcomes may not accurately reflect real-world physiological responses and (ii) not all patients respond the same to a pathological condition. We believe that exposing all levels of healthcare providers to a simulation environment that provides the highest fidelity of responses along with having the ability to provide differential responses to reflect the population provides the best training environment.

PBM in Research

Researchers use PBM extensively to understand human physiology. The development of specific models allows investigators to mathematically relate current knowledge on a topic, explore system interactions, test hypotheses, and develop new experiments to test hypotheses. In this way, the modeling development and testing is an iterative process. This allows the developer to fine-tune the model, providing greater insight into the underlying interactions. There are extensive studies using finite element analysis (FEA) in tissue engineering. Computational fluid dynamics (CFD) have been used in understanding tissue specific blood flows, such as cerebral [52] or coronary circulations [53]. CFD has been used for airflow and particle deposition in the lungs [54]. In this section, we concentrate on the use of PBM in physiological models, in cases where the model elucidates a mechanism that is difficult to observe in a laboratory. The cardiovascular system is one area of research that has relied extensively on modeling to understand the underlying physiological mechanisms, particularly when specific measurements cannot be made due to technical limitations. An example of this are studies to determine the mechanisms by with baroreceptor nerve activation leads to a fall in blood pressure [55]. Renal sympathetic nerve activation results in sodium retention leading to an increase in blood pressure. Baroreceptor activation inhibits systemic and renal sympathetic activation, decreasing blood pressure. However, renal denervation does not abolish the fall in blood pressure that occurs with baroreceptor stimulation, suggesting a minimal role for renal sympathetic activation in the control of blood pressure. In an attempt to understand the mechanisms responsible for the lack of a blood pressure fall with baroreceptor stimulation Iliescu and Lohmeier [56] performed a series of

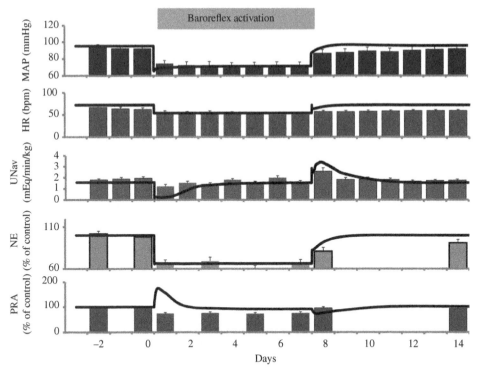

FIGURE 10.3 Simulation (black lines) and experimental responses to baroreflex stimulation. Experimental response to a baroreflex stimulation device in dogs was compared to a human simulation (HumMod) to explore the mechanisms behind chronic blood pressure reduction. The studies identified factors that correlated with positive response. (Adapted from Lohmeier and Iliescu [54].)

simulations using a version of HumMod (Fig. 10.3). The simulations predicted that two, technically difficult to measure factors, atrial natriuretic peptide and renal venous pressure, contribute to the increase in renal excretory capability and lowering of blood pressure. A consequence of the activation of the natriuretic systems is enhanced volume retention.

Hallow et al. [31] expanded the model of Karaaslan et al. [32, 33], itself an extension of Guyton's model, to include the influence of renal sympathetic nerve activity on renin control to understand antihypertensive therapies. This model was calibrated and validated against a series of clinical trials. The results of the simulations suggest that a particular mechanism responsible for the hypertension can influence the response to a particular treatment, suggesting that a hypertensive person that is sensitive to renin angiotensin blockers may lose sensitivity to a hydrochlorothiazide diuretic. These simulations potentially provide an understanding as to why combination therapy may be needed to decrease the blood pressure in hypertensive patients.

PBM in Clinical Practice

The goal of any biomedical research is to improve treatment options for patients, improving outcomes, reducing comorbidities, raising quality of life, and making health care more efficient. The necessity of translating basic science to clinical applications is a challenge. Bench research requires complete control over the subject, requiring the use of animal or tissue models that may not mimic the human response. Recently, questions about the applicability of basic science techniques in immunology to human medicine have been raised [57]. While the methodology of this particular study has been questioned [58], the point that it raises is reasonable. Basic scientists observe fundamental processes at a cellular or tissue level in one animal model and make inferences about the importance of those mechanisms in other models. Each model comes with its own assumptions, and the patchwork of suppositions necessary for drawing conclusions from complex combinations of factors makes generalization difficult and fraught with opportunities for honest error. This issue highlights the difficulties of understanding how basic science translates into clinical utility.

Another hurdle to integrating basic science into clinical utility is the inability to quantify complex combinations of effects successfully. Cristini et al. say that

> In spite of abundant experimental and clinical data surrounding molecular and cellular phenomena, it is difficult to quantify their aggregate effect on gross tumor-scale behavior using conventional methods that, for the most part, investigate isolated mechanisms ([59], p. S121)

This is the paradox of basic science as it is practiced today; effort is exerted to understand mechanisms in complete isolation without balancing that energy with equal effort understanding how mechanisms integrate to yield changes on the level of the tissue, the system, or the organism. PBMs offer a rigorous path for converting basic science into clinically useful results. For example, by integrating multiple models into multiscale constructions linking geometry, cell signaling, and metabolism, modelers have provided oncologists with a variety of tools that explain counterintuitive results, maximize the efficiency of therapy, and provide tantalizing clues about future targets for therapy.

Mathematical modeling of cancer began in the 1960s with simple tumor growth models and PK/PD models [60, 61]. Research turned almost immediately to predictive modeling of tumor response to therapy [62, 63]. Similarly, mathematical modeling of cancer addressed the distribution of therapeutic agents throughout the body [64]. These themes would dominate early efforts to use models as tools to bridge the laboratory-clinical gap. By 1973, the first modern model of cancer biology was presented, explicitly linking measurements of cell motility from the laboratory with those obtained from a clinical cohort. The model was developed to mimic the clinical protocol [65, 66]. This early effort introduced many themes that continue in the best efforts today including an evolving population of cancer cells with a nonhomogeneous distribution.

The number of mathematical models used in oncology research is staggering; 1750 indexed papers appear in PubMed as of the writing of this chapter. While much of the literature uses statistical, rather than mechanistic methodology, PBMs are still an important and large segment of the literature. For the purposes of summary, we will reference reviews of modeling efforts rather than the models themselves, with a few exceptions. The major classes of PBMs used today in oncology are models of tumor size and growth as reviewed in Refs. [67–69], metastasis [70–72], models of physical characteristics of solid tumors [73–75], tumor cell cycle [76], and analyses of various treatment regimens on specific cancer types [24, 77–79].

While the physical basis for modeling in oncology has always been present in the form of receptor-agonist kinetics and intracellular signaling in cancerous cells, and blood flow analysis in tumors, a new application of physics and modeling to treatment of breast cancer has emerged recently. A promising new treatment method for early stage breast cancer is radio frequency ablation of small tumors [80, 81]. However, small tumors are deformable, which makes precise the placement of a needle for conducting the ablation challenging. Early simulation results on force profiles necessary for needle insertion into soft tissue were obtained [82]. Combined with a PBM designed for an educational virtual reality environment for simulated palpation, multiple robotic needle placement instruments were designed for clinical use [83, 84]. This technology blends robotics, PBM, and a device intervention to provide a minimally invasive, maximally effective treatment.

Modelers, working in conjunction with physicians, developed other clinically useful. These include patient-specific CFD models of congenital heart disease [85], biofeedback-driven dialysis with integrated mathematical model control [86], and physiological control of body temperature for surgical patients [87]. The potential for PBM to create patient-specific, predictive, or information collating tools show their importance in creating the digital patient.

PBM in Regulatory Science

Regulatory science is the study of the scientific and technical foundations upon which regulations are based. In our context, we refer to the evaluation of new pharmaceutical products and devices by the Food and Drug Administration (FDA). This review is for the sake of safety and efficacy; success means that a product may be marketed. Because of the high cost of creating and testing new drugs and devices, manufacturers are constantly looking for ways to streamline the regulatory process.

The clinical trial is the most significant test of a treatment's efficacy, be it a pharmaceutical agent or a medical device. As such, it lies in the intersection of research and clinical practice, the domain of regulatory science. Every drug must receive a series of clinical trials to establish efficacy and safety. Clinical trials for new pharmaceutical drugs or devices are costly and require a long development time. Even then, the drug or device may not ever come to market due to unexpected adverse outcomes. Is there a way is which physics-based simulation can play a role in clinical trials?

Robust mathematical simulation may be one way in which costs can be defrayed and risk averted, but no official guidance has been issued for conducting or supplementing clinical trials with simulation. However, Section 115 of the FDA Modernization Act of 1997 stated "…based on relevant science, data from one adequate and well-controlled clinical investigation and confirmatory evidence (obtained prior to or after such investigation) are sufficient to establish effectiveness…" This statement has been interpreted to require not two clinical trials, but a single clinical trial and confirmatory evidence consisting of a mathematical model [88].

Because of the differences in how PBMs are used in devices and in pharmacological agents, we consider the two separately.

Device Side

PBM have been used by sponsors of devices for decades. The link between device engineering and model design is intuitively clear; engineers use mathematics to test the specifics of all kinds of projects in almost every sphere. Models provide the ability to maximize device response and minimize failure rates by optimizing all aspects of the design process, from material choice and geometry to device implementation. The FDA has acknowledged and welcomed PBM to the design and regulatory process, issuing specific guidance about fluid dynamics, solid mechanics, optics, ultrasound, and heat

TABLE 10.1 An Overview of FDA Requirements for Computer Modeling and Simulation (CM&S) Submissions for Device Approval

FDA Guidance on CM&S Reports	
System aspect	Required validation material
System configuration	System components and software
Governing equations	All constitutive laws with rationale; explanation of assumptions and simplifications
System properties	Biological, chemical, and physical properties of the studied system, including material properties with variability and tolerances
System conditions	Initial, boundary, and loading conditions; models constraints, and rationale for all choices made
Numerical implementation	System discretization and implementation methodology
Validation	Accuracy of the computational models, including experimental validation protocols

The emphasis is on reproducibility and clear identification of all assumptions.

transfer models for device submissions. Some aspects of the requirements for the computational modeling and simulation (CM&S) component of a device submission are shown in Table 10.1. This official move toward consolidating CM&S reports is a sign of a new attitude within the agency toward modeling's role in the design, submission, and evaluation process, and demonstrates their understanding of the ability of models to make device design safer, less time-consuming, and less expensive.

Currently FEA and CFD simulation technology is used extensively for medical device development, such as vascular implants, orthopedic implants, stents, heart valves, blood oxygenators, and left-ventricular-assist device (LVAD). The use of simulation can assist with development, but there are challenges with these technologies as reported in 2012 [89]. Twenty-eight groups used CFD to analyze flow through a specific geometry and the simulations demonstrated considerable variation from each other and from the experimental data. The authors recommended that validations studies "be performed on the device under review."

Drug Design

With the development of medical devices, controlled bench validation studies can be performed and compared to simulation results. However, pharmaceutical studies are more challenging and do not allow controlled validation studies to be performed. Pharmaceutical development is initially based on results from cell culture or animal studies. Pharmacokinetic/ pharmacodynamic (PK/PD) modeling describes the time course and directed effect of the pharmacologic response. Phase I and II clinical trials are designed to test safety, identify safe dosage, and identify side effects. Due to the limitation in human studies, it is not feasible to make all the possible physiological and clinical measurements to verify that the pharmaceutical agent is acting only in the way it was designed.

The pharmaceutical side of the FDA has not been as clear as has the device side with its intentions toward modeling. No global guidance for the use of CM&S in drug design or testing has been adopted, although the importance of including (PK/PD) modeling in drug development was asserted in a critical publication on retooling the regulatory pathway [90]. While guidance has been lacking, model-based drug development, first championed by Sheiner [91], has grown into a widely accepted tool for streamlining the development process [92].

PBM are used at three very different points in the product design cycle for drugs. First, it can be used to create the drugs themselves, which can occur in two distinct ways. First, biological modeling of intracellular pathways allows targets to be tested for effectiveness. This step culls molecules on heavily redundant pathways from being targeted. Second, likely agents can be tested for efficacy based on the physical shape and charge distribution of the molecules and their targets. One specification of this concept is integrating chemical and biological information into a coherent description of the structure of molecules believed to heterogeneous to well-studied molecules. The endpoint is to determine the nature and size of preclinical trials necessary to develop "follow-up" drug products based on molecular similarity. This approach has been singled out for study by the FDA due to its potential for streamlining the drug development process, as well as its foundation in established physics and chemistry [93]. The nature of this problem suggests that comprehensive model validation might be attained, and success could radically shorten the length of the development cycle.

Secondly, PK/PD modeling is used to refine dose selection and clinical trial design. Early drug trials are restricted in duration and sample size; modeling can augment the information available by leveraging what is known, such as information about the drug target and clearance mechanisms, as well as physical characteristics of the patient, into reduced observation uncertainty. Understanding how to effectively differentiate between drugs to ensure ample powering of a study is a critical step in the trial design process, and one in which PK/PD modeling plays a vital role [94] (Fig. 10.4). The endpoint is a link between dose, concentration, and exposure and other surrogate measures of drug efficacy such as adverse events and efficacy metrics. By using small numbers of individuals to parameterize an initial model, trial design, and dose scheduling can be optimized.

Population PK/PD, which are PK/PD models with additional relationships between patient covariates such as age and sex, allow development strategies and population trial design to be assessed before the trial goes forward. These techniques allow exposure in variability to be tested, and uncertainty associated with covariates to be measured explicitly. With a mechanistic, PBM, one can answer specific questions about peak dosage, peak effect, and the accrual of known risks secondary to the treatment.

Finally, population PK/PD have been extended to stochastic simulations that include drug progression models to measure drug efficacy at different stages of a disease and social models such as patient drop-out or compliance issues to explicitly measure the effects of these factors on study power. Because the models are based on physical mechanisms, much more information can be generalized from them than from earlier empirical studies [95]. In particular, physiological or pharmacological biomarkers can be proposed from model behavior, giving the model another influence on trial design and drug assessment.

In a success story, Pfizer used model-based drug development [96], which combined statistical and mechanistic modeling to streamline the drug development process, and in this case save valuable resources and time by rejecting a nonviable solution before Phase II trials began. Searching for a therapy to alter estrogen concentration to alleviate pain from endometriosis, a gonadotropin-releasing hormone (GnRH) analog was developed. These substances decrease estrogen, causing menopause-like symptoms and bone mineral loss. A proof-of-concept study would not be sufficiently long to

(a)

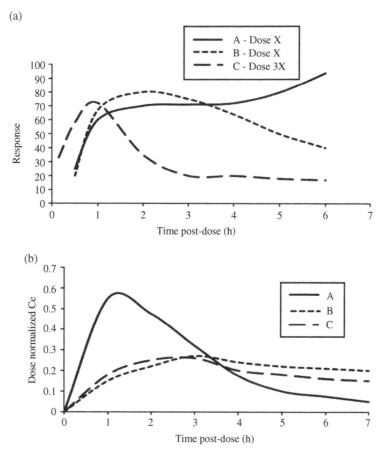

(b)

FIGURE 10.4   A. The pharmacological response to three compounds as measured in a bench experiment. B. The effect of Shiener's method of effect compartment modeling on normalizing the response to allow interpretation of the pharmacodynamic properties of the compounds relative to one another. (Adapted from Miller et al. [94].)

differentiate changes in bone mineral density, preventing the trial from addressing safety concerns. Moreover, questions about the optimal range of estrogen levels, and whether GnRH analogs could maintain estrogen within those ranges, could not be answered. An integrated model consisting of a mathematical model of female reproductive hormones [10] and a model of bone metabolism [97] were used to form a relationship between lumbar bone mineral density and circulating estrogen, with inputs from nafareline, the GnRH analog. The time course of bone markers and bone metabolism was simulated as a dose–response relationship with nafareline. This was combined with a logit relationship between endometriosis symptoms index score and circulating estrogen, to produce a study of the safety of nafareline at therapeutic doses. However, the endocrine model predicted challenges in maintaining estrogen within the safe range, which caused the cessation of the study. This measure demonstrated that a compound could not safely meet its efficacy and safety endpoints without risk to patients, and saved significant time and money. Similar strategies have streamlined Pfizer's production timetable and reduced costs [96] (Fig. 10.5).

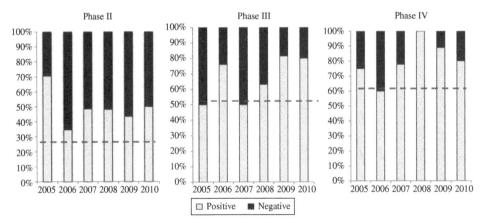

FIGURE 10.5   Model-based drug development (MBDD) at Pfizer. MBDD can be applied at all stages of drug development, and it impacts the success rates of trials at every stage after the simulation work was done. The dotted lines show the expected success rate assuming no change from 2004 levels [98]. (Adapted from Milligan et al. [96].)

FUTURE CHALLENGES

While the applications of physics based models to the digital patient are exciting and varied, several challenges face the community. The two most critical needs are connecting the top-down and bottom-up model projects. The problem is that the modeling languages have been established separately, and so the community must spend valuable time and effort replicating work already done by other groups. This represents a gross inefficiency in the development process, and hampers cooperation between groups. It is our belief that market forces represented for instance by the industry–academia–regulatory agency consortia such as Avicenna (http://avicenna-isct.org/) and Medical Device Innovation Consortium (http://mdic.org/) will provide the force to consolidate these efforts into a unified whole.

The more troubling challenge is that of rigorous model validation. While in the rarified space of reductionist models, validation is a well-defined concept. The assumptions that underlie the model induce a standard for evaluating the model. In the case of a larger target, tissue, organ, or an entire individual, validation becomes a more difficult concept to define. Intense intersubject variations exist in humans; a person even demonstrates different physiological at different ages, so even the existence of a data set that represents a target for validation is in question. Population modeling may be the key: by generating many individuals, a class of subjects similar to a given patient might be selected over a collection of observable variables. Consideration of differences in that population may suggest other observations to make in the patent, establishing an iterative process for matching an individual to a reasonable model. This challenge is not unique to biological models; it exists across all nonlinear dynamic models, and no systematic solution has been accepted [99]. Until this step is completed, the usefulness of the digital patient in the clinical setting is in doubt.

CONCLUSION

This chapter introduced the fundamentals of physics-based modeling and simulation in the medical and health sciences from the academic, industrial, and regulatory aspects. We summarized the efforts of multiple consortia dedicated to implementing the digital human in PBM form. We provided multiple examples of the use of PBM for advancing the goals of basic science, clinical utility, and for streamlining drug and medical device development. We introduced physics-based population modeling for the study of the human physiome with an eye towards understanding factors that contribute to the range of responses seen to simple perturbations in humans, and for predicting which individuals will respond which way. Finally, we discussed challenges that face the PBM community as we look toward realizing and employing the digital patient in science, industry, and education.

ACKNOWLEDGMENTS

This work is supported by NSF EPSCoR 0903787 and NIH P01HL051971.

Conflicts of interest: HumMod is licensed by HC Simulation, LLC from the University of Mississippi Medical Center. Dr. Hester is President of HC Simulation, LLC.

REFERENCES

1   Awh E, Barton B, and Vogel EK. Visual working memory represents a fixed number of items regardless of complexity. *Psychol Sci* 18: 622–628, 2007.

2   Guyton AC, Coleman TG, and Granger HJ. Circulation: overall regulation. *Annu Rev Physiol* 34: 13–46, 1972.

3   Cowley AW, Jr. and Guyton AC. Baroreceptor reflex effects on transient and steady-state hemodynamics of salt-loading hypertension in dogs. *Circ Res* 36: 536–546, 1975.

4   Guyton AC, Abernathy B, Langston JB, Kaufmann BN, and Fairchild HM. Relative importance of venous and arterial resistances in controlling venous return and cardiac output. *Am J Physiol* 196: 1008–1014, 1959.

5   Guyton AC, Coleman TG, Bower JD, and Granger HJ. Circulatory control in hypertension. *Circ Res* 27 (Suppl): S135–S147, 1970.

6   Guyton AC, Lindset AW, and Kaufmann BN. Effect of mean circulatory filling pressure and other peripheral circulatory factors on cardiac output. *Am J Physiol* 180: 463–468, 1955.

7   Guyton AC, Polizo D, and Armstrong GG. Mean circulatory filling pressure measured immediately after cessation of heart pumping. *Am J Physiol* 179: 261–267, 1954.

8   Knowlton FP and Starling EH. The influence of variations in temperature and blood-pressure on the performance of the isolated mammalian heart. *J Physiol* 44: 206–219, 1912.

9   Pruett WA and Hester RL. Parathyroid hormone secretion by multiple distinct cell populations, a time dynamic mathematical model. *Physiol Rep* 2: e00231, 2014.

10   Chaplain MA and Anderson AR. Mathematical modelling, simulation and prediction of tumour-induced angiogenesis. *Invasion Metastasis* 16: 222–234, 1996.

11   Edwards A and Layton AT. Calcium dynamics underlying the myogenic response of the renal afferent arteriole. *Am J Physiol Renal Physiol* 306: F34–F48, 2014.

12   Perley JP, Mikolajczak J, Harrison ML, Buzzard GT, and Rundell AE. Multiple model-informed open-loop control of uncertain intracellular signaling dynamics. *PLoS Comput Biol* 10: e1003546, 2014.

13   Tan WH, Popel AS, and Mac GF. Computational model of Gab1/2-dependent VEGFR2 pathway to Akt ctivation. *PLoS One* 8: e67438, 2013.

14   Tan WH, Popel AS, and Mac GF. Computational model of VEGFR2 pathway to ERK activation and modulation through receptor trafficking. *Cell Signal* 25: 2496–2510, 2013.

15   Hambli R. Micro-CT finite element model and experimental validation of trabecular bone damage and fracture. *Bone* 56: 363–374, 2013.

16   Liu XS, Wang J, Zhou B, Stein E, Shi X, Adams M, Shane E, and Guo XE. Fast trabecular bone strength predictions of HR-pQCT and individual trabeculae segmentation-based plate and rod finite element model discriminate postmenopausal vertebral fractures. *J Bone Miner Res* 28: 1666–1678, 2013.

17   Verhulp E, Van RB, Muller R, and Huiskes R. Micro-finite element simulation of trabecular-bone post-yield behaviour: effects of material model, element size and type. *Comput Methods Biomech Biomed Eng* 11: 389–395, 2008.

18   Webster D, Wirth A, van Lenthe GH, and Muller R. Experimental and finite element analysis of the mouse caudal vertebrae loading model: prediction of cortical and trabecular bone adaptation. *Biomech Model Mechanobiol* 11: 221–230, 2012.

19   Schmitz JP, Vanlier J, van Riel NA, and Jeneson JA. Computational modeling of mitochondrial energy transduction. *Crit Rev Biomed Eng* 39: 363–377, 2011.

20   Shorten PR, Pleasants TB, and Upreti GC. A mathematical model for mammary fatty acid synthesis and triglyceride assembly: the role of stearoyl CoA desaturase (SCD). *J Dairy Res* 71: 385–397, 2004.

21   Shorten PR and Upreti GC. A mathematical model of fatty acid metabolism and VLDL assembly in human liver. *Biochim Biophys Acta* 1736: 94–108, 2005.

22   Simpson SJ and Raubenheimer D. Obesity: the protein leverage hypothesis. *Obes Rev* 6: 133–142, 2005.

23   Wagner PD. Muscle O_2 transport and O_2 dependent control of metabolism. *Med Sci Sports Exerc* 27: 47–53, 1995.

24   Shafirstein, G and Baeumler, W. Use of lasers in dermatology. *Int J Hyperthermia* 27: 739–740, 2011.

25   Coveney PV and Fowler PW. Modelling biological complexity: a physical scientist's perspective. *J R Soc Interface* 2: 267–280, 2005.

26   Du P, O'Grady G, Gao J, Sathar S, and Cheng LK. Toward the virtual stomach: progress in multiscale modeling of gastric electrophysiology and motility. *Wiley Interdiscip Rev Syst Biol Med* 5: 481–493, 2013.

27   Hatzikirou H, Chauviere A, Bauer AL, Leier A, Lewis MT, Macklin P, Marquez-Lago TT, Bearer EL, and Cristini V. Integrative physical oncology. *Wiley Interdiscip Rev Syst Biol Med* 4: 1–14, 2012.

28   Paomedia. Sauro Lab: Networks, Control and Software. Retrieved August 19, 2014 from http://sourceforge.net/projects/jdesigner/ (accessed on November 17, 2014).

29   HumanSim. 2014. Retrieved from http://www.humansim.com/solutions/technologies. (accessed on November 17, 2014).

30   Sauro Lab: Networks, Control and Software. Retrieved August 19, 2014 from http://sys-bio.org (accessed on November 17, 2014).

31   Hallow KM, Lo A, Beh J, Rodrigo M, Ermakov S, Friedman S, de LH, Sarkar A, Xiong Y, Sarangapani R, Schmidt H, Webb R, and Kondic AG. A model-based approach to investigating the pathophysiological mechanisms of hypertension and response to antihypertensive therapies: extending the Guyton model. *Am J Physiol Regul Integr Comp Physiol* 306: R647–R662, 2014.

32   Karaaslan F, Denizhan Y, and Hester R. A mathematical model of long-term renal sympathetic nerve activity inhibition during an increase in sodium intake. *Am J Physiol Regul Integr Comp Physiol* 306: R234–R247, 2014.

33   Karaaslan F, Denizhan Y, Kayserilioglu A, and Gulcur HO. Long-term mathematical model involving renal sympathetic nerve activity, arterial pressure, and sodium excretion. *Ann Biomed Eng* 33: 1607–1630, 2005.

34 Moss R, Grosse T, Marchant I, Lassau N, Gueyffier F, and Thomas SR. Virtual patients and sensitivity analysis of the Guyton model of blood pressure regulation: towards individualized models of whole-body physiology. *PLoS Comput Biol* 8: e1002571, 2012.

35 Hester RL, Brown AJ, Husband L, Iliescu R, Pruett D, Summers R, and Coleman TG. HumMod: A modeling environment for the simulation of integrative human physiology. *Front Physiol* 2: 12, 2011.

36 Hempleman SC, Adamson TP, Begay RS, and Solomon IC. CO_2 transduction in avian intra-pulmonary chemoreceptors is critically dependent on transmembrane Na^+/H^+ exchange. *Am J Physiol Regul Integr Comp Physiol* 284: R1551–R1559, 2003.

37 Bartlett M. On theoretical models for competitive and predatory biological systems. *Biometrika* 44: 27–42, 1957.

38 Higdon D, Gattiker J, Williams B, and Rightley M. Computer model calibration using high-dimensional output. *J Am Stat Assoc* 103: 570–583, 2008.

39 Pruett WA, Husband LD, Husband G, Dakhlalla M, Bellamy K, Coleman TG, and Hester RL. A population model of integrative cardiovascular physiology. *PLoS One* 8: e74329, 2013.

40 Cooper JB and Taqueti VR. A brief history of the development of mannequin simulators for clinical education and training. *Postgrad Med J* 84: 563–570, 2008.

41 Rosen KR. The history of medical simulation. *J Crit Care* 23: 157–166, 2008.

42 Smith NT, Zwart A, and Beneken JE. Interaction between the circulatory effects and the uptake and distribution of halothane: use of a multiple model. *Anesthesiology* 37: 47–58, 1972.

43 Zwart A, Smith NT, and Beneken JE. Multiple model approach to uptake and distribution of halothane: the use of an analog computer. *Comput Biomed Res* 5: 228–238, 1972.

44 Hardman JG, Bedforth NM, Ahmed AB, Mahajan RP, and Aitkenhead AR. A physiology simulator: validation of its respiratory components and its ability to predict the patient's response to changes in mechanical ventilation. *Br J Anaesth* 81: 327–332, 1998.

45 Jonathan GH. The Nottingham Physiology Simulator. Retrieved September 1, 2005 from http://www.hardman01.plus.com/index_files/nps.htm (accessed on November 17, 2014).

46 Schwid HA and O'Donnell D. The Anesthesia Simulator-Recorder: A Device to Train and Evaluate Anesthesiologists' Responses to Critical Incidents. *Anesthesiology* 72: 191–197, 1990.

47 Coleman TG and Randall JE. Human: a comprehensive physiological model. *Physiologist* 26: 15–21, 1983.

48 Abram SR, Hodnett BL, Summers RL, Coleman TG, and Hester RL. Quantitative circulatory physiology: an integrative mathematical model of human physiology for medical education. *Adv Physiol Educ* 31: 202–210, 2007.

49 Lejus C, Magne C, Brisard L, Blondel P, Asehnoune K, and Pean D. What is the accuracy of the high-fidelity METI human patient simulator physiological models during oxygen administration and apnea maneuvers? *Anesth Analg* 117: 392–397, 2013.

50 Schebesta K, Hupfl M, Rossler B, Ringl H, Muller MP, and Kimberger O. Degrees of reality: airway anatomy of high-fidelity human patient simulators and airway trainers. *Anesthesiology* 116: 1204–1209, 2012.

51 Pettit BH, Norfleet J, and Descheneaux CR. Task specific simulations for medical training: fidelity requirements compared with levels of care. Proceedings of the Interservice/Industry Training, Simulations, and Education Conference, November 30–December 3, 2009, Orlando, FL.

52 Moon JY, Suh DC, Lee YS, Kim YW, and Lee JS. Considerations of blood properties, outlet boundary conditions and energy loss approaches in computational fluid dynamics modeling. *Neurointervention* 9: 1–8, 2014.

53 Longest PW and Holbrook LT. In silico models of aerosol delivery to the respiratory tract: development and applications. *Adv Drug Deliv Rev* 64: 296–311, 2012.

54 Lohmeier TE and Iliescu R. Lowering of blood pressure by chronic suppression of central sympathetic outflow: insight from prolonged baroreflex activation. *J Appl Physiol* 113: 1652–1658, 2012.

55 Iliescu R and Lohmeier TE. Lowering of blood pressure during chronic suppression of central sympathetic outflow: insight from computer simulations. *Clin Exp Pharmacol Physiol* 37: e24–e33, 2010.

56 Tanaka G, Hirata Y, Goldenberg SL, Bruchovsky N, and Aihara K. Mathematical modelling of prostate cancer growth and its application to hormone therapy. *Philos Trans A Math Phys Eng Sci* 368: 5029–5044, 2010.

57 Seok J, Warren HS, Cuenca AG, Mindrinos MN, Baker HV, Xu W, Richards DR, McDonald-Smith GP, Gao H, Hennessy L, Finnerty CC, Lopez CM, Honari S, Moore EE, Minei JP, Cuschieri J, Bankey PE, Johnson JL, Sperry J, Nathens AB, Billiar TR, West MA, Jeschke MG, Klein MB, Gamelli RL, Gibran NS, Brownstein BH, Miller-Graziano C, Calvano SE, Mason PH, Cobb JP, Rahme LG, Lowry SF, Maier RV, Moldawer LL, Herndon DN, Davis RW, Xiao W, and Tompkins RG. Genomic responses in mouse models poorly mimic human inflammatory diseases. *Proc Natl Acad Sci USA* 110: 3507–3512, 2013.

58 Takao K and Miyakawa T. Genomic responses in mouse models greatly mimic human inflammatory diseases. *Proc Natl Acad Sci USA* 112(4): 1167–1172, 2014.

59 Sanga S, Frieboes HB, Zheng X, Gatenby R, Bearer EL, and Cristini V. Predictive oncology: a review of multidisciplinary, multiscale in silico modeling linking phenotype, morphology and growth. *Neuroimage* 37 Suppl 1: S120–S134, 2007.

60 Priore RL. Using a mathematical model in the evaluation of human tumor response to chemotherapy. *J Natl Cancer Inst* 37: 635–647, 1966.

61 Summers WC. Dynamics of tumor growth: a mathematical model. *Growth* 30: 333–338, 1966.

62 Duchatellier M and Israel L. Growth fraction, resistance, schedule: doubling time relationship sequential versus simultaneous combinations, as evaluated by a mathematical model of response to chemotherapy. *Eur J Cancer* 7: 545–549, 1971.

63 Slack NH, Blumenson LE, and Bross ID. Therapeutic implications from a mathematical model characterizing the course of breast cancer. *Cancer* 24: 960–971, 1969.

64 Zaharko DS, Dedrick RL, Bischoff KB, Longstreth JA, and Oliverio VT. Methotrexate tissue distribution: prediction by a mathematical model. *J Natl Cancer Inst* 46: 775–784, 1971.

65 Blumenson LE and Bross ID. Use of a mathematical model to bridge the clinic-laboratory gap: local spread of endometrial cancer. *J Theor Biol* 38: 397–411, 1973.

66 Chen Y and Lowengrub JS. Tumor growth in complex, evolving microenvironmental geometries: a diffuse domain approach. *J Theor Biol* 361C: 14–30, 2014.

67 Cross SS and Cotton DW. Chaos and antichaos in pathology. *Hum Pathol* 25: 630–637, 1994.

68 Michelson S and Leith JT. Host response in tumor growth and progression. *Invasion Metastasis* 16: 235–246, 1996.

69 Sanga S, Frieboes HB, Zheng X, Gatenby R, Bearer EL, and Cristini V. Predictive oncology: a review of multidisciplinary, multiscale in silico modeling linking phenotype, morphology and growth. *Neuroimage* 37 Suppl 1: S120–S134, 2007.

70 Roblitz S, Stotzel C, Deuflhard P, Jones HM, Azulay DO, van der Graaf PH, and Martin SW. A mathematical model of the human menstrual cycle for the administration of GnRH analogues. *J Theor Biol* 321: 8–27, 2013.

71 Martins FC, Santos JL, and de Oliveira CF. Microdialysis: improving local chemotherapy in cancer using a mathematical model. *Front Biosci* (Elite Ed) 4: 401–409, 2012.

72   Perumpanani AJ, Sherratt JA, Norbury J, and Byrne HM. Biological inferences from a mathematical model for malignant invasion. *Invasion Metastasis* 16: 209–221, 1996.

73   Chaplain M and Anderson A. Mathematical modelling of tumour-induced angiogenesis: network growth and structure. *Cancer Treat Res* 117: 5175, 2004.

74   Chaplain MA. Mathematical modelling of angiogenesis. *J Neurooncol* 50: 37–51, 2000.

75   Voutouri C and Stylianopoulos T. Evolution of osmotic pressure in solid tumors. *J Biomech* 47(14): 3441–3447, 2014.

76   Elias J, Dimitrio L, Clairambault J, and Natalini R. The p53 protein and its molecular network: modelling a missing link between DNA damage and cell fate. *Biochim Biophys Acta* 1844: 232–247, 2014.

77   LaDisa JF, Jr., Dholakia RJ, Figueroa CA, Vignon-Clementel IE, Chan FP, Samyn MM, Cava JR, Taylor CA and Feinstein JA. Computational simulations demonstrate altered wall shear stress in aortic coarctation patients treated by resection with end-to-end anastomosis. *Congenit Heart Dis* 6: 432–443, 2011.

78   Martins FC, Santos JL, and de Oliveira CF. Microdialysis: improving local chemotherapy in cancer using a mathematical model. *Front Biosci* (Elite Ed) 4: 401–409, 2012.

79   Roeder I and Glauche I. Pathogenesis, treatment effects, and resistance dynamics in chronic myeloid leukemia–insights from mathematical model analyses. *J Mol Med* 86: 17–27, 2008.

80   Nguyen T, Hattery E, and Khatri VP. Radiofrequency ablation and breast cancer: a review. *Gland Surg* 3: 128–135, 2014.

81   Waaijer L, Kreb DL, Fernandez Gallardo MA, Van Rossum PS, Postma EL, Koelemij R, Van Diest PJ, Klaessens JH, Witkamp AJ, and Van HR. Radiofrequency ablation of small breast tumours: evaluation of a novel bipolar cool-tip application. *Eur J Surg Oncol* 40: 1222–1229, 2014.

82   DiMaio SP and Salcudean SE. Interactive simulation of needle insertion models. *IEEE Trans Biomed Eng* 52: 1167–1179, 2005.

83   Kobayashi, Y, Suzuki, M, Konishi, K, Hashizume, M, and Fujie, MG. Development of a novel approach, "palpation based needle insertion" for breast cancer treatment. Proceedings of the 2008 IEEE International Conference on Robotics and Biomimetics (ROBIO), 22-25 February 2009 (Rescheduled from December 2008). Institute of Electrical and Electronics Engineers (IEEE): 505–511, 2009.

84   Ottermo, MV, Stavdahl, O, and Johansen, TA. Palpation instrument for augmented minimally invasive surgery. IEEE/RSJ International Conference on Intelligent Robots and Systems, Institute of Electrical and Electronics Engineers (IEEE), September 28–October 2, Sendai, Japan, IEEE, XX. Vol. 4, pp. 3960–3964, 2004.

85   Pennati G, Corsini C, Hsia TY, and Migliavacca F. Computational fluid dynamics models and congenital heart diseases. *Front Pediatr* 1: 4, 2013.

86   Santoro A, Ferramosca E, and Mancini E. Biofeedback-driven dialysis: where are we? *Contrib Nephrol* 161: 199–209, 2008.

87   Fiala D, Psikuta A, Jendritzky G, Paulke S, Nelson DA, Lichtenbelt WD, and Frijns AJ. Physiological modeling for technical, clinical and research applications. *Front Biosci* (Schol Ed) 2: 939–968, 2010.

88   Lalonde RL, Kowalski KG, Hutmacher MM, Ewy W, Nichols DJ, Milligan PA, Corrigan BW, Lockwood PA, Marshall SA, Benincosa LJ, Tensfeldt TG, Parivar K, Amantea M, Glue P, Koide H, and Miller R. Model-based drug development. *Clin Pharmacol Ther* 82: 21–32, 2007.

89   Stewart SFC, Paterson EG, Burgreen GW, Hariharan P, Giarra M, Reddy V, Day SW, Manning KB, Deutsch S, Berman MR, Myers MR, and Malinauskas RA. Assessment of CFD performance in simulations of an idealized medical device: results of FDA's first computational interlaboratory study. *Cardiovas Eng Technol* 3: 139–160, 2012.

90   FDA. Innovation Stagnation: Challenge and Opportunity on the Critical Path to New Medical Products. Food and Drug Administration Report, March 2004. Retrieved from http://www.fda.gov/ScienceResearch/SpecialTopics/CriticalPathInitiative/CriticalPathOpportunitiesReports/ucm077262.htm (accessed on August 19, 2015), 2004.

91   Sheiner LB. Learning versus confirming in clinical drug development. *Clin Pharmacol Ther* 61: 275–291, 1997.

92   Holford NH, Kimko HC, Monteleone JP and Peck CC. Simulation of clinical trials. *Annu Rev Pharmacol Toxicol* 40: 209–234, 2000.

93   FDA RFA 14-082: Development of an Integrated Mathematical Model for Comparative Characterization of Complex Molecules. Department of Health and Human Services. RFA 14-082. Retrieved from http://grants.nih.gov/grants/guide/rfa-files/RFA-FD-14-082.html (accessed on August 19, 2015), May 19, 2014.

94   Miller R, Ewy W, Corrigan BW, Ouellet D, Hermann D, Kowalski KG, Lockwood P, Koup JR, Donevan S, El-Kattan A, Li CS, Werth JL, Feltner DE, and Lalonde RL. How modeling and simulation have enhanced decision making in new drug development. *J Pharmacokinet Pharmacodyn* 32: 185–197, 2005.

95   Danhof M, Alvan G, Dahl SG, Kuhlmann J, and Paintaud G. Mechanism-based pharmaco-kinetic-pharmacodynamic modeling-a new classification of biomarkers. *Pharm Res* 22: 1432–1437, 2005.

96   Milligan PA, Brown MJ, Marchant B, Martin SW, van der Graaf PH, Benson N, Nucci G, Nichols DJ, Boyd RA, Mandema JW, Krishnaswami S, Zwillich S, Gruben D, Anziano RJ, Stock TC, and Lalonde RL. Model-based drug development: a rational approach to efficiently accelerate drug development. *Clin Pharmacol Ther* 93: 502–514, 2013.

97   Peterson MC and Riggs MM. A physiologically based mathematical model of integrated calcium homeostasis and bone remodeling. *Bone* 46: 49–63, 2010.

98   Ledford H. Translational research: 4 ways to fix the clinical trial. *Nature* 477: 526–528, 2011.

99   Barlas Y. Formal aspects of model validity and validation in system dynamics. *System Dynamics Rev* 12: 183–210, 1998.

11

MODELING AND UNDERSTANDING THE HUMAN BODY WITH SwarmScript

SEBASTIAN VON MAMMEN[1], STEFAN SCHELLMOSER[1], CHRISTIAN JACOB[2], AND JÖRG HÄHNER[1]

[1] *Organic Computing Institute, University of Augsburg, Augsburg, Germany*

[2] *Department of Biochemistry and Molecular Biology and Department of Computer Science, University of Calgary, Calgary, Alberta, Canada*

INTRODUCTION

It is well known that generic medical advice and therapy may have adverse effects on the patient's health [1–3] as well as on the health care system as a whole, see for example, Ref. [4]. The other way round, individualized treatment has been shown to be more effective, less invasive, and reducing therapeutic side effects [5–7]. As a consequence, the patient would gain double from an individualized approach to medical treatment. From the technological perspective, individualized medicine can be supported in different ways, for instance, by making accurate predictions about the course of a disease or a treatment based on high-fidelity simulation of high-resolution models [8]. It is no less important to convey a comprehensive picture of the state and the development of a patient's health, using visual analytics methods [9] and means of interactive exploration of the physiological processes across the whole human body [9, 10]. The path toward comprehensive computational support for individualized medicine still bears numerous challenges, for instance, concerning the legal frameworks, technological limitations onsite, or a lack in computational predictive capabilities. Gradually, various pieces are falling into place, which makes it possible to retrieve an extensive digital fingerprint of a patient's predisposition and his current condition. Independently, the combination of high-resolution imaging techniques, for example, based on charged-coupled devices, computerized tomography [11], or magnetic resonance [12], with the predictive power of large-scale, multiscale simulation is paving the road for comprehensive individualized medical prevention and therapy. Big strides have been made toward this ambitious goal in terms of important stand-alone benchmarks—for instance, in terms of big data analysis [13], predictions at the level of protein interactions [14], or proteome analysis [15]. Yet, in order to comprehensively harness the potential of a digital patient, a tremendous need for the integration of diverse technologies remains.

In this chapter, we especially consider the integration of the computational representations used as well as the computational processes taking place during the phases of system M&S and exploration and analysis. Our according efforts have culminated in SwarmScript, an approach to interactively model and simulate physiological systems. We have designed SwarmScript to allow domain experts from the health sciences to translate seamlessly between biological and computational models. The uniqueness of each component of a model has to be properly represented, components be organized into subsystems and systems, and their interactions concerted across all scales. SwarmScript addresses this challenge of large heterogeneous model domains by means of an interaction-based representation and simulation algorithm. It provides a networked, hierarchical view of interdependencies and interactions for model and process analysis. It also enables the amalgamation of extensive model bases into an optimized approximative model during runtime. As a consequence of the diverse requirements that SwarmScript has been built on, it can be presented and understood at different levels: (i) at the formal, representational level; (ii) at the algorithmic level, that is, the execution model; (iii) at the level of user interaction, that is, the description and analysis of physiological models; and (iv) at the level of model abstraction. The latter is typically in the hands of the human modeller but increasingly taken over by automated optimisation mechanisms [16–18].

For the remainder of this chapter, we focus on the user perspective of SwarmScript, which provides the best conceptual point of entry to our approach. SwarmScript allows a user (i) to model a particular physiological system and (ii) to explore its evolution over time. The process of M&S is iterative—once the workings of a particular model, including its model entities, their parameters, and relationships have been understood, the user might want to either refine his model to better match his interests or to alter it to find out more about its complexities [19]. In case this tandem of observation and alteration happens seamlessly and at a fast pace (at real time), one speaks of interactive simulation. Visualization has been playing an enormous role in making interactive simulations accessible ever since their conception the 1980s [20]. Accordingly, we describe our approach in the light of various renderings immediately taken from SwarmScript runs. In the following section, we present scientific works related to SwarmScript from the field of agent-based M&S, focusing on visualization and visual programming related to SwarmScript. Afterward, we introduce the basic vocabulary and how to phrase sentences in the SwarmScript modeling language. This knowledge is put to the task in the next section where we demonstrate the application of SwarmScript by tracing a previously published agent-based model of the secondary human immune response [21]. We then discuss the current challenges of SwarmScript and we outline its short-term and long-term potential for accessible M&S of physiological systems. We conclude this chapter with a short summary of our contribution.

RELATED WORK

Complex systems can be formalized by means of agent-based modeling techniques, whereas the systems' individual parts are represented as (software) agents that interact based on their states and an internal behavioural logic. As this modeling approach is easily comprehensible, also for domain experts outside of the realm of mathematics or computer science, it has received a lot of attention from fields as diverse as economics, the social sciences, and the life sciences [22–24]. In this section, we introduce preceding works that nourished the conception of SwarmScript. It comprises a basic definition of an agent, and introduces aspects of visual agent-oriented or agent-based programming environments. In particular, it underlines aspects of the formulation of behavioural rules, it outlines the basic vocabularies used by related visual agent-based environments next to their execution models, and it briefly touches on different ways of agent organizations.

Agents and Their Representation

Agents representing the parts of a complex system have certain properties and behaviors [25]. The properties typically refer to the data that is stored with an agent, whereas the behaviors describe the system changes that the agent will introduce in specific situations. Accordingly, an agent Ag can be defined as a quadruple Ag = fSit; Act;Dat; fAgg, whereas Sit is the set of a possible situations, Act the set of possible actions, Dat represents the set of the agent's internal data, and fAg is the agent's decision function that maps the agent's states to its actions [26]. While this definition allows for arbitrarily complex blueprints of agents, our elaborations focus on reactive biological agents [27] whose behaviours are relatively simple as they do not communicate with each other directly, but they coordinate indirectly by changing and reacting to the environment. The value of agent-based models across disciplines [28] has motivated efforts toward accessible agent-based M&S frameworks [29]. To some great extent, their designers have been quite aware of the need for understandable visualization techniques [30] and accessible user interfaces [31]. As a result, some concurrent agent-based modelling frameworks offer visual programming interfaces that resemble block diagram environments that are also found in modeling toolkits such as LabVIEW and Simulink [32, 33]. In the 1990s, scientists from MIT developed a programmable LEGO brick that allowed to build robots from LEGO parts [34]. The programmable brick connects sensors with effectors, for example, bumper sensors or light sensors with electronic engines. Researchers were quick to develop LEGOsheets, a user-friendly visual programming environment in which graphical icons representing sensors and effectors were connected to the programmable brick [35]. The behavior of the programmable brick that processed the incoming sensory data and directed the engines' activity was configured by means of if-then rules in a separate editor. LEGOsheets is a specialized visual programming environment based on the more generic AgentSheets framework [36]. Here, too, objects are considered agents whose behaviors are expressed through sets of behavioral rules composed of basic operators (conditions such as see or stacked as well as actions such as transport or set). However, neither the application domain nor the application types, for example, simulations or games, are predefined in AgentSheets.

An application model in AgentSheets is composed of several agents, whereas not only the active parts of a modelled system (e.g., *Escherichia coli* bacteria) are represented as agents but also reactants such sugar, and even user-interaction elements such as buttons that activate gravity—an according simulation that predicts the waste production of *E. coli* bacteria in zero gravity is part of AgentSheets' examples library. For configuring operators, AgentSheets offers drop-down menus to choose from available parameters and agent types. Hereby, it makes extensive use of icons that depict spatial relationships and graphical states of the simulation: For instance, an offset dot in a rectangle depicts an agent's relative position and arrows in eight directions from that dot refer to its adjacent neighbors. SeSAm is another agent-based modeling and simulation environment that offers visual programming [37]. Here, the agents' behaviors are declared in activity graphs: diagrams derived from Unified Modeling Language (UML) that show the agents' states and indicate their state transitions. In each state, a sequence of interactions is performed. Since an entry in this list can be another activity graph, SeSAm allows the modeller to define behavioural hierarchies from bottom-up. Some visual programming environments do not model the control flow implicitly through the connections in a diagrammatic fashion. Instead, they provide comprehensive sets of basic programming statements, including those responsible for control flow, as visual jigsaw pieces, whereas fitting pieces imply a syntactically correct sequence of statements. Examples are LEGO/Logo [38], StarLogoTNG [31], and Scratch [39].

MULTIAGENT ORGANIZATION

Actor-lab presents an approach to agent-based programming of robotic systems that is slightly different from LEGOsheets and its various related software frameworks [40]. In Actor-lab, several agents share and process the information available to a robot and determine its actions. Here, input, agents, control events, and output are visually organized in separate views of the model editor, but they are connected with each other to define the flow of information. Typically, sets of agents receive and process sensory signals or controller events and drive the activation of effectors. Again, the agents behave according to sets of rules that are exposed when inspecting the respective model component. The organization of agents in the Actor-lab environment emphasizes the idea of a team of agents that collaborates to reach a given goal, that is, steering a robot. Alternative organizations in multiagent systems are, for instance, coalitions which may form, if several agents agree to collaborate on common, temporary (sub-)goals. Groups of agents may also be organized in hierarchical structures that reflect an order of command among the agents and emphasize the higher-level agents' responsibilities as supervisors of lower-level groups. A comprehensive survey on common organizational structures in multiagent systems is provided in Ref. [41]. Hierarchical agent organizations are often used to express their spatial arrangement, which is of great importance given the fact that interactions happen locally [42]. Hierarchical organizations are also a means to integrate multiple spatiotemporal model scales [43].

DESIGNING INTERACTIVE AGENTS

The agent-based modeling paradigm has received a lot of attention also from the field of computer graphics and the entertainment industry. Maya and Blender, for instance, are three-dimensional (3D) modeling environments in which 3D meshes can be crafted and equipped with physical properties as well as individual behaviors to produce physically realistic and behaviorally motivated animations [44, 45]. Blender, for instance, offers a visual Logic Editor that allows to model agents and their behaviors. Although such applications provide means to introduce behaviors, they focus on rendering, and the behavioral mechanisms mostly facilitate the production of animations or generative, parametric 3D structures.

   Modeling interactive agents that can change their environment and be subject to change move into the focus of attention of frameworks targeting the design and development of games and interactive simulations [46]. Visual programming interfaces are sometimes part of the respective IDEs or can be added as plug-ins, as for instance, the Antares VIZIO

Visual Logic Editor for the game engine Unity3D [47]. Primarily, these frameworks provide high-level access to rudimentary physics calculations and computer graphics functions including 3D asset management and scene graph organization. As SwarmScript draws from this functionality as well, we have chosen jMonkeyEngine for its implementation— an actively maintained, free and open-source Java-based framework that supports interactive simulation [48].

SPEAKING SwarmScript

The development of a domain-specific language promises the basic foundation to integrate various system models into one comprehensive multiscale simulation of human physiology, as outlined in Ref. [9] and [10]. The standardization accompanying the modeling process further allows to deploy automated, self-adaptive model optimization routines [16]. Its most immediate benefit, however, can be making computational modeling accessible to domain experts with limited knowledge of mathematics or algorithmics. This goal by itself is rather difficult, and it requires elaborate decisions about which programming elements, that is, which data structures and which control flow statements, should be made accessible and in which way. In this section, we recap the agile design process of SwarmScript, which also entails the description of its most recent implementation.

ANSWERING DEMAND: THE DESIGN OF SwarmScript

In numerous interviews with domain experts from the health sciences who are closely affiliated with our research groups, we inferred that models are described by means of rule-based behaviors associated to individual biological or chemical agents. This reaffirmed the demand for agent-based, rule-based modeling referenced in Section 1.2. The translation of verbally expressed rules into computational statements is not trivial. Considering a rule to consist of a conditional part and an action, we found that contextual referencing, that is, referencing specific or unspecific objects or sets of objects in either or both parts of a rule poses a difficult task. Similarly, an agent's ownership of a behavioral rule or of sets of rules cannot be associated easily in general.

GRAPH-BASED RULE REPRESENTATION

Motivated by grammatical substitution rules that guide the interactions in developmental simulation models [49], we were initially pursuing a graph-based approach to the representation of behavioral rules [50]. As can be seen in Figure 11.1, antecedence and consequence of a rule were represented as two graphs with star topologies of depth 1, encircling a node representing the acting agent. Matching the antecedence in the global state graph of the simulation implied its substitution with the given consequence. The advantage of this representation lies in (a) the inclusion of the acting agent into the behavioral rule and (b) the clear separation between querying and altering the state of a simulation. However, this representation needed considerable modifications to become usable in day-to-day modeling tasks.

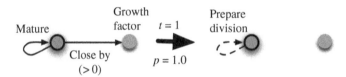

FIGURE 11.1 One of a set of graph rewriting rules that describe the proliferation behavior of a cell.

(a)   (b)

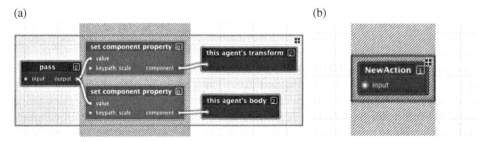

FIGURE 11.2 Screenshots from the implementation of the Source-Action-Target representation of SwarmScript. (a) Several operators can be selected by means of the enclosing rubber band and wrapped into (b) a high-level operator.

THE SOURCE–ACTION–TARGET

In order to maintain the clear separation of state queries on the one hand and state changes on the other hand, we introduced a new rule representation, similar to the input-actor-output triple used in Actor-Lab [40]. In particular, the next iteration of SwarmScript connected chains of operators (command objects without "needing any detailed knowledge of how the rest of the program works" [51]) that query the given state of a simulation to action operators that would introduce changes to the system. We distinguished between two different semantics of the chains of query operators: Those that provide data to trigger and to inform state-changing actions (sources) and those that identify the targets of any of those introduced changes (targets). Only if both types of query chains delivered valid results, the associated action operators would be actualized, that is, their effects be introduced to the simulation. Figure 11.2a shows the trisection of operators: Source queries that process data and trigger actions are shown on the left-hand side of the dashed area. Target queries that identify the objects that would be changed are shown on the right-hand side of the gray area. Actions that cause the change, if both sides deliver proper results are situated on the dashed strip itself. The Source–Action–Target representation of SwarmScript also addressed the need for modularization [52] (see Fig. 11.2b), scope (preceding calculations could trigger or skip sections downstream in a chain), and pre-processing data to determine the effected changes. However, although references were explicitly resolved, the ownership of the coded behavior was not clearly assignable. In addition, the strict separation between source and target queries did not mitigate the inconvenience of potentially redundant expression of references, in cases where sources and targets were identical (which is often the case).

SwarmScript INTO3D

The latest version of SwarmScript, SwarmScript INTO3D, lifts the separation between sources and target query chains, it introduces loops denominating an iteration variable for wrappers (now called "circuits"), and it allows to join actions into sequences to specify an

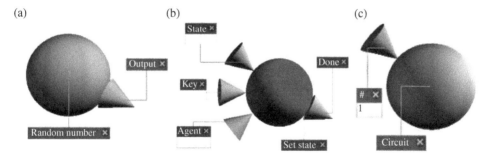

FIGURE 11.3 Instances of (a) query, (b) action, and (c) circuit operators. The spherical shapes allow for a consistent view in 3D space, the attached cones convey the flow of information between operators. The depictions include label windows that the user can create clicking the respective UI elements. Labels of input connectors contain a text field that presents the currently received input and allows the user to assign a constant value.

execution order. In order to establish clarity about the ownership of a behavior, it puts forward another novelty: The behavior is projected right into the visualization of the simulated world, logical circuitry is embedded in the context of simulated physical and geometrical bodies, relationships are explicitly drawn to potential interaction partners. This projection eliminates the distinction between modeling environment and simulation space. Figure 11.3 depicts instances of queries and action operators as well as of circuit operators. The spheres represent the operators themselves; the attached cones depict input and output connectors, pointing toward and away from the operator spheres' centers, respectively.

We decided on spherical operators as they provide consistent visual cues and interaction surfaces, independent of the user's perspective in a 3D modeling/simulation scene. The conic connector shapes intuitively reflect the flow of information between operators—as in functional diagrammatic programming environments, the results of an operator's execution are passed on to downstream connected command objects, where they serve as parameter inputs. Action operators drive the simulation process, as they alone introduce state changes. On screen, we visually reflect their important role. Query operators, on the other hand, which do not affect the simulation state, are usually rendered on-screen in less-obtrusive yellow shades. Circuits are visualized on screen in blue so as to convey their distinct function of semantically neutral operator containers.

Operators are nested and connected by means of simple drag and drop interactions. A complete behavioral rule is phrased as soon as values/connections are provided for all inbound connectors of an action operator. Figure 11.4 shows a simple example of a random number query being passed into a log action. In general, connectors may maintain n:m connections, whereas the data from its n inbound connections would get aggregated into a collection and its m outbound connections would spread its data.

A SwarmScript DIALOGUE

In this section, we present and explore a simple SwarmScript model. Instead of designing an agent-based biological model from scratch, we rely on preceding work by one of the authors, which traces the secondary human immune response to infection with the Influenza A virus [21, 53, 54]. Reconstructing an established agent-based biological model, we can direct the focus of our presentation toward the behavioral logic and model visualization of SwarmScript INTO3D.

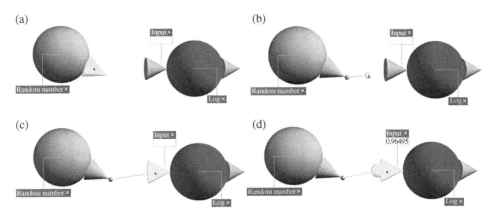

FIGURE 11.4 (a) Dragging across an output connector creates a new edge, (b) whose head is navigated by the user, (c) to be dropped onto an input connector of another operator. (d) The new connection has established a properly phrased behavioral rule. Therefore, the action operator now receives and processes input information as seen in the input connector's label window.

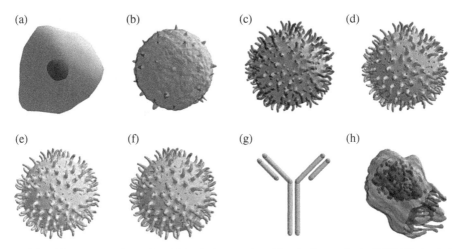

FIGURE 11.5 Visualizations of the biological agents that drive the SwarmScript INTO3D simulation of the secondary human immune response to Influenza A. (a) Epithelial cells. (b) Influenza A virus. (c) Dendritic cell. (d) B cell. (e) T cell. (f) Killer T cell. (g) Antibody. (h) Macrophage.

The domain model itself stages several types of agents (Fig. 11.5) that react based on spatial collisions and internal states. Epithelial cells (Fig. 11.5a) that constitute lung tissue are susceptible to infection by Influenza A viruses (Fig. 11.5b). When infected (at 0.1% chance upon collision with a virus), the epithelial cell is destroyed after an incubation time of 200 time steps, and it releases five new viruses into its environment. In Ref. [21], a comprehensive set of behavioral constants are presented that reliably retrace the progression of the immune response. After exposure to the viruses, dendritic cells (Fig. 11.5c), which are scarcely spread across the lung tissue, migrate to the lymphatic system to activate B (Fig. 11.5d) and T cells (Fig. 11.5e). Some of those mature into cytoxic killer T cells (Fig. 11.5f) and destroy infected epithelial cells, terminating the viral spread. B cells boost the production of antibodies (Fig. 11.5g) that attach to the viruses—such opsonized viruses are then destroyed by macrophages (Fig. 11.5h). Long-lived B cells hold the key for a fast secondary immune response releasing great numbers of antibodies as soon as the pathogens are re-entering the system.

In Ref. [21], the secondary human immune response simulation was staged in the context of the whole human body. Aiming at interactive multiscale simulation of physiological processes, this context deems all the more important as two scenes were intertwined—the infection of lung tissue and the recruitment of B and T cells by the dendritic cells in the lymph nodes. In SwarmScript INTO3D, this visual multiscale view translates into an algorithmic multiscale perspective (see Fig. 11.6). Providing the global context, that is, the human body, one can dive into the simulation grounds inside the virtual patient's lungs, and recurse ever deeper into any nested components and their behaviors (Fig. 11.7).

Each visual object that represents a biological agent (Fig. 11.5) is augmented with the according SwarmScript behavior as seen in Figure 11.8.

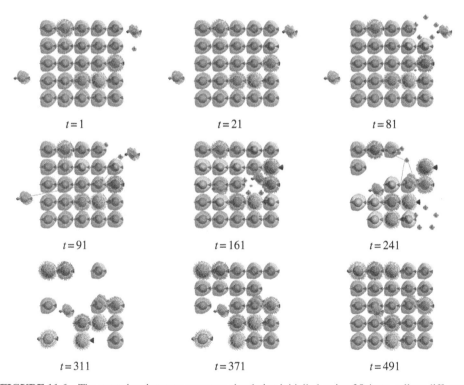

$t=1$ $t=21$ $t=81$

$t=91$ $t=161$ $t=241$

$t=311$ $t=371$ $t=491$

FIGURE 11.6 The secondary immune-response simulation initially hosting 25 tissue cells at different time steps t. The progression shows the initial infection, the reaction of the macrophages, the differentiation and recruitment of lymphocytes, the viral spread, the production of antibodies, and the eventual recovery of healthy tissue. Please note that the behavioral logic described earlier is algorithmically and visually translated into temporary relationships and interactions (edges) among the agents. At any point of the simulation, the user can dive into and reconfigure the agents' behaviors.

(a)

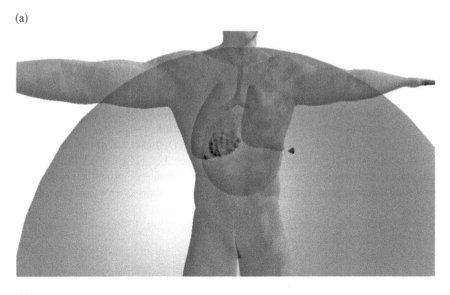

(b)

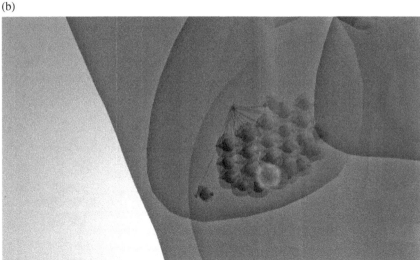

FIGURE 11.7 Gray spheres indicate the embedded SwarmScript INTO3D agents and their logic. (a) The lung inside the human body and (b) containing the infected tissue.

Floating labels provide clarity about the operators' and connectors' semantics. Configuring the involved operators and combining them into behaviors works directly in 3D space using intuitive drag and drop interaction tasks, as shown in Figure 11.4. Virtual reality provides virtually infinite space for modeling individual biological agents and multiscale behavioral modules. In the scope of this chapter, we can only present a rather limited view on the visually modeled behaviors (Fig. 11.8). Based on a set of primitive query and action operators, the given domain model has been prototyped: The agents' behaviors are wrapped in circuit operators; they interact through connectors feeding information from and to their environment. Individual operators can be specifically configured and re-used at different locations, as can be modular behaviors, for example, the "MoveToClosest" operator in Figure 11.8f, which calculates the distances to a set of other agents, moves its owner toward the closest neighbor, and yields a Boolean flag that indicates whether it has reached its target ("closeToTarget"). The modeled high-level operators can be stored alongside primitive operators for convenient reuse and refinement (also exported as generic XML files). Figure 11.9 shows the according selection window at the center, next to the heads-up display menu that allows the user to direct the modeling procedures and simulation processes at the top and the view for introspecting an operator on the right.

Here, constants could be entered for any inbound connectors, the name of the operator could be changed to match the semantics assigned by the user, and individual connectors could be removed or added to circuit operators.

(a)

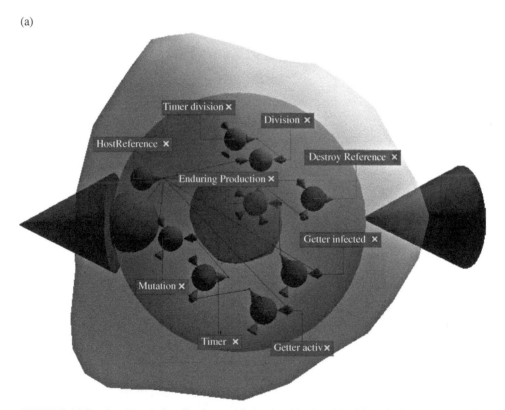

FIGURE 11.8 Combined visualization and behavioral logic of the biological agents that drive the presented SwarmScript INTO3D simulation of the human immune system. (a) Epithelial cells. (b) Influenza A virus. (c) Dendritic cell. (d) B cell. (e) T cell. (f) Killer T cell. (g) Antibody. (h) Macrophage. In (f), a nested operator of one of the agents is magnified (conic overlay).

(b)

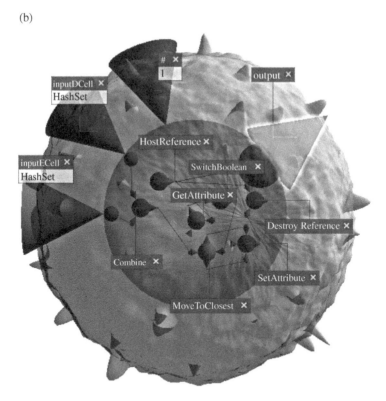

(c)

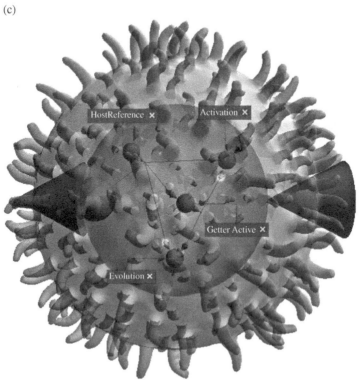

FIGURE 11.8 (Continued)

(d)

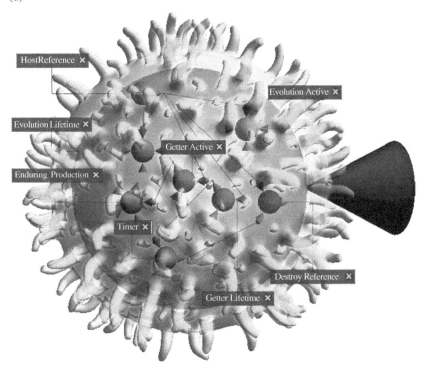

(e)

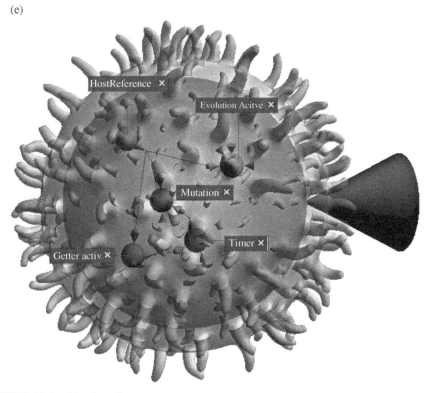

FIGURE 11.8 (Continued)

(f)

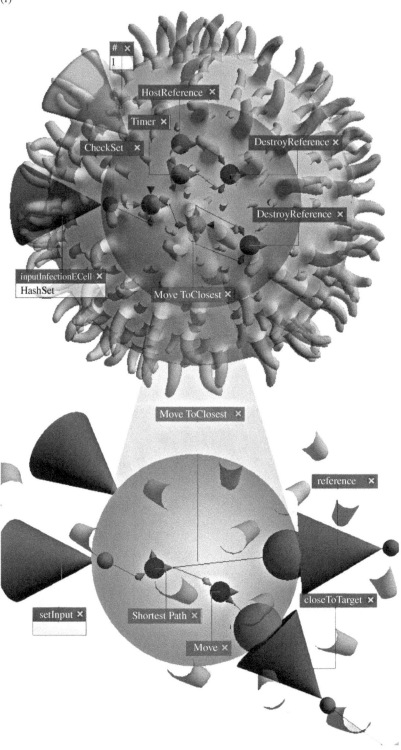

FIGURE 11.8 (Continued)

(g)

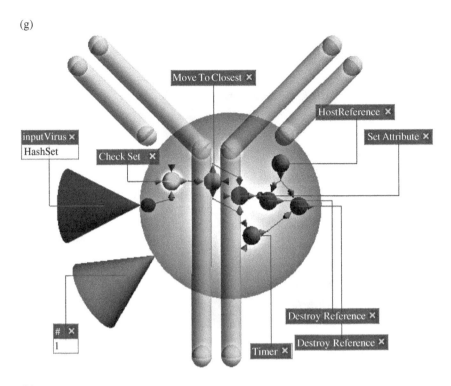

(h)

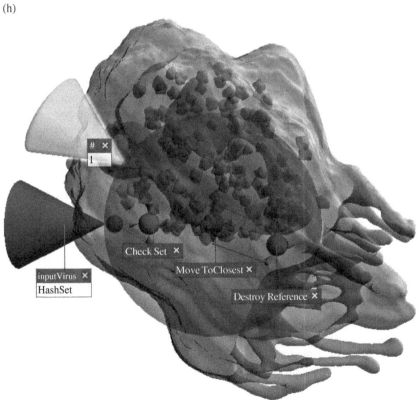

FIGURE 11.8 (Continued)

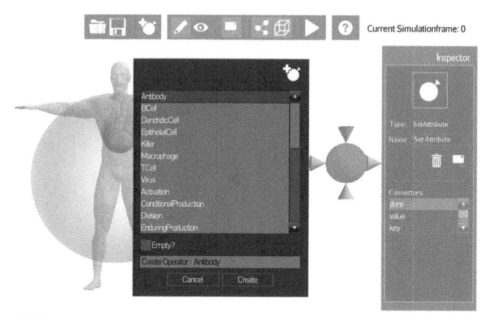

FIGURE 11.9 The headsup display for navigating the modeling and simulation phases with SwarmScript INTO3D (top), for selecting and deploying previously stored operators in the current scene (center), and to configure the currently selected operator (right).

DISCUSSION

From its graph-based predecessors [50], SwarmScript has evolved into a 3D modeling and simulation approach. It has consequently been extended to meet demands from domain experts, thereby becoming increasingly flexible and expressive. It has also established a close connection between model visualisation and behavior. However, despite its simplicity in terms of control flow and modularization, its novelties have also given rise to new challenges. On the one hand, there are challenges in terms of the modeling syntax, its support for semantics, the simulation performance, and its support for optimization. On the other hand, there are challenges associated with visual programming in 3Ds. In this chapter, we briefly discuss both directions.

The SwarmScript Language

The goal of SwarmScript is to provide accessible software for developing, presenting and exploring models of interacting biological agents at multiple scales. It is nurtured by the general bottom-up perspective on biological and physiological phenomena, see for instance Refs. [42] and [27]. As a consequence, SwarmScript is first and foremost a language that provides the means to express agent-centric, interaction-based behavior. It differs from similar, agent-based languages in numerous ways, for instance, regarding its means to connect operators horizontally and at the same time to allow the construction of modules hierarchically. Only SeSAm addresses these aspects in a similar context relying on UML-based state diagrams combined with lists of activities [37]. In contrast, SwarmScript provides a one-stop solution that amalgamates (a) concrete algorithmic calculations, (b) state-based modeling (via querying and setting state attributes), and (c) the expression of rule-based behaviors. In order to improve the clarity of SwarmScript M&S, different criteria can be considered to classify its semantics [55]. In SwarmScript, all variables that are queried or modified can be modeled explicitly. For instance, the operator HostReference (e.g., in Fig. 11.8a) provides an explicit reference to the agent a specific behavior belongs to. Abiding to a strict guideline for explicit variable usage, the query–action dualism provides a starting point for a clear axiomatic definition as only action operators introduce change to the actual system state. In our current implementation, there are still some primitive operators that are reducible to more basic definitions. For instance, the rather basic SetAttribute and GetAttribute operators, which occur frequently in Figure 11.8, in combination with various arithmetic operators could be utilised to model a Move operator that changes an agent's location based on a given velocity. In this way, a clear extensible definition could be established. SwarmScript's strength lies in its operational semantics as the execution of interactions can be meticulously traced during the simulation, in terms of conditional relationships, subsequent actions, and state changes. Yet, it could be furthered by the integration of numerous visualization techniques, including, for instance, a broadly applied colouring schematic for the agents' internal states.

SwarmScript Programming in 3D

Currently, SwarmScript-coded behavior is projected onto a surface parallel to the camera frustum. This simplifies the user interaction through devices such as monitors and mice. Effectively working in 3D virtual space, for example, placing operators and connecting them, necessitates the utilization of novel human–computer interaction methods. This can happen through rendering various depth cues (through shadows and grids on the floor) and projection of the user's body posture into the scene [56], or through immersion of the user into virtual space, for instance, tracking his body and fingers and displaying the scene stereoscopically. The latter full-body virtual reality systems could increase the naturalness of the interaction language of the SwarmScript INTO3D interface [57]. They would also allow for the natural exploration of the multiscale display of the simulated systems—diving in and out of a system, rearranging, rewiring its components. Making the shaping of 3D form accessible (consider early studies [58] combined with novel technologies [59]), they could bridge the gap between modeling of form and modeling of function, and let the bioagents' physical shape determine their interactions—not only at the microscopic protein-shape level but potentially also in terms of variation at greater levels of organisation, for instance, considering variations of organs. Blending between 3D visualization and behavioral relationships requires the user to navigate in 3Ds for the purpose of modeling alone. This by itself bears several challenges. For instance, the speed of the camera movement relative to the level of magnification has to be adjusted in accordance with the user's needs: Diving several levels deep into a multiscale model should happen fast, ensuring that the user is aware of the global context. When the user wants to adjust the camera to capture the synchronised interactions of two neighboring cells, the camera adjustment needs to be very sensitive. When exploring 3D space, it is also important to easily travel and to return to specific locations—all these issues need to be incorporated into a 3D visual modeling and simulation environment as well. Prezi, a vector-based presentation software demonstrate how such "location"-management functionality can be implemented in an accessible fashion [60].

Although 3D rendering conveys a great appeal and naturalness, a hybrid approach to visualisation would be advantageous that makes the model accessible in different modes depending on the information sought [61]. The combination of heads-up displays for navigation and introspection as seen in Figure 11.9 already addresses the need for hybrid display modalities to a very limited extent. Similar to the rich options provided by visual analytics [9], increasing the number of modeling modalities might prove useful in the context of SwarmScript-based models.

SUMMARY

In this chapter, we provided some background in agent-based modeling and visual agent-based programming, emphasizing the often-underrated feature of agent interactivity. We then familiarized the reader with the foundational challenges SwarmScript has been addressing since its inception—starting from graph-based behavioral rules over source–action–target triples to INTO3D. Finally, we demonstrated the mechanics of SwarmScript INTO3D retracing an agent-based model of the secondary human response to Influenza A infection. Based on these elaborations, we discussed the achievements of SwarmScript INTO3D and immediate leeway for its improvement. SwarmScript represents an approach to accessible modeling and simulation of biological agent-based systems. It offers an expressive model representation that originates from a spatial, interaction-based modelling mindset. SwarmScript INTO3D bridges the gap between modelling and simulation spaces, making every model aspect accessible during simulation, providing a truly interactive simulation experience. The design of SwarmScript has been motivated by the needs of a multidisciplinary enterprise. Input from domain experts (teachers, scientists, and practitioners) from the health sciences has informed its evolution, as has research into agent representation, visual programming, and interactive simulation. As a result, it integrates technologies and concepts from a diverse range of disciplines to take the unification of system modeling and simulation one step further toward teachers and students in the health sciences as well as doctors, health care personnel, and patients.

REFERENCES

1 I. R. Edwards and J. K. Aronson. Adverse drug reactions: definitions, diagnosis, and management. *The Lancet*, 356(9237):1255–1259, 2000.

2 A. Trotti, A. D. Colevas, A. Setser, V. Rusch, D. Jaques, V. Budach, C. Langer, B. Murphy, R. Cumberlin, C. N. Coleman, et al. Ctcae v3.0: development of a comprehensive grading system for the adverse effects of cancer treatment. In J. E. Tepper et al., eds. Seminars in Radiation Oncology, volume 13. Elsevier, Amsterdam, 2003, pp. 176–181.

3 J. P. Vandenbroucke and B. M. Psaty. Benefits and risks of drug treatments: how to combine the best evidence on benefits with the best data about adverse effects. *JAMA*, 300(20):2417–2419, 2008.

4 C. Steenholdt, J. Brynskov, O. Ø. Thomsen, L. K. Munck, J. Fallingborg, L. A. Christensen, G. Pedersen, J. Kjeldsen, B. A. Jacobsen, A. S. Oxholm, et al. Individualised therapy is more cost-effective than dose intensification in patients with Crohn's disease who lose response to anti-TNF treatment: a randomised, controlled trial. *Gut*, 63(6):919–927, 2014.

5 M. Eichelbaum, M. Ingelman-Sundberg, and W. E. Evans. Pharmacogenomics and individualized drug therapy. *Annual Review of Medicine*, 57:119–137, 2006.

6 W. E. Evans and M. V. Relling. Moving towards individualized medicine with pharmacogenomics. *Nature*, 429(6990):464–468, 2004.

7   B. Shastry. Pharmacogenetics and the concept of individualized medicine. *The Pharmacogenomics Journal*, 6(1):16–21, 2005.

8   R. O. Dror, R. M. Dirks, J. Grossman, H. Xu, and D. E. Shaw. Biomolecular simulation: a computational microscope for molecular biology. *Annual Review of Biophysics*, 41:429–452, 2012.

9   D. A. Keim, F. Mansmann, J. Schneidewind, J. Thomas, and H. Ziegler. Visual analytics: scope and challenges. In Simoff, S. J., Böhlen, M. H., and Mazeika, A. Visual Data Mining, vol. 4404. Lecture Notes in Computer Science. Springer, Berlin/Heidelberg, 2008, pp. 76–90.

10 C. Jacob, S. von Mammen, T. Davison, A. Sarraf-Shirazi, V. Sarpe, A. Esmaeili, D. Phillips, I. Yazdanbod, S. Novakowski, S. Steil, C. Gingras, H. Jamniczky, B. Hallgrimsson, and B. Wright. LINDSAY Virtual Human: Multi-scale, Agent-based, and Interactive, volume 422 of Advances in Intelligent Modelling and Simulation: Artificial Intelligence-based Models and Techniques in Scalable Computing. Springer Verlag, Berlin/Heidelberg, 2012, pp. 327–349.

11 J. Hsieh. Computed Tomography: Principles, Design, Artifacts, and Recent Advances. SPIE, Bellingham, WA, 2009.

12 P. A. Bandettini. Twenty years of functional MRI: the science and the stories. *Neuroimage*, 62(2):575–588, 2012.

13 D. Heller. Combined search in structured and unstructured medical data. In Plattner, H. and Schapranow, M-P. eds. High-Performance In-Memory Genome Data Analysis. Springer, XX, 2014, Springer International Publishing, Cham, Switzerland, pp. 181–206.

14 Y. Matsuzaki, N. Uchikoga, M. Ohue, T. Shimoda, T. Sato, T. Ishida, and Y. Akiyama. Megadock 3.0: a high-performance protein–protein interaction prediction software using hybrid parallel computing for petascale supercomputing environments. *Source Code for Biology and Medicine*, 8:18, 2013.

15 N. Neuhauser, N. Nagaraj, P. McHardy, S. Zanivan, R. Scheltema, J. Cox, and M. Mann. High performance computational analysis of large-scale proteome data sets to assess incremental contribution to coverage of the human genome. *Journal of Proteome Research*, 12(6):2858–2868, 2013.

16 S. von Mammen and J.-P. Steghöofer. In Pitt, J. ed. The Computer After Me: Awareness and Self-Awareness in Autonomic Systems, Chapter Bring it on, Complexity! Present and Future of Self-Organising Middle-Out Abstraction. World Scientific Publishing, Singapore, 2014.

17 A. Sarraf Shirazi, T. Davison, S. von Mammen, J. Denzinger, and C. Jacob. Adaptive agent abstractions to speed up spatial agent-based simulations. *Simulation Modelling Practice and Theory*, 40:144–160, 2014.

18 A. S. Shirazi, S. von Mammen, and C. Jacob. Abstraction of agent interaction processes: towards large-scale multi-agent models. *Simulation*, 89(4):524–538, 2013.

19 F. A. C. Polack. Proposals for validation of simulations in science. In S. Stepney, P. H. Welch, P. S. Andrews, A. T. Sampson, eds. Proceedings of the 2010 Workshop on Complex Systems Modelling and Simulation, August 19–23, 2010, Odense, Denmark. Luniver Press, Frome, pp. 51–74.

20 S. Narayanan and L. Rothrock. Human-in-the-Loop Simulations: Methods and Practice. Springer, London, 2011.

21 V. Sarpe and C. Jacob. Simulating the decentralized processes of the human immune system in a virtual anatomy model. *BMC Bioinformatics*, 14:1–18, 2013.

22 L. Tesfatsion. agent-based computational economics: a constructive approach to economic theory. In L. Tesfatsion and K. L. Judd, eds. Handbook of Computational Economics, volume 2. Elsevier, Amsterdam, 2006, pp. 831–880.

23 N. Gilbert and P. Terna. How to build and use agent-based models in social science. *Mind & Society*, 1(1):57–72, 2000.

24 S. Camazine, J.-L. Deneubourg, N. R. Franks, J. Sneyd, G. Theraulaz, and E. Bonabeau. Self-Organization in Biological Systems. Princeton Studies in Complexity. Princeton University Press, Princeton, NJ, 2003.

25 M. J. Wooldridge. An Introduction to MultiAgent Systems. John Wiley and Sons Ltd, West Sussex, 2nd edition, 2009.

26 J. Denzinger and C. Winder. Combining coaching and learning to create cooperative character behavior. In G. Kendall and S. Lucas, eds. IEEE Symposium on Computational Intelligence and Games, April 4–6, 2005. Essex University, Colchester, Essex.

27 J. Fisher, D. Harel, and T. A. Henzinger. Biology as reactivity. *Communications of the ACM*, 54(10):72–82, 2011.

28 R. Axelrod. Agent-based modeling as a bridge between disciplines. In L. Tesfatsion and K. L. Judd, eds. Handbook of Computational Economics, volume 2. Elsevier, Amsterdam, 2006, pp. 1565–1584.

29 S. F. Railsback, S. L. Lytinen, and S. K. Jackson. Agent-based simulation platforms: Review and development recommendations. *Simulation*, 82(9):609–623, 2006.

30 D. Kornhauser, U. Wilensky, and W. Rand. Design guidelines for agent based model visualization. *Journal of Artificial Societies and Social Simulation*, 12(2), 1–27, 2009.

31 E. Klopfer, H. Scheintaub, W. Huang, and D. Wendel. Starlogo TNG: making agent-based modeling accessible and appealing to novices. In A. Adamatzky and M. Komosinski, eds, Artificial Life Models in Software. Springer, Dordrecht/Heidelberg/London/New York, 2009, pp. 151–182.

32 G. W. Johnson. LabVIEW Graphical Programming: Practical Applications in Instrumentation and Control, 2nd edition. McGraw-Hill School Education Group, New York, 1997.

33 J. B. Dabney and T. L. Harman. Mastering SIMULINK 4, 1st edition. Prentice Hall PTR, Upper Saddle River, NJ, 2001.

34 M. Resnick, F. Martin, R. Sargent, and B. Silverman. Programmable bricks: toys to think with. *IBM Systems Journal*, 35(3.4):443–452, 1996.

35 J. Gindling, A. Ioannidou, J. Loh, O. Lokkebo, and A. Repenning. Legosheets: a rule-based programming, simulation and manipulation environment for the lego programmable brick. In V. Haarslev, ed. Proceedings of the 11th IEEE International Symposium on Visual Languages, September 5–9, 1995, Darmstadt, Germany. IEEE Computer Society Press, Los Alamos, pp. 172–179.

36 A. Repenning. Agentsheets: a tool for building domain-oriented visual programming environments. In S. Ashlund, K. Mullet, A. Henderson, E. Hollnagel, and T. White, eds. Proceedings of the INTERACT '93 and CHI '93 Conference on Human Factors in Computing Systems, April 24–29, 1993, Amsterdam, the Netherlands. ACM Press, New York, pp. 142–143.

37 F. Klügl, R. Herrler, and M. Fehler. Sesam: implementation of agent-based simulation using visual programming. In AAMAS '06: Proceedings of the Fifth International Joint Conference on Autonomous Agents and Multiagent Systems, May 8–12, 2006. ACM Press, New York, pp. 1439–1440.

38 M. Resnick, S. Ocko, and S. Papert. Lego, logo, and design. *Children's Environments Quarterly*, 5(4):14–18, 1988.

39 M. Resnick, J. Maloney, A. Monroy-Hern´andez, N. Rusk, E. Eastmond, K. Brennan, A. Millner, E. Rosenbaum, J. Silver, B. Silverman, and Y. Kafai. Scratch: programming for all. *Communications of the ACM*, 52(11):60–67, 2009.

40 P. Whalley. Representing parallelism in a control language designed for young children. In IEEE Symposium on Visual Languages and Human-Centric Computing, 2006, September 4–8, 2006, Brighton, pp. 173–176. IEEE Computer Society, Los Alamos.

41 B. Horling and V. Lesser. A survey of multi-agent organizational paradigms. *Knowledge Engineering Review*, 19(4):281–316, 2004.

42 A. Spicher, O. Michel, and J.-L. Giavitto. Interaction-based simulations for integrative spatial systems biology. In W. Dubitzky, J. Southgate, and H. Fuß, eds, Understanding the Dynamics of Biological Systems. Springer New York, 2011, pp. 195–231.

43   S. Picault and P. Mathieu. An interaction-oriented model for multi-scale simulation. In T. Walsh, ed. 22nd International Joint Conference on Artificial Intelligence, Barcelona, Catalonia, Spain, July 16–22, 2011. AAAI Press, Menlo Park, CA.

44   J. Sharpe, C. Lumsden, and N. Woolridge. In silico: 3D animation and simulation of cell biology with Maya and MEL. Morgan Kaufmann, Burlington, MA, 2008.

45   T. Mullen. Mastering blender. John Wiley & Sons, Indianapolis, IA, 2009.

46   S. Marks, J. Windsor, and B. Wünsche. Evaluation of game engines for simulated surgical training. In Proceedings of the Fifth International Conference on Computer Graphics and Interactive Techniques in Australia and Southeast Asia, GRAPHITE '07, December 1–4, 2007, Perth, Australia. ACM Press, New York, pp. 273–280.

47   Antares Universe. Antares universe vizio. Available at: http://www.antares-universe.com/ (accessed on August 11, 2015), March 2014.

48   K. Vainer, E. S. Heggen, B. S., N. Hansen, R. Kusterer, R. Bouquet, P. Speed, and B. Owens. The jMonkeyEngine java game engine. Available at: http://jmonkeyengine.org/ (accessed on August 11, 2015), January 2013.

49   S. von Mammen and C. Jacob. The evolution of swarm grammars: growing trees, crafting art and bottom-up design. IEEE Computational Intelligence Magazine, 4. IEEE Press, New York, pp. 10–19, August 2009.

50   S. von Mammen, D. Phillips, T. Davison, and C. Jacob. A graph-based developmental swarm representation and algorithm. In M. e. a. Dorigo, ed. Swarm Intelligence, volume 6234 of Lecture Notes in Computer Science. Springer Verlag, Brussels, 2010, pp. 1–12.

51   J. W. Cooper. Using design patterns. *Communications of the ACM*, 41(6):65–68, 1998.

52   J. Vlissides and R. Helm. Pattern hatching: compounding command. C++ Report. Industrial Logic Inc., Berkeley, CA, April 1999, pp. 47–52.

53   C. Jacob, J. Litorco, and L. Lee. Immunity through swarms: agent-based simulations of the human immune system. In G. Nicosia, V. Cutello, P. J. Bentley, and J. Timmis. Artificial Immune Systems. Springer, Berlin/Heidelberg, 2004, pp. 400–412.

54   C. Jacob, S. Steil, and K. Bergmann. The swarming body: simulating the decentralized defenses of immunity. In H. Bersini and J. Carneiro, eds. Artificial Immune Systems. Springer, Berlin/Heidelberg, 2006, pp. 52–65.

55   A. Aho, M. Lam, R. Sethi, J. Ullman. Compilers: Principles, Techniques, and Tools, Pearson Education Limited, Essex, 2006.

56   A. Jaimes and N. Sebe. Multimodal human–computer interaction: a survey. *Computer Vision and Image Understanding*, 108(1):116–134, 2007.

57   J. D. Foley, V. L. Wallace, and P. Chan. The human factors of computer graphics interaction techniques. *Computer Graphics and Applications, IEEE*, 4(11):13–48, 1984.

58   X. Liu, Y. Xiong, and E. A. Lee. The Ptolemy II framework for visual languages. In Proceedings of the IEEE Symposia on Human-Centric Computing Languages and Environments, September 5–7, 2001 Stresa, Italy. IEEE Press, New York, pp. 50–51.

59   F. Weichert, D. Bachmann, B. Rudak, and D. Fisseler. Analysis of the accuracy and robustness of the leap motion controller. *Sensors*, 13(5):6380–6393, 2013.

60   B. E. Perron and A. G. Stearns. A review of a presentation technology: Prezi. *Research on Social Work Practice*, 21(3):376–377, 2011.

61   M. S. John, M. B. Cowen, H. S. Smallman, and H. M. Oonk. The use of 2D and 3D displays for shape-understanding versus relative-position tasks. *Human Factors: The Journal of the Human Factors and Ergonomics Society*, 43(1):79–98, 2001.

12

USING AVATARS AND AGENTS TO PROMOTE REAL-WORLD HEALTH BEHAVIOR CHANGES

SUN JOO (GRACE) AHN

Department of Advertising and Public Relations, Grady College of Journalism and Mass Communication, University of Georgia, Athens, GA, USA

INTRODUCTION

Fluid, dynamic, and infinitely replicable, virtual worlds have been an enticing yet prohibitively costly platform for health behavior researchers in the past decade. What difficulties that the researchers of the past have faced in incorporating virtual worlds in primary and secondary prevention and intervention programs have dramatically decreased in the recent years with unprecedented advancement in digital media technology [1], and virtual worlds are enjoying a newfound surge of popularity in both academic and clinical environments. Digital devices that simulate vivid sensory information, allowing users in virtual worlds to experience visceral environmental cues, have now become much more affordable and accessible, opening up new horizons for incorporating virtual reality technology in people's everyday lives, outside of sophisticated laboratories.

This chapter reviews the past and current trends of one particularly intriguing aspect of virtual worlds—virtual representations commonly known as avatars—in the context of health behavior change. Despite the growing interest in the influence of virtual representations on health behaviors, there has been a surprising dearth of research exploring the use of virtual representations as a direct and central vehicle of behavior change. State-of-the-art findings on the use of virtual representations to promote behavior change will be discussed first, followed by a more detailed discussion of recent studies that specifically target health behavior change using virtual representations.

AVATARS AND AGENTS

The word "avatar" originates from the Sanskrit word *avatara*, which means "descent" to describe an incarnation or a bodily manifestation of an immortal being in Hinduism. In much the same way, users interact in the virtual world in the form of embodied virtual identities that mark their presence in the virtual environment [2]. In the past, avatars typically served as simplistic and static visual markers (e.g., a simple chat icon on AOL or Yahoo Messenger), much like the virtual equivalent of horse players use to represent themselves in board games. Over time, avatars have become significantly more complex, rendered in three-dimensional forms with an extensive range of dynamic movements, photorealistic appearances, naturalistic language, and even the ability to mimic empathy when interacting with users. The avatars of today are still works in progress—the humanoids that have evolved to feel and express naturalistic emotions as are often depicted in popular media are yet figments of imagination. However, the speed at which avatars have gained technical sophistication forecasts that more realistic, natural, and affordable avatars may soon become a reality in the near future.

Agents are another form of virtual representation that shares similar features and capabilities with an avatar, but the two forms are distinguished by the element of control: avatars are controlled by human users, whereas agents are controlled by computer algorithms [3]. Although seemingly similar in their specifications, agents and avatars yield meaningfully different influences in their interactions with human users [4]. Research studies have demonstrated that the mere *perception* of interacting with another human (vs. a computer algorithm) meaningfully affects whether a virtual representation is successful at influencing an individual's attitude and behaviors even when the agents and avatars are performing identical tasks at the same level [5, 6].

A recent meta-analysis examining 32 studies that compared the influence of agents against avatars concluded that the mere perception of human control elicited stronger social responses from humans than the perception of machine control [7]. In particular, this agency effect was stronger when humans were required to form a certain degree of relationship with the virtual representations by engaging in a competitive or cooperative task, rather than a neutral task. The effect of agency was also stronger when the virtual representations were actually controlled by a human rather than a machine, regardless of perceived agency.

Designing Agents and Avatars for Health Programs

These findings have important implications for the design and implementation of virtual representations in health prevention and intervention programs. First, avatars that are controlled by humans are likely to have stronger impacts on health behavior change than agents that are controlled by machines. Thus, rather than an agent providing a heavily scripted intervention, an avatar delivering naturalistic responses is likely to be much more effective in changing health behaviors.

Having an actual person control, a virtual representation may be useful in a variety of health contexts. For instance, a rich collection of literature points to the fact that individuals often judge others based on nonverbal cues such as physical appearance or behavior [8–10]. Indeed, people are often drawn to others perceived as similar to themselves [11, 12] or simply familiar (e.g., celebrities) [13, 14]. Because virtual representations afford labor- and cost-effective means of adopting almost a limitless option of physical appearances and behaviors that may be different from the actual self, human controllers behind the virtual representation may flexibly adapt to tailor their avatars for each respective interactant.

Such a scenario is then possible: an Asian female health care provider is controlling an avatar. A patient of different sex and ethnicity walks in. The health care provider may then select a male avatar of the patient's ethnicity and interact with the patient through the male avatar to elicit positive responses based on perceived similarity. Similarity is not necessarily confined to physical appearances; the health care provider may also mimic the behavior of the patient. Behavioral mimicry has been found to increase a host of favorable attitudes toward the interaction partner, including liking [15]. Alternatively, the avatar could take on the physical appearance of a well-known celebrity to deliver health messages, and the perceived familiarity triggered by the avatar may favorably impact persuasion as demonstrated in earlier studies [14].

Despite earlier findings that indicate the superiority of avatars over agents in a persuasion context, having human controllers positioned for each and every avatar is likely a costly option. A more labor- and cost-effective solution may be to implement computer-controlled agents. Although the initial development and setup of the agent might be costly, once the infrastructure is established, agents can continue to work at the same speed and efficiency without the need to eat or rest. These agents may be infinitely replicable, which would allow patients to receive equal and uniform care across all health care facilities. Also, for sensitive topics of discussion (e.g., sexual history), patients may prefer to interact with a machine-controlled agent rather than a human-controlled avatar for greater perceived privacy.

Thus, both agents and avatars are viable options for incorporation in health prevention and intervention programs, and the choice to use one over the other should be made after a careful cost-effectiveness analysis [16]. Although research demonstrates that avatars are more effective in promoting desired behaviors than agents, the associated costs in employing a human controller may be prohibitive in a large-scale program. On the other hand, if the program calls for strong and impactful interventions that are more likely to elicit behavior change, avatars may be well worth the costs. The following section discusses representative case studies on the systematic investigation of using agents and avatars in the context of health behavior change to consider the costs and benefits associated with each type of virtual representative.

USING AGENTS AND AVATARS TO PROMOTE HEALTH BEHAVIOR CHANGES

Virtual representations offer a set of novel characteristics that allow researchers and practitioners to implement new strategies to approach health behavior change that were difficult or not possible with traditional tools and platforms. These characteristics include the virtual acceleration of time [17], wherein agents and avatars are able to transcend temporal boundaries of the physical world to digitally depict events in the past or future from the present point in time. Another major characteristic that distinguishes virtual representations from traditional media platforms is high interactivity, or the medium's capacity that allows users to influence the form and/or content of the mediated experience in real time [18]. It is generally agreed that the best interactive medium mimics the interactive dynamics of face-to-face communication [19]. Using interactive virtual representations that afford naturalistic social interactions is likely to heighten users' engagement and involvement [20], as well as foster more positive attitudes or liking toward the interaction content [21].

The initial scientific foray into using agents and avatars to impact behavior in the physical world began with the Proteus Effect [22, 23], which found that when individuals are aware of the visual characteristics and traits of an avatar that he or she is embodying, and understand what others will expect of their behaviors based on those characteristics and traits [24], the experience of embodying that particular avatar will encourage them to continue to engage in the expected behaviors in the physical world. For example, when individuals were given tall avatars to embody in a virtual world, they were more aggressive during a negotiation task in the physical world than individuals who were given shorter avatars. This is likely a result of conforming to normative expectations that taller people are more confident and more likely to be in positions of power [25].

Combined with the novel media characteristics that afford users some experiences that were difficult or impossible with traditional media platforms, the ability of agents and avatars to influence behaviors in the physical world introduces new horizons for research on the incorporation of virtual representations in health promotion campaigns as vehicles of behavior change. The implication is that even the most creative and fantastical virtual experiences with agents and avatars may yield effects that transfer into the physical world to affect individuals' attitudes and behaviors, giving researchers the freedom to explore any health context of their desires. Despite such potentials, few studies have systematically investigated agents and avatars in the context of health behavior change. Among the collection of literature on agents and avatars in the health realm, the following sections review some of the representative and state-of-the-art studies that specifically focus on how interactions in the virtual world with virtual representatives affect health behaviors in the physical world.

Vicariously Experiencing Future Negative Health Consequences through Agents and Avatars

Individuals are likely to hold a "rosy view" of distant futures, conceptualizing their futures in a positive light. Kahneman and Lovallo [26] attribute this overly optimistic assessment of future outcomes to an isolation error: people tend to think of the future as an isolated event, independent of past and present events, and base their forecasts of the future on plans and scenarios of success rather than on accurate past results. Greater temporal distance of an event, relative to the present, enhances the perceived positivity toward it [27]. Because future negative health consequences may take some time to manifest following present behaviors, the large temporal distance is likely to encourage unrealistic and inaccurate levels of optimism in thinking about the health issue. For instance, smoking a cigarette today will not immediately lead to lung problems the next day; rather, the detrimental effect of smoking may require years to manifest. The temporal distance between the cause (smoking) and effect (lung problems) renders this relationship abstract and opaque, leading individuals to assume an optimistic outlook for their own health in the future. Consequently, this "rosy view" phenomenon is one major barrier to successfully communicating health risks and changing present health behaviors.

One solution to the rosy view phenomenon is personal experience. Studies have demonstrated that going through the actual experience at the moment reduces the unrealistic level of optimism that individuals perceive about future events [28], and that recent experiences are given more weight in deciding one's susceptibility to risk than distant experiences [29]. However, with future negative health consequences, it would be unrealistic to prescribe personal experiences of negative health outcomes (e.g., lung problems) to reduce overly optimistic future forecasts. These negative health outcomes are often irrevocable or fatal.

Using agents and avatars to digitally' render future negative health consequences allows individuals to vicariously, but vividly, experience negative outcomes without having to incur actual damages to their physical and mental health. In the virtual world, time becomes a more fluid concept; once created, an agent or an avatar may be digitally manipulated to dynamically shift their appearances. For example, a virtual representation of an individual in his or her 20s may be created and then rapidly aged to depict the same person in his or her 60s [30]. Although 40 years has passed in the virtual world, this may take only a few seconds in the physical world. More importantly, these virtual experiences are sufficiently realistic to influence behaviors in the physical world.

In one of the first studies to observe how using agents and avatars to virtually depict future negative health consequences may influence health relevant behaviors in the physical world, participants were asked to watch a virtual simulation of an agent with photorealistic resemblance to themselves gain weight by eating candy or lose weight by eating carrots [31]. After watching the virtual simulation, participants were subjected to an unobtrusive measure of candy consumption in the physical world. Candy consumption was influenced by an interaction of two variables: sex and *presence*, or the degree to which participants felt that they were right there in the virtual world [32]. Male participants who felt high presence ate more candy, whereas female participants who felt high presence suppressed this behavior and ate less candy. The authors posited that this finding was a result of virtual imitation, wherein participants modeled the behavior he or has observed from his or her agent, particularly when the perceived presence was high. However, as the agents were shown to eat both candies and carrots, it was not clear which observed virtual behavior was affecting candy consumption in the physical world.

Building on these preliminary results, a recent set of studies investigated the transfer of virtual world effects to physical world behaviors in the context of soft drink consumption [33, 34]. If the earlier study posited that individuals would model and imitate the behaviors observed by the agent, this set of studies argued that agents and avatars may be used to reduce two types of psychological distances—temporal and social. Reducing the perceived temporal distance between the present health behavior and the future negative health consequence is likely to render the causal relationship concrete [35]. Also, reducing the perceived social distance between the individual and the given health issue is likely to promote perceived personal relevance and involvement with the issue [35].

The results from this set of studies revealed that perceived social distance could be successfully reduced by tailoring the information to the audience [33]. Tailoring may be as simple as changing the verbiage in a traditional pamphlet to create the illusion that the pamphlet was created specifically to target an individual. In virtual worlds, an agent or an avatar may be tailored to bear photorealistic resemblance to an individual, so that the individual may feel as if the vicarious virtual experiences are actually happening to him or her. Tailoring in both modalities reduced social distances, increased levels of involvement with the health issue at hand, and ultimately led to greater intentions to adopt the desired health behavior (i.e., reducing soft drink consumption) immediately following experimental treatments [33].

The results also revealed that perceived temporal distance could be successfully reduced by coupling traditional health pamphlets with virtual simulations that feature agents and avatars depicting future negative health consequences [33]. A virtual simulation was created to show an agent dynamically gaining weight as it continued to consume soft drinks in a virtual world, wherein 2 min of virtual time was equivalent to 2 years of physical time. By accelerating the passage of physical time in the virtual world, participants who were exposed to the virtual simulation perceived shorter temporal distances between their present health behaviors and future health consequences. The reduced temporal distance, in turn, increased the perceived imminence of risks related with soft drink consumption, ultimately leading to lower consumption of soft drinks 1 week following the experimental treatment compared to participants who were not exposed to the virtual simulation. At this point, the effect of tailoring that was observed immediately following experimental treatments dissipated, and only the effect of watching the virtual simulation remained influential.

A following study explored the effect of *virtual doppelgängers* [36], agents with photo-realistic resemblance to individuals, to investigate the underlying mechanisms driving health behavior change in the same context of soft drink consumption [34]. Virtual doppel-gängers create an interesting social phenomenon wherein a virtual entity that has photore-alistic resemblance to an individual may look like an individual but not act like him or her because the agent is being controlled by an algorithm. Participants in the study were exposed to a virtual simulation showing either virtual doppelgängers or an unfamiliar agent gaining weight as a result of consuming soft drinks regularly for 2 years, depicted in 2 min in the virtual world. Results indicated that virtual doppelgängers were more effective than unfamiliar agents in increasing the perception of presence as well as self-relevant thoughts in the virtual simulation. Watching an agent that looks like the self consume soft drinks and become obese made participants feel as if he or she were truly undergoing the experience and encouraged them to think about themselves in the context of soft drink consumption. Heightened presence and self-relevant thoughts, in turn, led to increased personal relevance to the issue of soft drink consumption and obesity.

Finally, different modalities used to deliver a health message about soft drink consumption and obesity were compared to determine the most effective message modality in the promotion of health behaviors [33]. Results indicated that compared to strictly statistical information, print narratives, and pictures, the virtual simulation of an agent gaining weight as a result of soft drink consumption over the years was best able to highlight the risks involved with soft drink consumption and actually reduce consumption one week following experimental treatments.

Taken together, these studies indicate that agents and avatars may serve as a powerful vehicle of health behavior change by depicting future negative health consequences. Without incurring actual harm to personal health, individuals are able to observe suffi-ciently realistic simulations of what the future might have in store for them if they were to continue their present health behaviors. The observation of accelerated changes in the virtual representations' health is able to meaningfully reduce the temporal and social distances perceived between the health risk and the self. Consequently, individuals feel that the risk may be more imminent and more personally relevant than they had originally thought, and ultimately adopt desirable health behaviors in the physical world.

Interactive Agents and Avatars for Health Behavior Change

If merely observing the vicarious experience of future negative health consequences occur-ring to agents and avatars are powerful enough to change health behavior, the ability to directly interact with the agent or avatar is likely to amplify these favorable effects. In one of the earliest studies looking at how interactions with avatars could lead to differences in health behaviors in the physical world, participants were given either a photorealistically similar self-avatar or an unfamiliar avatar to interact with in a virtual world [37]. When the participants exercised in the physical world, the avatar exercised with them using synchronous head and body movements in the virtual world. Results indicated that when participants interacted with a self-avatar that exercised with them, they engaged in more exercising than when they interacted with an unfamiliar avatar. These effects persisted for up to 24 h following the experimental treatments.

In the past, such studies had to be conducted in a highly controlled laboratory setting to deliver interactive experiences with a virtual representation because the experimental setup required state-of-the-art digital devices to track and render participants' movements. Recently, however, the development of consumer grade electronics, such as video game consoles, has gradually increased the accessibility and affordability of interactive media, allowing individuals to interact with virtual representations in the comforts of their own living rooms [38]. The newer video game consoles such as the Microsoft Kinect Xbox and the Nintendo Wii are equipped with sensors and accelerometers that allow players to use naturalistic body movements to control their avatars in the game. This development has introduced a novel genre of gaming called exergames, which require players to use body movements to progress through the game [39]. Several recent studies have demonstrated that interacting with the avatars in these exergames results in increased physical activity [40] as well as weight reduction [41], particularly when playing with others rather than playing alone. Although exergames still contribute to the overall number of hours individuals spend in front of screens, which is positively linked to negative health outcomes [42], they help to substitute what would otherwise have been completely sedentary screen time with low to moderate levels of physical activity [43].

Although the bulk of studies looking at agents and avatars fail to reflect this, not all virtual representations are required to take on human forms. In one of the few studies that explored the effect of nonhuman virtual representations on health behaviors in the physical world, researchers investigated the potential of using a virtual pet to promote physical activity in children [44]. The American Heart Association released a scientific statement in 2013 regarding pet ownership and cardiovascular risk [45], noting that owing a pet, a dog in particular, significantly increases physical activity levels of the pet's owner, thereby reducing the risks for cardiovascular diseases and obesity.

Guided by the framework of social cognitive theory [46], the virtual pet was a dog designed to systematically promote physical activity in children through goal setting, vicarious experiences, and positive reinforcement. In the study, children's physical activity was measured with an activity monitor that was synchronized with each virtual dog so that each child was paired with a unique pet displayed on a television screen mounted on a kiosk. The kiosk setup allows for the virtual pet to be mobile, following the children wherever needed rather than the children having to come to a specified location to participate in the program.

The underlying logic was that as children engaged in physical activity in the physical world, the virtual dog would also stay active with them in the virtual world, reaping the health benefits. When compared with children in the control group who were given an identical computer system with the same functionalities but without the virtual dog, children who interacted with the virtual dog engaged in approximately 1.09 more hours of physical activity daily. Self-report survey data revealed that interacting with the virtual dog led children to feel confident about their abilities to set and meet physical activity goals, which in turn, heightened their beliefs that physical activity is good for them. The increase in physical activity belief ultimately led to an increase in physical activity.

CONCLUSION

In an era of digital media technology, people consume health information in ways that are very different from the past. For young people, in particular, the Internet is one of the most sought out sources for health information [47]. Atkin [48] argues that choosing a channel appropriate for a specifically targeted audience will maximize the effect of health information. With the increasing ubiquity of interactive and mobile digital technology in our homes, it may be a timely endeavor to reexamine not just the content of health information but also *how* it is being disseminated.

Agents and avatars offer a dynamic yet highly controllable means to deliver health information in a novel, involving way. Offering a wide range of strategic tools that take advantage of novel media characteristics, such as the virtual acceleration of time and inter-activity, agents and avatars yield powerful impacts in the virtual world that transfer to the physical world to change health behaviors. Observing and interacting with these virtual representations allows individuals to feel as if they are genuinely present in the situation [31, 33, 34], heightens their confidence about achieving health goals [44], and encourages them to think of the health risk as a personally relevant, important, and imminent event [33, 34]. Ultimately, these underlying mechanisms drive desired health behaviors that persist longer over time than the same health information delivered through more traditional channels, such as statistical information, print, or pictures [31, 33, 34, 37, 44]. These efforts may even be combined with gaming mechanisms to replace overall sedentary time with physical activity while playing video games [39–41].

As agents and avatars offer different strengths and weaknesses, researchers and practitioners should administer an extensive analysis of cost-effectiveness to select the more appropriate form of virtual representation in the given context. An alternative option would be to consider an agent-avatar hybrid, which capitalizes the strength of programmable features and algorithms of agents while still being guided by a human controller [49, 50]. This crossover design would offer health interventions that have greater impact on human behavior but remain cheaper to operate and manage.

There is still much work to be done to harness the dynamic flexibility that agents and avatars offer to implement systematic primary and secondary prevention and intervention programs. However, the state-of-the-art research introduced in this chapter confirms the potential of virtual representations to serve as a vehicle of health behavior change. Health issues often involve an intricate and complex web of individual and environmental factors, and avatars and agents may not be a panacea for all these issues. Yet, with the rapid advancement of digital technology transforming our traditional norms and patterns of communication, these virtual representations, whether they are human or animal form, hold much potential in the realm of health interventions that has yet to be discovered.

REFERENCES

1 Schnipper M. The state of virtual reality. *The Verge.* 2014. http://www.theverge.com/a/virtual-reality/intro (accessed on August 10, 2015).

2 Ahn SJ, Fox J, Bailenson J. Avatars. In: Bainbridge WS, ed. Leadership in Science and Technology: A Reference Handbook. Thousand Oaks, CA: SAGE Publications; 2011: pp. 695–702.

3 Bailenson J, Blascovich J. Avatars. In: Bainbridge WS, ed. Encyclopedia of Human–Computer Interaction. Great Barrington, MA: Berkshire; 2014: pp. 64–68.

4 Blascovich, J. Social influence within immersive virtual environments. In: Schroeder R, ed. The Social Life of Avatars: Presence and Interaction in Shared Virtual Environments. London: Springer-Verlag; 2002: pp. 127–145.

5   Lim S, Reeves B. Computer agents versus avatars: Responses to interactive game characters controlled by a computer or other player. *International Journal of Human-Computer Studies.* 2010; 68: 57–68.

6   Okita SY, Bailenson JN, Schwartz DL. The mere belief in social interaction improves learning. In: Proceedings of the Twenty-Ninth Meeting of the Cognitive Science Society, August 1–4, Nashville, TN, USA.

7   Fox J, Ahn SJ, Janssen J, Yeykelis L, Segovia K, Bailenson JN. Avatars versus agents: A meta-analysis quantifying the effect of agency. *Human Computer Interaction.* 2015; 30: 401–432.

8   Sigelman L, Sigleman CK, Fowler C. A bird of a different feather? An experimental investigation of physical attractiveness and the electability of female candidates. *Social Psychology Quarterly.* 1987; 50: 32–43.

9   Rosenberg SW, McCafferty P. The image and the vote: Manipulating voter's preferences. *Public Opinion Quarterly.* 1987; 51: 31–47.

10 Todorov A, Mandisodza AN, Goren A, Hall CC. Inferences of competence from faces predict election outcomes. *Science.* 2005; 308: 1623–1626.

11 Baumeister R. The self. In: Gilbert DT, Fiske ST, Lindzey G, eds. The Handbook of Social Psychology. Boston, MA: McGraw-Hill; 1998: pp. 680–740.

12 Bailenson JN, Iyengar S, Yee N, Collins NA. Facial similarity between voters and candidates causes influence. *Public Opinion Quarterly.* 2008; 72: 935–961.

13 Zajonc RB. Mere exposure: A gateway to the subliminal. *Current Directions in Psychological Science.* 2001; 10: 224–228.

14 Tanner RJ, Maeng A. A tiger and a president: Imperceptible celebrity facial cues influence trust and preference. *Journal of Consumer Research.* 2012; 39: 769–783.

15 Chartrand TL, Bargh JA. The chameleon effect: The perception-behavior link and social interaction. *Journal of Personality and Social Psychology.* 1999; 76: 893910.

16 Tan-Torres ET, Baltussen R, Adam T, Hutubessy R, Acharya A, Evans DB, Murray CJL. Making Choices in Health: WHO Guide to Cost-Effectiveness Analysis. World Health Organization, Geneva; 2003.

17 Ahn SJ, Fox J, Dale KR, Avant JA. Framing virtual experiences: Effects on environmental efficacy and behavior over time. *Communication Research.* 2015; 42(6): 839–863.

18 Heeter C. Interactivity in the context of designed experiences. *Journal of Interactive Advertising.* 2000; 1.

19 Rafaeli S. Interactivity: From new media to communication. In: Hawkins RP, Wiemann JM, Pingree S, eds. Sage Annual Review of Communication Research: Advancing Communication Science: Merging Mass and Interpersonal Processes, vol. 16. Beverly Hills: Sage; 1988: pp.110–134.

20 Fortin DR, Dholakia RR. Interactivity and vividness effects on social presence and involvement in a web-based advertisement. *Journal of Business Research.* 2005; 58: 387–396.

21 Sundar SS, Kim J. Interactivity and persuasion: Influencing attitudes with information and involvement. *Journal of Interactive Advertising.* 2005; 5(2): 6–29.

22 Yee N, Bailenson JN. The proteus effect: The effect of transformed self-representation on behavior. *Human Communication Research.* 2007; 33: 271–290.

23 Yee N, Bailenson JN, Ducheneaut N. The proteus effect: Implications of transformed digital self-representation on online and offline behavior. *Communication Research.* 2009; 36: 285–312.

24 Bem DJ. Self-perception theory. *Advances in Experimental Social Psychology.* 1972; 6: 1–62.

25 Young TJ, French LA. Height and perceived competence of U.S. presidents. *Perceptual and Motor Skills.* 1996; 82: 1002.

26 Kahneman D, Lovallo D. Timid choices and bold forecasts: A cognitive perspective on risk taking. *Management Science.* 1993; 39: 17–31.

27 Trope Y, Liberman N, Wakslak C. Construal levels and psychological distance: Effects on representation, prediction, evaluation, and behavior. *Journal of Consumer Psychology.* 2007; 17: 83–95.

28   Mitchell TR, Thompson L, Peterson E, Cronk R. Temporal adjustments in the evaluation of events: The "rosy view." *Journal of Experimental Social Psychology*. 1997: 33; 421–448.

29   Murdock, BB Jr. The serial position effect in free recall. *Journal of Experimental Psychology*. 1962; 64: 482–488.

30   Hershfield HE, Goldstein DG, Sharpe WF, Fox J, Yeykelis L, Carstensen LL, Bailenson JN. Increasing saving behavior through age-progressed renderings of the future self. *Journal of Marketing Research*. 2011; 48: S23–S37.

31   Fox J, Bailenson JN, Binney J. Virtual experiences, physical behaviors: The effect of presence on imitation of an eating avatar. *Presence: Teleoperators and Virtual Environments*. 2009; 18: 294–303.

32   Lombard M, Ditton T. At the heart of it all: The concept of presence. *Journal of Computer-Mediated Communication*. 1997; 3.

33   Ahn SJ. Incorporating immersive virtual environments in health promotion campaigns: A construal level theory approach. *Health Communication*. 2015; 30(6): 545–556.

34   Ahn SJ, Fox J, Hahm JM. Using virtual doppelgängers to increase personal relevance of health risk communication. *Lecture Notes in Computer Science*. 2014; 8637: 1–12.

35   Trope Y, Liberman N. Construal-level theory of psychological distance. *Psychological Review*. 2010; 117: 440–463.

36   Fox J, Bailenson JN. The use of doppelgängers to promote health behavior change. *CyberTherapy & Rehabilitation*. 2010; 3: 16–17.

37   Fox J, Bailenson JN. Virtual self-modeling: The effects of vicarious reinforcement and identification on exercise behaviors. *Media Psychology*. 2009; 12: 1–25.

38   Blascovich J, Bailenson JN. Infinite Reality – Avatars, Eternal Life, New Worlds, and the Dawn of the Virtual Revolution. New York: William Morrow; 2011.

39   Biddiss E, Irwin J. Active video games to promote physical activity in children and youth: A systematic review. *Archives of Pediatrics and Adolescent Medicine*. 2010; 164: 664–672.

40   Peng W, Crouse J. Playing in parallel: The effects of multiplayer modes in active video game on motivation and physical exertion. *Cyberpsychology, Behavior, and Social Networking*. 2013; 16: 423–427.

41   Staino AE, Abraham AA, Calvert SL. Adolescent exergame play for weight loss and psychosocial improvement: A controlled physical activity intervention. *Obesity*. 2013; 21: 598–601.

42   Hu FB, Li TY, Colditz GA, Willett WC, Manson JE. Television watching and other sedentary behaviors in relation to risk of obesity and type 2 diabetes mellitus in women. *The Journal of the American Medical Association*. 2003; 289: 1785–1791.

43   Peng W, Crouse J, Lin J-H. Using active video games for physical activity promotion: A systematic review of the current state of research. *Health Education & Behavior*. 2013; 40: 171–192.

44   Ahn SJ, Johnsen K, Robertson T, Moore J, Brown S, Marable A, Basu A. Using virtual pets to promote physical activity in children: An application of the youth physical activity promotion model. *Journal of Health Communication*.

45   Levine GN, Allen K, Braun L, Christian HE, Friedmann E, Taubert KA et al. Pet ownership and cardiovascular risk: A scientific statement from the American Heart Association. *Circulation*. 2013; 127: 2353–2363.

46   Bandura A. Social Foundations of Thought and Action: A Social Cognitive Theory. Englewood Cliffs, NJ: Prentice-Hall. 1986.

47   Gray NJ, Klein JD, Noyce PR, Sesselberg TS, Cantrill JA. Health information-seeking behaviour in adolescence: The place of the internet. *Social Science & Medicine*. 2005; 60: 1467–1478.

48   Atkin C. Impact of Public Service Advertising: Research Evidence and Effective Strategies. Kaiser Family Foundation, Menlo Park, CA. 2001.

49   Benford S, Bowers J, Fahlén LE, Greenhalgh C, Snowdon D. Embodiments, avatars, clones, and agents for multi-user, multi-sensory virtual worlds. *Multimedia Systems*. 1997; 5: 93–104.

50   Gerhard M, Moore DJ, Hobbs DJ. Continuous presence in collaborative virtual environments: Towards a hybrid avatar-agent model for user representation. In Intelligent Virtual Agents. Berlin: Springer; 2001: pp. 137–155.

13

VIRTUAL REALITY AND EATING, DIABETES, AND OBESITY

JESSICA E. CORNICK AND JIM BLASCOVICH

Department of Psychological and Brain Sciences, University of California, Santa Barbara, CA, USA

INTRODUCTION

As computer processing increases in power and affordability, more and more research has surfaced addressing the influence of digital avatars, agents, and virtual environments on user behavior. An important aspect of digital virtual environments is that researchers can exert complete control over environmental variables and tailor them to suit experimental goals. This feature is enormously important when creating environments designed to help users address health concerns such as excess body weight, disordered eating behavior, and diabetes management. Here, we describe digital virtual environment technology as well as applications for exercise, eating, and diabetes interventions.

VIRTUAL REALITY

Although virtual environments can be experienced without technology (e.g., via books, imagination, and art), the rapid rate of technological advancements over the past few decades has markedly increased the use of digital virtual environments in both daily life and research arenas [1]. Virtual environments can be accessed via many technologies including phones, televisions, movies, CAVES [2, 3], head-mounted displays (HMDs), and even headphones [4, 5]. Importantly, digital virtual environments vary along a spectrum from nonimmersive to immersive [6]. Technologically, an immersive digital virtual environment is one that provides a continuous stream of stimuli and is relatively omnipresent [1]. Such virtual environments provide powerful immersion experiences that have, for example, been shown to reduce severe pain, providing

The Digital Patient: Advancing Healthcare, Research, and Education, First Edition.
Edited by C. Donald Combs, John A. Sokolowski, and Catherine M. Banks.
© 2016 John Wiley & Sons, Inc. Published 2016 by John Wiley & Sons, Inc.

a novel but powerful approach to pain management for individuals suffering from serious injuries and life-threatening illnesses [7–10].

Digital virtual environments also boast other advantages over "grounded reality"—physical environments—that make them ideal for human research. For example, using digital immersive virtual environments allows researchers to achieve nearly complete control over all aspects and variable in experimental environments, thereby reducing the influence of extraneous variables and their potential influences on outcomes of interest [1]. Additionally, once created, digital virtual environments can be saved and catalogued, facilitating replication attempts because the digital files comprising the virtual world can be sent anywhere instantly. Their shareable nature reduces the influence of unpublished "lab lore" on study procedures and allows studies to be conducted on more diverse samples [4]. Finally, digital virtual environments free researchers to conduct studies in laboratory settings that would otherwise be impossible due to issues such as safety, money, space, etc.

For example, researchers [11] interested in the formation of false memories brought young children into the laboratory and immersed them in a digital virtual environment where they swam with whales. Five days later, the children were asked if they remembered swimming with whales in "the real world." Children immersed in the digital virtual environment reported more false memories than those in the control condition. In another study, users walked on the edge of a digital virtual cliff while being watched and supported by their romantic partner, a situation that would be very difficult to simulate or safely conduct in a more traditional laboratory space [12]. Research applications like these highlight the unique features of digital immersive virtual environments and reinforce their utility as a research tool.

Digital virtual environments utilize technologies—hardware and software—that automatically collects users' physical and communicative behaviors (i.e., body and head movements) and renders them within the digital environment. Digital virtual environment implementations vary in "immersibility." The Kinect PlayStation interface and online environments such as Second Life are regarded as more and less immersible, respectively. The Kinect sensor projects infrared light on the body of the user and monitors its reflection allowing tracking of physical movements, body position, head pose, and facial expression [13]. Online digital environments such as Second Life do not collect any information regarding the user's body movements, instead relying on users conscious input of a series of mouse and keyboard selections to control their digital representation (i.e., avatar) and interact with others [14]. Studies incorporating such digital environments demonstrate that user's avatars are representative of the user's personality [15]. Over time, users continue to develop social networks within digital environments such as Second Life demonstrating that even less technologically immersive environments quite powerful [14].

One key to implementation of more immersive digital virtual environments is the inclusion of a digital HMD allowing users to view and experience virtual environment stereoscopically. Another is tracking of users' physical movements. Head (roll, pitch, and yaw) and body (x, y, z position) movements are tracked in real time sending user location information and gaze direction to the controlling computer so it can update the user's avatar movements and provide the appropriate field of view to the user [1].

Importantly, multiple users can be tracked simultaneously in real time within an immersive virtual environment. Recently, HMD costs have decreased by two orders of magnitude (i.e., $30,000–$300). As of this writing, one such HMD is the Oculus Rift, boasting a lightweight frame allowing more researchers and home users to venture into the world of digital immersive virtual environment technology [16]. Many other tech companies are scrambling to produce their own versions of inexpensive HMDs.

In the past, relatively low computer processing power resulted in notable time lags between a user's movements and the updating of virtual visual fields causing disorientation and "cybersickness." However, as the technology has continued to improve and become more affordable, digital environments can be rendered with minuscule lag time resulting in perceptually unbroken visual perception within immersive virtual worlds for users.

All virtual environments, regardless of immersibility and functionality, exert some level of influence whereby users feel temporarily transported and enveloped by the environment [17]. In terms of social environments, multiple users, or a single user and one or more apparent others (i.e., digital agents) can simultaneously inhabit the same immersive virtual world. Their influence upon each other is explained by the threshold model of social influence [4, 18–20]. The most recent instantiation of this model [20] specifies five variables that influence virtual humans within a virtual environment, including three mediating variables and at least two moderating variables.

The mediating variables include perceived *agency* levels of the virtual other present, *communicative realism* of these virtual human representations, and *users' response system* level. The moderating variables include *self-relevance* to the user of the virtual social environment and *context* (see Fig. 13.1) [20].

Agency involves users' theory of mind or attributions regarding other human appearing users and vary as a function of the degree to which users believe that virtual human

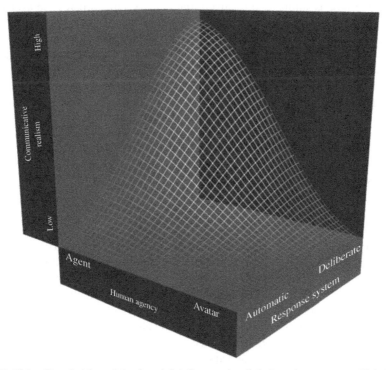

FIGURE 13.1 Threshold model of social influence in digital environments at high levels of self-relevance.

representations are being completely controlled in real time by another person (i.e., an avatar), one completely controlled by a computer (i.e., an agent), or some combination thereof [19].

Users treat avatars in virtual environments similar to how they treat humans in the physical world or "grounded reality" [21] as evidenced, for example, by maintaining greater interpersonal distance as a function of mutual gaze between users and agents [22]. Additionally, user reactions to social cues vary during interactions with avatars and agents. Surprisingly, one study demonstrated that smiles from a digital agent counselor increased empathy ratings while empathy ratings for smiling digital avatar counselors decreased empathy ratings [23]. These authors argue that there needs to be a match between how realistic the avatar/agent appears and how similar to humans they behave; when mismatches occurs, liking is decreased.

Agency levels and communicative realism together influence users' perceptions and reactions to digital virtual humans. The communicative realism of a virtual human is transmitted via movement, anthropomorphic, and photo realism, the interaction of which determines the perceived authenticity of the virtual representation as a human and, in turn, its influence on users' subsequent behaviors. For example, when conversing with digital others, users respond differentially during text compared to animated face interfaces, presenting themselves in the latter situation more positively and reporting more arousal. This behavior underscores the importance of communicative realism driven by the visual presence of "others" that incorporate movement, anthropomorphic and photo realism [24].

The response system level of the user is also critical for determining the threshold of social influence within an immersive virtual environment. At the unconscious or automatic level, the threshold is similar and relatively flat (e.g., whether a perceived avatar or perceived agent emits a sudden loud noise, the user will exhibit a startle response). However, if higher-level processes are at work, the threshold is relatively steep (see Fig. 13.1) [4]. Hence, a user is less likely to try to persuade an agent about something than an avatar. Finally, the level of self-relevance of the virtual situation greatly influences the social influence threshold, as in the minimally self-relevant situations in which users do not differ in terms of their interactions with people or agents; for example, withdrawing money from a bank via an actual teller or a digital agent such as an ATM. In these cases, the threshold is flat. Conversely, the threshold will be rather steep in highly relevant situations (e.g., job interviews and falling in love) where the extent of communicative realism is very important. Together, these five variables interact to determine the level of social influence that occurs in digital immersive virtual worlds.

Transformed Social Interactions

Although many digital virtual social environments are nearly identical to their counterparts in grounded reality, such environments can be transformed to alter social interaction experiences for users facilitating what are labeled as "transformed social interactions" (TSIs) [25, 26]. Because digital virtual environments can be independently rendered for users simultaneously, unique views and experiences can be generated for each. More specifically, transformed social interactions are created by altering sensory abilities, situational contexts, and/or self-representations in order to create environments that are truly altered in ways that are not possible in grounded reality.

When their sensory abilities are altered, users can access recent archival information about their own behaviors as well as those of other users (i.e., avatars) or agents. For example, virtual environments can be designed so that users are privy to information about the activities of themselves and others in the virtual environment. A study employing teachers using virtual environments to interact with their students demonstrated that when teachers received feedback about the amount of their own eye contact given to each student, they were better able to apportion gaze amongst the entire class [27]. Relatedly, researchers can implement augmented gaze algorithms in which the gaze of an agent speaker can be rendered uniquely for each user among members of a group such that it appears that the speaker is gazing only at that user, but for every user in the environment. Women interacting with didactic agents using augmented gaze find the agents to be more persuasive, and men remember more of the information they provided [28].

Situational contexts within digital immersive virtual environments can also be manipulated such that facets like space or time are altered to be other than that which one would experience in grounded reality. For example, the passage of time can be sped up, paused, or slowed to increase the efficiency and comprehension for students [25]. Additionally, the physical space within the virtual environment can be altered in many ways. Research on optimizing learning spaces demonstrates that virtual classrooms can be rendered so that each student experiences sitting in the center of the teacher's field of view: a virtual classroom position that has been shown to increase learning [27].

In addition to transformations to context and sensory abilities in digital virtual environment research, transformations to self-representations have been commonly used [25]. When self-representations are transformed, the behavior or appearance of the user is decoupled from the behavior and appearance of their avatar. For example, when users see their own avatars aged as though they are elderly, they allocate more money toward retirement accounts [29]. Another study demonstrated that users knowingly embodied by Black avatars reported greater implicit racial bias than users embodied by White avatars [30]. Another common method for manipulating self-representations involves slight shifts in user appearance and behavior to inform the appearance and behavior of the avatar. For example, users who were immersed in a digital virtual environment with an agent who mimicked their head movements on a 4-second delay rated the agent more positively and as more persuasive than agents that exhibited generic pre-recorded movements [31].

The Proteus Effect

As demonstrated by self-representation transformations, digital humans can directly influence the perceptions and experiences of users. Extending this idea further, the Proteus Effect (based on self-perception theory) demonstrates that people can infer their attitudes and behaviors by observing the behavior of their own avatar [32–34]. For example, users assigned more attractive avatars were more intimate with confederates than users assigned to less attractive avatars, and users with taller avatars behaved more confidently in a negotiation task [33].

This effect has been extended to branding and marketing; users who identified with their avatar preferred brands worn by their avatars [35]. Importantly, distinctions have been drawn regarding how and when avatars most influence users. Researchers report that being embodied by an avatar in real time compared to watching an independent avatar perform actions results in greater behavioral changes such as maintaining decreased personal distance between themselves and other ostensible users' avatars as well as choosing more attractive partners [36]. Additionally, individuals who were embodied by digital avatar representing the self liked their avatar more, walked physically closer to it in a virtual environment, and were more willing to commit an embarrassing act suggesting increased intimacy than if that avatar was embodying someone else [37]. Hence, embodied avatars represent a unique way to directly influence attitudes and behaviors of users with the ultimate goal of encouraging beneficial behaviors.

OBESITY AND WEIGHT STIGMA

During the past few decades, concerns over rising rates of obesity in the United States peaked when the World Health Organization declared obesity a global epidemic [38]. In 2007, over 32% of men and 35% of women in the United States were obese [39]. Obesity forecasts estimate that 51% of the population will be obese by 2030 [40]. At the time this chapter was written, individuals above a "body mass index" (BMI) of 25 are labeled overweight and those above 30, obese [41].

Research continues to emphasize the importance of nutritional education and increases in physical activity to combat obesity [42]. According to the Center for Disease Control (CDC), less than half of US adults perform the recommended amount of daily exercise to maintain health [43]. National surveys conducted between 1988 and 2010 indicate that the proportion of adults reporting no physical activity rose from 19 to 51% in women and 11 to 43% in men [44]. Nationally representative samples show that obesity levels have continued to rise in all US counties during the 2000s but no overall increase in the percentage of adults exercising [45].

Importantly, obesity does not affect all types of people equally; approximately 45% of African American adults are obese compared to 30% of Caucasian adults [46]. Additionally, obesity affects men and women differently. Compared to normal weight individuals, overweight and mildly obese women report poorer physical health, but only moderately obese men report poorer perceived health [47]. The authors suggest that these disparities are driven by weight-related stigma, discrimination, and body image concerns that are greater for women than men [47]. Indeed, the desire to lose weight (a proxy for body image concerns) is a stronger predictor of sick days than actual BMI [48].

Results of many lines of research converge on the conclusion that the psychological stress associated with weight stigma leads to increased stress responses that decrease psychological and physical health and well-being (this pattern is especially pronounced in cultures who value thinness) [49]. Obesity-related stigma often stems from the belief that an individual's weight is completely within their control and, if they are overweight, it is only because they are lazy, sloppy, or noncompetent [50]. Furthermore, overweight and obese individuals experience discrimination in a many settings including education, healthcare, employment, and interpersonal relationships [50, 51].

Experiencing weight stigma leads to negative effects such as increased eating, decreased exercise, decreased self-regulatory ability, decreased self-reported health, and heightened future risk of obesity [52–54]. Indeed according to the Cyclic Obesity/Weight-Based Stigma (COBWEBS) model, weight stigma leads to weight gain by increasing stress, thereby increasing eating and cortisol levels [55]. These and other findings have caused backlash to media campaigns with messages stigmatizing weight [56, 57].

To escape the crushing influence of socially driven weight stigma, obese individuals can turn to digital platforms and environments. Recent research suggests that people express their ideal selves by using thinner avatars, underreporting weight and age, and profiles that primarily reflect positive traits and idealized versions of the self [58–64].

Using an avatar reflecting an ideal self increases immersion as well as perceived interactivity of the avatar [65]. However, digital immersive virtual environments could be a powerful tool in addressing the growing obesity epidemic.

VIRTUAL REALITY AS A TOOL FOR COMBATTING HEALTH ISSUES

The use of digital platforms for health and well-being interventions is not new [1]. Importantly, as technology has continued to become more powerful and simultaneously more affordable, more health-related experimental research has been conducted using both immersive and non-immersive virtual environments. An impressive body of literature supports the use of virtual environments to increase levels of exercise, regulate eating behavior, and help those with diabetes improve healthful behavior adherence.

Exercise

Exercising regularly is important for maintaining physical health and normal weight and to prevent future weight gain [66]. The CDC recommends that adults perform at least 2.5 h of aerobic physical activity (i.e., fast-paced walking) weekly, yet only half of adults do [43]. Even small amounts of exercise can reduce risks of cardiovascular morbidity and mortality [67]. Unsurprisingly, research indicates that more weekly exercise is needed to lose significant amounts of weight (more than 250 min per week) compared to maintaining or losing modest amounts of weight (150–250 min per week) [66]. Given rising levels of obesity and declining levels of exercise, researchers and clinicians have sought new ways to increase adult exercise.

With mass-market distribution of gaming consoles, game developers and clinicians found a new tool to encourage exercise in a fun, engaging manner. Exergames (i.e., active video games) track players' body movements and incorporate the movements as part of the game [68–70]. Some of the earliest instantiations of exergames included Dance Dance Revolution (1998) in which users dance on a pressure sensitive platform that collects foot movement information and the Sony Playstation EyeToy (2004) that utilizes a camera to gather user movement information. In 2006, Nintendo released the Wii that utilized a camera and a motion sensitive controller to record user movement. In 2007, Nintendo released a peripheral device (known as the Wii fit board) which records pressure information and has been shown to stimulate light-to-moderate physical activity in children and adults [71, 72]. Nintendo created games that require the use of more of the body (thereby increasing exercise levels).

In a similar manner, Microsoft's created the Kinect sensor bar for its Xbox console that projects an infrared array onto the user to map body movements, as well as incorporating a microphone and camera [70]. The Kinect system differs from the Wii dramatically because it does not require a controller to operate; the user is the controller via a series of gestures to advance and play games.

Finally, immersive digital virtual environments and games have been created in laboratories across the country for research purposes. For example, Astrojumper is a game in which participants move their entire body to avoid colliding with planets they see in the HMD. A study employing this game revealed increased heart rate levels post game play [73]. These platforms represent current advancements in exergame technology; but as sensors become more portable and less invasive, it will be easier to collect and utilize body motion information to encourage increased exercise levels in users.

A wealth of research exists highlighting the benefits of exergame platforms [74]. Generally, employing digital virtual environments presents advantages over exercising in grounded reality as they allow users to easily review their physical movements (via features like pause and rewind) as well as view their avatar from a third person perspective. In two studies, immersion in a digital virtual environment increased accuracy of newly learned exercise movements compared to users who were not immersed and unable to review their movements [75].

Perhaps of most interest to clinicians and researchers, exergames can be used to increase exercise intensity and duration. Two decades of research demonstrates that when users are immersed in a digital virtual environment and interact with a virtual other (i.e., a coach), they exercise more intensively and report higher intrinsic motivation [76]. Similarly, after observing a virtual representation of the self-running on a treadmill, participants completed significantly more exercise in the following 24-h period than did participants observing a virtual representation of another person [77]. A follow-up study revealed higher levels of skin conductance (physiological arousal) while watching a virtual representation of the self-running on a treadmill which is hypothesized to be the reason for subsequent increased exercise behavior [78].

Many exergame studies employ bicycles as the preferred method of exercise in immersive virtual environments because they allow users to remain seated, thereby reducing the risk of injury. In one study, participants cycled on a stationary bike while playing or not playing video games. Those who played while cycling exhibited increased VO_2 max and decreased resting systolic blood pressure [79]. In similar studies, participants pedaled a stationary bike attached to a computer and monitor (or projector) displaying an exergame that either provided information about pedaling speed and distance or no such feedback. Results indicated that participants exposed to more realistic exergames exhibited increased pedaling intensity, cycling endurance, and energy expenditure [80, 81].

Innovations in digital virtual environment exercise research have focused on interweaving behavior in virtual environments with exercise in grounded reality. To this end, researchers created exergames that rely on daily exercise totals, which are measured via peripheral devices such as pedometers, phone applications, and palm pilots. In an attempt to engage children, researchers created a video game in which children can exercise, play with, and train a virtual pet using their own daily exercise as input (i.e., number of steps taken) for the game. They found that children given the opportunity to play the game increased exercise levels [82].

Similarly, participants playing Neverball must navigate a large ball through a maze in a given amount of time. Importantly, participants can earn extra game time by exercising more in grounded reality. Players increased their exercise time by 20% when exposed to the Neverball platform [83]. In another novel design, NEAT-o-Games developers created an avatar for each player that would meet in the virtual environment daily and compete in a foot race. The speed of the participant's avatar depended on how much exercise the participant completed throughout the day, which was automatically tracked using a palm pilot carried by the participant. Results indicate that engaging with the game increased the time and intensity of the participant's aerobic activity [84].

Finally, research employing the Proteus Effect demonstrates that behavior of avatars in digital virtual environments can influence users' grounded reality behaviors. Using Second Life, researchers confirmed that users whose avatars engage in healthy behaviors in Second Life are more likely to engage in exercise and other active behavior than users who have avatars that are less physically active [85].

Exergames can also influence more than just physical behavior. Several studies have shown that exergames platforms increase positive mood in participants and reduce fatigue across different exercise types and immersion levels [86–90]. Importantly, for individuals with high body image dissatisfaction, exergames increase negative effect. Participants with high body image dissatisfaction who saw their avatars while exercising reported less enjoyment, lower positive mood, and lowered exercise self-efficacy [91]. In a follow-up study, the researchers recruited participants with either high or low body image dissatisfaction to play an exergame in which they boxed with a computer agent using a generic avatar. Findings indicate that those with high body image dissatisfaction enjoyed the exergame more than those with low body image dissatisfaction and exhibited a larger decrease in social physique anxiety [92]. The difference in results between the two studies could be due to using a generic avatar instead of a weight and gender specific avatar as in study 2. Participant's self-awareness was likely lessened allowing them to exercise with lower concerns for weight stigma.

Eating Behavior

Although physical activity is admittedly only one approach to losing and maintaining a healthy weight, other research employing digital immersive virtual environments aims to help people choose better foods, gain healthy eating knowledge, and provide novel, personalized treatment methods for those with eating disorders.

Digital virtual environments are ideally suited to helping people make better food choices because virtual environments can be transformed to present an environment unlike that which users experience regularly. In one study, the apparent size of the food consumed by the user was transformed in an attempt to better understand how peripheral cues influence indicators of satiety. In this study, participants came to the laboratory on three occasions and ate actual Oreo cookies while immersed in a digital virtual environment. Crucially, the virtual environment allowed the researchers to change the apparent size of the cookie being eaten such that one day it appeared original size (33 mm), one day 67 times the normal size (22 mm) and one day, 1.5 times the normal size (50 m). Findings indicate that users ate significantly more cookie when they ate the visually smaller cookie compared to the larger cookie [93].

In another study, researchers immersed participants in a virtual environment in which their avatar's weight either changed to reflect the effect of what the avatar ate or did not eat. The researchers subsequently assessed the amount of candy the participant ate. Results demonstrated that participants with changing avatars reported higher levels of presence (the feeling that the virtual environment is real and that their actions in grounded reality are linked to the virtual environment) that differentially influenced eating behavior of men and women. Women who had low levels of presence and men with high levels of presence ate more candy than women with high presence or men with low presence [94].

Another important advantage of digital virtual environments is that clinicians and researchers can create environments in which users learn and practice healthful behaviors with the goal of translating the new virtual behaviors to behaviors in grounded reality. For example, in Second Life, a special island called "Club One" was created to get users to attend virtual health, exercise, and nutrition classes that encouraged weight loss [95]. Club One Island represents a novel approach to tackling weight loss as it allows individuals with limited funds or access to gyms to get the support needed to make lifestyle changes. After a 12-week intervention program, Club One Island participants showed increased levels of exercise and fruit and vegetable consumption while a control group who completed a standard face-to-face weight loss intervention showed no such improvements. Similar results were found when participants completed a 3-month weight loss intervention program either face-to-face or in Second Life. After 3 months, participants in the face-to-face intervention showed greater weight loss but those in the Second Life condition showed significantly greater weight maintenance [96].

Importantly, health knowledge gained in digital virtual environments can spread through families to improve the health of multiple individuals. Overweight and obese mothers received information about their child's environmental and genetic risk of becoming obese and family health history and were then immersed in a digital virtual environment created to look like a buffet. The mothers were then instructed to select virtual foods and drink for their child's lunch. Mothers receiving information (relative to control groups) created plates with 45 fewer calories on average [97]. Communicating health information to participants and allowing them to practice healthful behaviors in digital virtual environments represents a novel approach to health education.

In the past decade, digital environments have become more popular in clinical settings as a method for delivering targeted and personalized therapy for issues such as eating disorders and body image disturbances [98, 99]. Studies show that using virtual environments as stress management tools is effective for individuals with emotional eating concerns. Immersing individuals in virtual environments lowers anxiety levels below those from imagining or DVD-based stress management systems [100, 101]. Similarly, immersion in virtual environments can improve body image for those who are obese or have eating disorders [102, 103]. For example, obese patients were assigned to either a virtual environment treatment condition or a standard therapy group. Exposure to a therapeutic virtual environment improved body image satisfaction, self-efficacy, and motivation for change and a reduction in problematic eating and social behaviors [104, 105].

Given the research above, virtual reality technologies have facilitated research and practices on eating disorders. Hence, it is not surprising that researchers [106] have concluded that virtual environments represent a novel approach for addressing the needs of a growing population of individuals with eating disorders or weight loss needs.

Diabetes Management

While utilizing virtual environments to address disordered eating, exercise, and eating behaviors is relatively novel,, even more recent applications have been pioneered, such as diabetes care and management. Like studies with patients with eating disorders, clinicians and researchers have created virtual environments with the goal of teaching patients with diabetes about self-care and disease management.

For example, a virtual environment, Second Life Impacts Diabetes and Education and Support (SLIDES), provides diabetes patients with access to health care providers as well as to other patients. Additionally, it allows patients to go through skill-building simulations and scenarios that will give them necessary tools to manage their disease in grounded reality [107]. In a recent study, researchers utilized SLIDES as a teaching tool with a group of patients who had had diabetes for an average of 12 years [108]. After 6 months, patients showed increases in self-reported social support for diabetes management, self-efficacy to perform management behaviors, and foot care (a critical disease management behavior). Other virtual environments target additional disease management behaviors such as selecting nutritious foods are the grocery store. Participants select products on the aisles of the virtual grocery store and researchers track how long they spend in each aisle, what packaging components they consider, and how factors such as shelf positioning and merchandising influence appeal [109]. This information allows researchers to design targeted intervention and information to help patients select the healthiest foods.

Finally, researchers have begun to utilize virtual environment walking systems designed for stroke patients in diabetes management programs. Exercise is a crucial component of managing diabetes, yet many patients (between 60 and 70%) do not get enough exercise. Researchers have suggested utilizing virtual environments that encourage walking on a treadmill or cycling on a stationary bike as methods for increasing physical activity levels in diabetes patients [110]. With virtual environment technology rapidly improving, innovative applications for disease management will soon be developed and implemented in hospitals and homes around the world.

CONCLUSION

This chapter reviews the fundamentals of digital virtual environments and their use in presenting users with augmented forms of grounded realty by transforming factors such as the situational context, self-representations, and sensory abilities. Importantly, by altering "reality" in these digital virtual environments, researchers can harness the influential nature of avatars on their human user counterparts to enact psychological and physical changes in the user (via the Proteus Effect). Using an avatar's to influence the user has enormous potential implications for addressing the growing obesity epidemic, as well as clinical concerns such as eating disorders and diseases such as diabetes. Digital virtual environments allow users to practice positive behaviors, learn new skills, and interact with others all within a safely built environment. The skills acquired in the virtual environment are then transferred to daily life in grounded reality, increasing the health and well-being of users.

Even with the recent declines in the cost of virtual reality hardware (e.g., the Kinect sensor bar and the Oculus Rift HMD), cost and computing power still limit the use of digital virtual environments on a large scale or in many research facilities. Given the current body of research highlighting the plethora of benefits of using virtual environment-based interventions, many more studies are needed to address gaps in the literature. Specifically, studies are needed address topics such as portion size, food marketing effects, applying learning in virtual environments to behaviors in grounded reality, creating exergames that maintain interest and significantly elevate heart rate, and incorporating information from peripheral devices (i.e., pedometers or phone applications) into exergames to further encourage grounded reality physical activity.

Overall, digital virtual environments, whether accessed via phones, computers, projectors or HMDs, represent a new frontier in research tools for addressing growing health care concerns. Going forward, health concerned users will find more and more relevant virtual environments. Hence, continuing research to understand influences on users' health is critical.

REFERENCES

1 Blascovich, J., Loomis, J., Beall, A.C., Swinth, K.R., Hoyt, C.L., & Bailenson, J.N. (2002). Immersive virtual environment technology as a methodological tool for social psychology. *Psychological Inquiry*, 13(2), 103–124.

2 Cruz-Neira, C., Sandin, D.J., & DeFanti, T.A. (1993). Surround-screen projection-based virtual reality: the design and implementation of the CAVE. In *Proceedings of the 20th Annual*

Conference on Computer Graphics and Interactive Techniques. August 2–6, 1993. Anaheim, CA: Association for Computing Machinery.

3 DeFanti, T.A., Dawe, G., Sandin, D.J., Schulze, J.P., Otto, P., Girado, J., Kuester, F., Smarr, L., & Rao, R. (2009). The StarCAVE, a third-generation CAVE and virtual reality OptIPortal. *Future Generation Computer Systems*, 25(2), 169–178.

4 McCall, C. & Blascovich, J. (2009). How, when, and why to use digital experimental virtual environments to study social behavior. *Social and Personality Psychology Compass*, 3(5), 744–758.

5 Blascovich, J. & Bailenson, J. (2011). Infinite Reality: Avatars, Eternal Life, New Worlds, and the Dawn of the Virtual Revolution. New York: Harper Collins.

6 Fox, J., Arena, D., & Bailenson J.N. (2009). Virtual reality: a survival guide for the social scientist. *Journal of Media Psychology*, 12, 95–113.

7 Dahlquist, L.M., McKenna, K.D., Jones, K.K., Dillinger, L., Weiss, K.E., & Ackerman, C.S. (2007). Active and passive distraction using a head-mounted display helmet: effects on cold pressor pain in children. *Health Psychology*, 26(6), 794.

8 Dede, C. (2009). Immersive interfaces for engagement and learning. *Science*, 323(5910), 66–69.

9 Gordon, N.S., Merchant, J., Zanbaka, C., Hodges, L.F., & Goolkasian, P. (2011). Interactive gaming reduces experimental pain with or without a head mounted display. *Computers in Human Behavior*, 27(6), 2123–2128.

10 Hoffman, H.G., Sharar, S.R., Coda, B., Everett, J.J., Ciol, M., Richards, T., & Patterson, D.R. (2004). Manipulating presence influences the magnitude of virtual reality analgesia. *Pain*, 111(1), 162–168.

11 Segovia, K.Y. & Bailenson, J.N. (2009). Virtually true: children's acquisition of false memories in virtual reality. *Media Psychology*, 12(4), 371–393.

12 Kane, H.S., McCall, C., Collins, N.L., & Blascovich, J. (2012). Mere presence is not enough: responsive support in a virtual world. *Journal of Experimental Social Psychology*, 48(1), 37–44.

13 Zhang, Z. (2012). Microsoft kinect sensor and its effect. *MultiMedia, IEEE*, 19(2), 4–10.

14 Harris, H., Bailenson, J.N., Nielsen, A., & Yee, N. (2009). The evolution of social behavior over time in second life. *Presence: Teleoperators and Virtual Environments*, 18(6), 434–448.

15 Bélisle, J.F. & Bodur, H.O. (2010). Avatars as information: perception of consumers based on their avatars in virtual worlds. *Psychology & Marketing*, 27(8), 741–765.

16 Desai, P.R., Desai, P.N., Ajmera, K.D., & Mehta, K. (2014). A review paper on oculus rift—a virtual reality headset. *International Journal of Engineering Trends and Technology*, 13(4), 175–179.

17 Lee, K.M. (2004). Presence, explicated. *Communication Theory*, 14(1), 27–50.

18 Blascovich, J. (2002). Social influence within immersive virtual environments. In R. Schroeder (Ed.), The Social Life of Avatars (pp. 127–145). London: Springer.

19 Bailenson, J.N. & Blascovich, J. (2004). Avatars. Encyclopedia of Human–Computer Interaction. Gt Barrington, MA: Berkshire Publishing Group, pp. 64–68.

20 Ryan, W.S., Cornick, J.E., Blascovich, J., & Bailenson, J.N. (in press). Virtual reality: whence, how and what for? In C. Rizzo & S. Bouchard (Eds.), Psychological and Neurocognitive Interventions (Vol. 2), in P. Sharkey (Ed.), Virtual Reality Technologies for Health and Clinical Applications. New York: Springer.

21 Zanbaka, C., Ulinski, A., Goolkasian, P., & Hodges, L.F. (2004). Effects of virtual human presence on task performance. In Proceedings of the International Conference on Artificial Reality and Teleexistance, November 30–December 2, 2004, Seoul, Korea. Coex: ICAT (pp. 174–181).

22 Bailenson, J.N., Blascovich, J., Beall, A.C., & Loomis, J.M. (2003). Interpersonal distance in immersive virtual environments. *Personality and Social Psychology Bulletin*, 29(7), 819–833.

23 Guadagno, R.E., Swinth, K.R., & Blascovich, J. (2011). Social evaluations of embodied agents and avatars. *Computers in Human Behavior*, 27(6), 2380–2385.

24 Sproull, L., Subramani, M., Kiesler, S., Walker, J.H., & Waters, K. (1996). When the interface is a face. *Human-Computer Interaction*, 11(2), 97–124.

25 Bailenson, J.N. (2006) Transformed social interaction in collaborative virtual environments. In P. Messaris and L. Humphreys (eds.), Digital Media: Transformations in Human Communication. New York: Peter Lang, pp. 255–264.

26 Bailenson, J.N., Yee, N., Blascovich, J., & Guadagno, R.E. (2008). Transformed social interaction in mediated interpersonal communication. *Mediated Interpersonal Communication*, 77–99.

27 Bailenson, J.N., Yee, N., Blascovich, J., Beall, A.C., Lundblad, N., & Jin, M. (2008). The use of immersive virtual reality in the learning sciences: Digital transformations of teachers, students, and social context. *The Journal of the Learning Sciences*, 17(1), 102–141.

28 Bailenson, J.N., Beall, A.C., Loomis, J., Blascovich, J., & Turk, M. (2005). Transformed social interaction, augmented gaze, and social influence in immersive virtual environments. *Human Communication Research*, 31(4), 511–537.

29 Hershfield, H.E., Goldstein, D.G., Sharpe, W.F., Fox, J., Yeykelis, L., Carstensen, L.L., & Bailenson, J.N. (2011). Increasing saving behavior through age-progressed renderings of the future self. *Journal of Marketing Research*, 48, S23–S37.

30 Groom, V., Bailenson, J.N., & Nass, C. (2009). The influence of racial embodiment on racial bias in immersive virtual environments. *Social Influence*, 4(3), 231–248.

31 Bailenson, J.N. & Yee, N. (2005). Digital chameleons automatic assimilation of nonverbal gestures in immersive virtual environments. *Psychological Science*, 16(10), 814–819.

32 Bem, D. (1972). Self perception theory. In L. Berkowitz (Ed.), Advances in Experimental Social Psychology (Vol. 6, pp. 2–57). New York: Academic Press.

33 Yee, N. & Bailenson, J. (2007). The Proteus effect: the effect of transformed self-representation on behavior. *Human Communication Research*, 33(3), 271–290.

34 Yee, N., Bailenson, J.N., & Ducheneaut, N. (2009). The Proteus effect: implications of transformed digital self-representation on online and offline behavior. *Communication Research*, 36 (2), 285–312.

35 Ahn, S.J. & Bailenson, J.N. (2011). Self-endorsing versus other-endorsing in virtual environments. *Journal of Advertising*, 40(2), 93–106.

36 Yee, N. & Bailenson, J.N. (2009). The difference between being and seeing: the relative contribution of self-perception and priming to behavioral changes via digital self-representation. *Media Psychology*, 12(2), 195–209.

37 Bailenson, J.N., Blascovich, J., & Guadagno, R.E. (2008). Self-representations in immersive virtual environments. *Journal of Applied Social Psychology*, 38(11), 2673–2690.

38 Callahan, D. (2013). Obesity: chasing an elusive epidemic. *Hastings Center Report*, 43(1), 34–40.

39 Flegal, K.M., Carroll, M.D., Ogden, C.L., & Curtin, L.R. (2010). Prevalence and trends in obesity among US adults, 1999–2008. *JAMA*, 303(3), 235–241.

40 Finkelstein, E.A., Khavjou, O.A., Thompson, H., Trogdon, J.G., Pan, L., Sherry, B., & Dietz, W. (2012). Obesity and severe obesity forecasts through 2030. *American Journal of Preventive Medicine*, 42(6), 563–570.

41 Houston, D.K., Nicklas, B.J., & Zizza, C.A. (2009). Weighty concerns: the growing prevalence of obesity among older adults. *Journal of the American Dietetic Association*, 109(11), 1886–1895.

42 Kaminsky, L.A., Arena, R., Beckie, T.M., Brubaker, P.H., Church, T.S., Forman, D.E., Franklin, B.A., Gulati, M., Lavie, C.J., Myers, J., Patel, M.J., Pina, I.L., Weintraub, W.S., & Williams, M.A. (2013). The importance of cardiorespiratory fitness in the United States: the need for a national registry a policy statement from the American Heart Association. *Circulation*, 127(5), 652–662.

43 Center for Disease Control. (2012). Vital Signs: More People Walk to Get Better Health (publication no. CS233690-B). Washington, DC: U.S. Government Printing Office.

44 Ladabaum, U., Mannalithara, A., Myer, P.A., & Singh, G. (2014). Obesity, abdominal obesity, physical activity, and caloric intake in US adults: 1988–2010. *The American Journal of Medicine*, 8, 717–727.

45 Dwyer-Lindgren, L., Freedman, G.D., Engell, R.E., Fleming, T.D., Lim, S.S., Murray, C.J., & Mokdad, A.H. (2013). Prevalence of physical activity and obesity in US counties, 2001–2011: a road map for action. *Population Health Metrics*, 11(1), 7.

46 Abraham, P.A., Kazman, J.B., Zeno, S.A., & Deuster, P.A. (2013). Obesity and African Americans: Physiologic and Behavioral Pathways. International Scholarly Research Notices, 2013, 1–8.

47 Azarbad, L. & Gonder-Frederick, L. (2010). Obesity in women. *Psychiatric Clinics of North America*, 33(2), 423–440.

48 Muennig, P., Jia, H., Lee, R., & Lubetkin, E. (2008). I think therefore I am: perceived ideal weight as a determinant of health. *American Journal of Public Health*, 98(3), 501.

49 Muennig, P. (2008). The body politic: the relationship between stigma and obesity-associated disease. *BMC Public Health*, 8(1), 128.

50 Puhl, R.M. & Heuer, C.A. (2009). The stigma of obesity: a review and update. *Obesity*, 17(5), 941–964.

51 Persky, S. & Eccleston, C.P. (2010). Medical student bias and care recommendations for an obese versus non-obese virtual patient. *International Journal of Obesity*, 35(5), 728–735.

52 Hoyt, C.L., Burnette, J.L., & Auster-Gussman, L. (2014). "Obesity is a disease" examining the self-regulatory impact of this public-health message. *Psychological Science*, 25(4), 997–1002.

53 Major, B., Hunger, J.M., Bunyan, D.P., & Miller, C.T. (2014). The ironic effects of weight stigma. *Journal of Experimental Social Psychology*, 51, 74–80.

54 Schafer, M.H. & Ferraro, K.F. (2011). The stigma of obesity does perceived weight discrimination affect identity and physical health? *Social Psychology Quarterly*, 74(1), 76–97.

55 Tomiyama, A.J. (2014). Weight stigma is stressful: a review of evidence for the cyclic obesity/weight-based stigma model. *Appetite*, 82, 8–15.

56 Puhl, R.M. & Heuer, C.A. (2010). Obesity stigma: important considerations for public health. *Health*, 24, 252.

57 Puhl, R., Luedicke, J., & Lee Peterson, J. (2013). Public reactions to obesity-related health campaigns: a randomized controlled trial. *American Journal of Preventive Medicine*, 45(1), 36–48.

58 Bessière, K., Seay, A.F., & Kiesler, S. (2007). The ideal elf: identity exploration in World of Warcraft. *CyberPsychology & Behavior*, 10(4), 530–535.

59 Ducheneaut, N., Wen, M.H., Yee, N., & Wadley, G. (2009, April). Body and mind: a study of avatar personalization in three virtual worlds. In *Proceedings of the SIGCHI Conference on Human Factors in Computing Systems*, April 4–9, 2009, Boston, MA. Anaheim, CA: Association for Computing Machinery (pp. 1151–1160).

60 Ellison, N., Heino, R., & Gibbs, J. (2006). Managing impressions online: self-presentation processes in the online dating environment. *Journal of Computer-Mediated Communication*, 11(2), 415–441.

61 Manago, A.M., Graham, M.B., Greenfield, P.M., & Salimkhan, G. (2008). Self-presentation and gender on MySpace. *Journal of Applied Developmental Psychology*, 29(6), 446–458.

62 Strano, M.M. (2008). User descriptions and interpretations of self-presentation through Facebook profile images. *Cyberpsychology: Journal of Psychosocial Research on Cyberspace*, 2(2), 5.

63 Thomas, A.G. & Johansen, M.K. (2012). Inside out: avatars as an indirect measure of ideal body self-presentation in females. *Cyberpsychology: Journal of Psychosocial Research on Cyberspace*, 6(3).

64 Vasalou, A. & Joinson, A.N. (2009). Me, myself and I: the role of interactional context on self-presentation through avatars. *Computers in Human Behavior*, 25(2), 510–520.

65 Jin, S.A.A. (2009). Avatars mirroring the actual self versus projecting the ideal self: the effects of self-priming on interactivity and immersion in an exergame, Wii Fit. *CyberPsychology & Behavior*, 12(6), 761–765.

66 Donnelly, J.E., Blair, S.N., Jakicic, J.M., Manore, M.M., Rankin, J.W., & Smith, B.K. (2009). American college of sports medicine position stand. Appropriate physical activity intervention strategies for weight loss and prevention of weight regain for adults. *Medicine and Science in Sports and Exercise*, 41(2), 459–471.

67 Dangardt, F.J., McKenna, W.J., Lüscher, T.F., & Deanfield, J.E. (2013). Exercise: friend or foe?. *Nature Reviews Cardiology*, 10(9), 495–507.

68 Lu, A.S., Kharrazi, H., Gharghabi, F., & Thompson, D. (2013). A systematic review of health videogames on childhood obesity prevention and intervention. *Games for Health: Research, Development, and Clinical Applications*, 2(3), 131–141.

69 Smith, B.K. (2005). Physical fitness in virtual worlds. *Computer*, 38(10), 101–103.

70 Tanaka, K., Parker, J.R., Baradoy, G., Sheehan, D., Holash, J.R., & Katz, L. (2012). A comparison of exergaming interfaces for use in rehabilitation programs and research. *Loading*, 6(9), 69–81.

71 Biddiss, E. & Irwin, J. (2010). Active video games to promote physical activity in children and youth: a systematic review. *Archives of Pediatrics & Adolescent Medicine*, 164(7), 664–672.

72 Graves, L.E., Ridgers, N.D., Williams, K., Stratton, G., & Atkinson, G.T. (2010). The physiological cost and enjoyment of Wii Fit in adolescents, young adults, and older adults. *Journal of Physical Activity & Health*, 7(3), 393–401.

73 Finkelstein, S. & Suma, E. (2011). Astrojumper: motivating exercise with an immersive virtual reality exergame. *Presence*, 20(1), 78–92.

74 Rizzo, A.S., Lange, B., Suma, E.A., & Bolas, M. (2011). Virtual reality and interactive digital game technology: new tools to address obesity and diabetes. *Journal of Diabetes Science and Technology*, 5(2), 256–264.

75 Bailenson, J., Patel, K., Nielsen, A., Bajscy, R., Jung, S.H., & Kurillo, G. (2008). The effect of interactivity on learning physical actions in virtual reality. *Media Psychology*, 11(3), 354–376.

76 Porcari, J.P., Zedaker, M.S., & Maldari, M.S. (1998). Virtual motivation. *Fitness Management*, 14(13), 48–51.

77 Fox, J. & Bailenson, J.N. (2009). Virtual self-modeling: the effects of vicarious reinforcement and identification on exercise behaviors. *Media Psychology*, 12(1), 1–25.

78 Fox, J., Bailenson, J.N., & Ricciardi, T. (2012). Physiological responses to virtual selves and virtual others. *Journal of CyberTherapy & Rehabilitation*, 5(1), 69–73.

79 Warburton, D.E., Bredin, S.S., Horita, L.T., Zbogar, D., Scott, J.M., Esch, B.T., & Rhodes, R.E. (2007). The health benefits of interactive video game exercise. *Applied Physiology, Nutrition, and Metabolism*, 32(4), 655–663.

80 Chuang, T.Y., Chen, C.H., Chang, H.A., Lee, H.C., Chou, C.L., & Doong, J.L. (2003). Virtual reality serves as a support technology in cardiopulmonary exercise testing. *Presence: Teleoperators and Virtual Environments*, 12(3), 326–331.

81 Ijsselsteijn, W.A., Kort, Y.D., Westerink, J.H.D.M., Jager, M.D., & Bonants, R. (2006). Virtual fitness: stimulating exercise behavior through media technology. *Presence: Teleoperators and Virtual Environments*, 15(6), 688–698.

82 Johnsen, K., Ahn, S.J., Moore, J., Brown, S., Robertson, T.P., Marable, A., & Basu, A. (2014). Mixed reality virtual pets to reduce childhood obesity. *IEEE Transactions on Visualization and Computer Graphics*, 20(4), 523–530.

83 Berkovsky, S., Freyne, J., Coombe, M., Bhandari, D., Baghaei, N., & Kimani, S. (2010). Exercise and play: earn in the physical, spend in the virtual. *International Journal of Cognitive Technology*, 15(1), 22.

84 Fujiki, Y., Kazakos, K., Puri, C., Buddharaju, P., Pavlidis, I., & Levine, J. (2008). NEAT-o-Games: blending physical activity and fun in the daily routine. *Computers in Entertainment (CIE)*, 6(2), 21.

85 Dean, E., Cook, S., Keating, M., & Murphy, J. (2009). Does this avatar make me look fat? Obesity and interviewing in Second Life. *Journal for Virtual Worlds Research*, 2(2), 3–11.

86 Legrand, F.D., Joly, P.M., Bertucci, W.M., Soudain-Pineau, M.A., & Marcel, J. (2011). Interactive-Virtual Reality (IVR) exercise: an examination of in-task and pre-to-post exercise affective changes. *Journal of Applied Sport Psychology*, 23(1), 65–75.

87 Lyons, E.J., Tate, D.F., Komoski, S.E., Carr, P.M., & Ward, D.S. (2012). Novel approaches to obesity prevention: effects of game enjoyment and game type on energy expenditure in active video games. *Journal of Diabetes Science and Technology*, 6(4), 839–848.

88 Russell, W.D. & Newton, M. (2008). Short-term psychological effects of interactive video game technology exercise on mood and attention. *Educational Technology & Society*, 11(2), 294–308.

89 Plante, T.G., Aldridge, A., Bogden, R., & Hanelin, C. (2003). Might virtual reality promote the mood benefits of exercise? *Computers in Human Behavior*, 19(4), 495–509.

90 Plante, T.G., Cage, C., Clements, S., & Stover, A. (2006). Psychological benefits of exercise paired with virtual reality: outdoor exercise energizes whereas indoor virtual exercise relaxes. *International Journal of Stress Management*, 13(1), 108.

91 Song, H., Peng, W., & Lee, K.M. (2011). Promoting exercise self-efficacy with an exergame. *Journal of Health Communication*, 16(2), 148–162.

92 Song, H., Kim, J., & Lee, K.M. (2014). Virtual vs. real body in exergames: reducing social physique anxiety in exercise experiences. *Computers in Human Behavior*, 36, 282–285.

93 Narumi, T., Ban, Y., Kajinami, T., Tanikawa, T., & Hirose, M. (2012). Augmented perception of satiety: controlling food consumption by changing apparent size of food with augmented reality. In *Proceedings of the SIGCHI Conference on Human Factors in Computing Systems*, May 5–10, 2012, Austin, TX. Anaheim, CA: Association for Computing Machinery (pp. 109–118).

94 Fox, J., Bailenson, J., & Binney, J. (2009). Virtual experiences, physical behaviors: the effect of presence on imitation of an eating avatar. *Presence: Teleoperators and Virtual Environments*, 18(4), 294–303.

95 Johnston, J.D., Massey, A.P., & DeVaneaux, C. (2012). Innovation in weight loss intervention programs: an examination of a 3D virtual world approach. In *45th Hawaii International Conference on System Science (HICSS)*, January 4–7, 2012, Maui: Curran Associates (pp. 2890–2899).

96 Sullivan, D.K., Goetz, J.R., Gibson, C.A., Washburn, R.A., Smith, B.K., Lee, J., Gerald, S., Fincham, T., & Donnelly, J.E. (2013). Improving weight maintenance using virtual reality (second life). *Journal of Nutrition Education and Behavior*, 45(3), 264–268.

97 McBride, C.M., Persky, S., Wagner, L.K., Faith, M.S., & Ward, D.S. (2013). Effects of providing personalized feedback of child's obesity risk on mothers' food choices using a virtual reality buffet. *International Journal of Obesity*, 37(10), 1322–1327.

98 Rizzo, A.A., Wiederhold, M.D., & Buckwalter, J.G. (1998). Basic issues in the use of virtual environments for mental health applications. *Studies in Health Technology and Informatics*, 21–42.

99 Myers, T.C., Swan-Kremeier, L., Wonderlich, S., Lancaster, K., & Mitchell, J.E. (2004). The use of alternative delivery systems and new technologies in the treatment of patients with eating disorders. *International Journal of Eating Disorders*, 36(2), 123–143.

100 Manzoni, G.M., Gorini, A., Preziosa, A., Pagnini, F., Castelnuovo, G., Molinari, E., & Riva, G. (2008). New technologies and relaxation: an explorative study on obese patients with emotional eating. *Journal of CyberTherapy and Rehabilitation*, 1(2), 182–192.

101 Riva, G., Manzoni, M., Villani, D., Gaggioli, A., & Molinari, E. (2008). Why you really eat? Virtual reality in the treatment of obese emotional eaters. *Studies in Health Technology and Informatics*, 132, 417.

102 Ferrer-Garcia, M., Gutierrez-Maldonado, J., & Riva, G. (2013). Virtual reality based treatments in eating disorders and obesity: a review. *Journal of Contemporary Psychotherapy*, 43(4), 207–221.

103 Riva, G. (2011). The key to unlocking the virtual body: virtual reality in the treatment of obesity and eating disorders. *Journal of Diabetes Science and Technology*, 5(2), 283–292.

104 Riva, G., Bacchetta, M., Baruffi, M., & Molinari, E. (2001). Virtual reality-based multidimensional therapy for the treatment of body image disturbances in obesity: a controlled study. *Cyberpsychology & Behavior*, 4(4), 511–526.

105 Riva, G., Bacchetta, M., Baruffi, M., Cirillo, G., & Molinari, E. (2000). Virtual reality environment for body image modification: a multidimensional therapy for the treatment of body image in obesity and related pathologies. *CyberPsychology & Behavior*, 3(3), 421–431.

106 Coons, M.J., Roehrig, M., & Spring, B. (2011). The potential of virtual reality technologies to improve adherence to weight loss behaviors. *Journal of Diabetes Science and Technology*, 5(2), 340–344.

107 Vorderstrasse, A., Shaw, R.J., Blascovich, J., & Johnson, C.M. (2014). A theoretical framework for a virtual diabetes self-management community intervention. *Western Journal of Nursing Research*, 36(9), 1222–1237.

108 Johnson, C., Feinglos, M., Pereira, K., Hassell, N., Blascovich, J., Nicollerat, J., Beresford, H.F., Levy, J., & Vorderstrasse, A. (2014). Feasibility and preliminary effects of a virtual environment for adults with type 2 diabetes: pilot study. *JMIR Research Protocols*, 3(2), 23–49.

109 Ruppert, B. (2011). New directions in the use of virtual reality for food shopping: marketing and education perspectives. *Journal of Diabetes Science and Technology*, 5(2), 315–318.

110 Deutsch, J.E. (2011). Using virtual reality to improve walking post-stroke: translation to individuals with diabetes. *Journal of Diabetes Science and Technology*, 5(2), 309–314.

14

IMMERSIVE VIRTUAL REALITY TO MODEL PHYSICAL: SOCIAL INTERACTION AND SELF-REPRESENTATION

Eric B. Bauman

Clinical Playground LLC, Madison, WI, USA

INTRODUCTION

Technological advancements have paved the way for new approaches to modeling, simulation, and visualization. Modeling now encompasses high degrees of complexity and holistic methods of data representation [1]. Clinicians can model physiology and body systems of a patient, while complex, on predictable algorithms. However, accurately modeling the inherently social nature of clinical encounters among clinicians and patients is much more difficult, but perhaps just as important. Collaboration and social interaction are symbiotic [2]. Further, all aspects of healthcare take place through collaboration and are necessarily distributive. This chapter reviews and discusses pedagogy to help educators frame learning opportunities to accurately model nontechnical or behavioral skills such as social interactions related to clinical education within immersive virtual reality environments.

THEORY FOR IMMERSIVE VIRTUAL LEARNING SPACES

The healthcare simulation paradigm most often embraces experiential learning theory to frame simulation-based learning encounters. Whether these simulations take place using standardized patients, mannikin-based simulators in situ, within simulation laboratories or within digital environments, they all take place within created environments [3]. Created environments provide the environmental fidelity that situates the learning encounter within the context of clinical education. Accurately situating the simulation-based learning

The Digital Patient: Advancing Healthcare, Research, and Education, First Edition.
Edited by C. Donald Combs, John A. Sokolowski, and Catherine M. Banks.
© 2016 John Wiley & Sons, Inc. Published 2016 by John Wiley & Sons, Inc.

experience allows learners to explore their roles as clinicians and members of the patient care team [4]. The most often cited experiential learning theory authors found within simulation literature include David Kolb, Donald Schön, and Patricia Benner. What is most interesting about the application of Kolb, Schön, and Benner to modern simulation is that their respective theories all predated contemporary mannikin-based simulation and most certainly the complex simulation occurring in immersive digital environments. Of the three only Benner, a nursing scholar, is a healthcare clinician.

The concept of Kolb's experiential learning theory is that of a continuous cycle that includes reflection, conceptualization and experimentation to create a concrete experience. Each concrete experience begins the cycle again [3, 5, 6]. Schön's model [7] of professional practice emphasizes the role of reflective cycles of internal dialogue that come to represent a learner's *reflection-on-action*. In Schön's theory the professional works through an internal dialog with a problematic situation [7]. This dialogue, or talk-back provides a form of feedback that helps guide and inform decision making [8, 9].

Benner's theory [10] focusing on the journey from novice to expert emphasizes the concept of *thinking-in-action*. Benner argued that nurses enter the profession as novices and that over time they accumulate situated experience that drives their practice. As novices obtain more experience within the practice of nursing or other healthcare professions, they are able to draw on past experiences to influence the quality of decisions made in day-to-day practice.

Contemporary Theory for Immersive Virtual Learning Spaces

Some argue that good pedagogy stands the test of time, and that there is no need to extrapolate beyond the experiential learning theories of the 1980s as identified above. However, Kolb, Schön, and Benner could not have anticipated how educators and clinicians would use their respective theories to support educational experiences taking place within virtual learning spaces. Virtual learning spaces often afford learners with more agency and afford instructors less formal control than in traditional bricks-and-mortar teaching spaces. In traditional learning spaces social and professional mores are well understood by teachers and students alike. In short, students know their role and place. Students view faculty and teachers as experts. Faculty and teachers in turn understand their roles as an authority figures.

Educators can best leverage digital immersive learning environments when they evaluate curriculum content for best fit within the digital environment and they craft lessons to unfold purposefully with these environments. In order to accomplish these tasks, educators should not only spend time in immersive environments, but they should also explore contemporary pedagogy specific to game-based learning and learning within immersive learning environments existing in total or in part digitally. The remainder of this chapter reviews three contemporary theories specific to digital, game-based, immersive virtual learning spaces. The three theories presented here are socially situated cognition, designed experiences, and the ecology of culturally competent design. The chapter's discussion assumes that clinical education and the healthcare professions are inherently social phenomena.

Socially Situated Cognition   Learning necessarily takes place as a social construct. Teachers carefully craft a syllabus with objectives that require the acquisition of knowledge, and facts that represent standards of practice. However, the ability for learners to recall knowledge and to apply learned behavior appropriately is situated within a material, social, and cultural world [11]. Teaching somebody to become a healthcare clinician and actually practicing as one is situated within a contextually specific environment with a host of values and expectations [3, 9, 12].

Immersive virtual environments digitally immerse students as player characters into future professional contexts. Immersive environments allow the learners to see themselves and participate in roles beyond the context of a medical or nursing student and allows faculty to evaluate students within these roles. Authentically situating learning experiences allow students to complete activities and to interact with others within the social construct and professional mores inherent to clinical practice. Immersion into virtual settings requires players to "try on" different identities [12–14]. This process provides the student with the opportunity to see clinical practice from multiple perspectives.

Immersive virtual environments provide a powerful tool for students to reflect acculturation processes. Acculturation is an important part of joining any profession. Students must learn what it means to become a nurse, physician or any other type of clinician. Acculturation provides a social and cultural imprinting process that identifies the expectations of practice for students. Immersive virtual environments that encourage or require students to assume future roles and responsibilities ask students to reflectively negotiate and reconcile their current status and identity as a student with the role they are assuming within the a socially situated virtual environment.

Gee [12] refers to this paradigm as the projective identity. In the real world the learner is clearly identified and known as a student with all of the social and professional constructs associated with the student role. In real-world clinical learning spaces medical and nursing students wear short white coats, school patches and nametags so they are easily identified as students. This branding serves to keep patients and students safe. However, it also limits the type of experiences that students will have during clinical and professional encounters. In immersive virtual learning spaces the students are asked to play the role they have assumed to the best of their ability. This requires that the students negotiate and reconcile who they are in the real world with the role they play in the virtual world.

The student's reflection on the projective identity represents a sophisticated and complex process that allows for cultural framing. A student's real-world progress and the development of an identity within a field of study usually progress in a linear, temporal manner. However, identities developed within immersive virtual environments are not bounded by time. Learners engaged in immersive virtual environments are encouraged to explore future roles and responsibilities generally not available to novices [9, 8, 12].

Designed Experience   Squire [15] in his discussion of the role that videogames can play in educational contexts, argues that educators and curriculum designers in particular should pay careful attention to videogames because they can provide "…designed experiences, in which participants learn through a grammar of doing and being." The designed experience frames educational opportunities as performance. Seeing learning as performance is of particular interest to healthcare professions such as medicine and nursing because it provides a familiar framework. Once students move out of the classroom and into clinical sites and clerkships everything they do is performance based. Students are evaluated not simply based on technical skills but also on nontechnical or behavioral skills.

Designed experiences embody structured activities in the environments where these activities take place. In the context of this chapter, the immersive virtual environment represents the created space where educators, designers and content experts have carefully crafted and scaffolded lessons for students. The lessons unfold in the situated immersive environment through student performance. The environment itself, as well as the narrative that drives the designed experience will provide cues and rules to encourage targeted and predictable behavior that should map back to curriculum objectives.

In short, educational designers should script specific interactions that create predictable types of experience for players (learners). However, educators must understand that virtual environments provide and encourage a safe place for students cocreate their own lived experiences. In other words, successful immersive virtual environments will provide created spaces where interesting interactions will take place (see Refs. [3, 15, 16.])

Embracing the designed experience within immersive virtual learning spaces provides a template and theoretical framework for curriculum design for the clinical health sciences. It allows content experts and educational designers to work together to address important educational lessons focused on acculturation to the clinical professions. Because learning is seen as performance, students are encouraged to act as a physician or a nurse. Faculty who monitor student progress within the immersive digital environment act as guides to provide just-in-time feedback to encourage desired behavioral outcomes. The virtual environment can be created to itself provide both just-in-time feedback and anytime feedback to students. Environments that provide feedback based on artificial intelligence provide appealing advantages to the learning paradigm unavailable during traditional clinical encounters or even existing in bricks-and-mortar simulation laboratories [16].

Ecology for Culturally Competent Design   The ecology for culturally competent design was specifically created to provide a template for educators, educational designers, and game designers to address concerns related to culture and acculturation of students studying clinical disciplines. The ecology of culturally competent design defines clinical disciplines to include healthcare, as well as professions such as teaching and protective services such as emergency medical services, firefighting and law enforcement (see Refs. [8, 9].)

Acculturation into a profession is vitally important because it moves beyond the tasks or psychomotor skills needed to join a given profession. Novices to clinical professions must learn the social and cultural norms required to gain full access to the profession in order realize their full potential. Benner [10] posited that it takes 7 years for nurses entering the profession to move from novice to expert. While Benner refers to the temporal experience required for nurses to make expert clinical decisions, it is clear that students make these decisions within the sociocultural context of what it means to be a nurse. Until one transitions from the role of pre-novice or student to a novice entering a clinical profession it is impossible to understand a given clinical profession's socio-cultural expectations. Because the practice of nursing and medicine takes place in an inherently social context, it is imperative that clinical educators find ways to introduce students to what it means to be a nurse or physician. In short, how can we begin the acculturation process for our students before they enter their professions?

The immersive virtual reality environment allows faculty to design experiences in virtual learning spaces that allow students explore the roles they hope to assume when they complete their training. Even more important, faculty can encourage students to play the part of other professions they will eventually work with. Interprofessional (IPE) education has been identified as an essential component in advancing education in healthcare professions [17]. Unfortunately, traditional bricks-and-mortar clinical experiences do not always provide the best opportunity for students to observe best practices associated with clinical professions. Leape [18] identifies disrespect among clinical professionals as a substantial barrier and threat to patient safety. Disrespect among the clinical professions also contributes to professional dissatisfaction and high rates of turnover among experienced staff [19]. Leape [20] also argues that IPE is key to redesign flawed processes to prevent harm to patients [21]. Unfortunately, much of the behavior that Leape identifies as disrespectful and disruptive is learned in hospitals and clinics found in contemporary practice. Assuming and understanding a new role is complex and stressful. To become a successful nurse, physician or any other type of clinician requires that the clinician come to understand their role within the context of many other disciplines. The provision of healthcare is by definition distributive. The immersive virtual environment provides the context and environment to explore the roles associated with self and other disciplines found within the healthcare arena.

We frame the ecology of culturally competent design by four elements: activities, context, narrative, and characters. The ecology of culturally competent design argues that all of the elements together provide rich educational experiences in virtual learning spaces not always available in traditional real-world teaching and learning situations. It is the nexus of these for elements (activities, context, narrative, and characters) occurring simultaneously in real time within the immersive virtual environment that engage students and authentically situate learning [8, 9].

Activities

Activity and interactivity found within a virtual immersive learning environment is essential to engaging students to promote learning objectives. The graphic esthetics of immersive virtual environments are becoming more and more appealing and realistic. However, without the ability of learners to engage in some sort of meaningful activity that maps back to the curricula, immersive virtual environments offer little to hold students' attention.

Contexts

Context grounds situational learning. For the novice, context is often a confounding variable. Learners can find it difficult to recognize important patterns that are situated contextually in new or unfamiliar situations when they have little past experience to draw from. In the real world optimal context may not be available to provide students with a safe place to explore ethical questions related to self and others. Educators must be prepared to provide feedback and mentorship on the behavior that students exhibit in virtual spaces. Students often have little genuine or authentic experience about the roles they hope to assume. We should not be surprised to see students modeling the experiences often seen during real-world clinical encounters. Students' misinterpretations and missteps should be seen as important opportunities for educational guidance and intervention.

Virtual learning spaces provide experiences educators can situate within the context of the clinical and professional spaces that students will come to occupy later in their own practice. Well-designed experiences taking place in created environments, immersive virtual environments provide authentic contexts that allow students to glean valuable cues related to pattern recognition to influence future decision making [9, 22, 23].

Narratives

Narratives provide meaning to lessons unfolding in digital spaces, whether those spaces are taking place during game play, in a videogame, or in an educational context within immersive virtual reality environments. When educators authentically situate narratives in immersive virtual environments students have the ability to imprint patterns learned in the virtual world for later recall and utility in the real world [8, 9, 24, 25]. Pattern recognition is a key component in the distinction among novices and experts.

Narratives provide the stage directions to guide designed experiences within virtual environments. Well-written overarching narratives allow educators and educational designers with the ability to seed the virtual environment with emerging and branching narratives based on the quality of students' decision making. A narrative may be as simple as providing learners with a virtual patient hand off or verbal report of a patient's history and physical exam. Narratives found within virtual learning spaces should map back to curriculum objectives from the context of the students perspective. In other words, the narrative has to make sense to the student; it defines the characters and the roles they will play within the virtual environment.

Characters

Players or students within virtual environment are represented by avatars. Individuals immersed in virtual worlds interact with their environment and others who occupy the virtual space by using avatars. Avatars also know as player-characters represent the embodiment of the person immersed within a virtual environment. Players exist and interact with the virtual environment through their avatars [16].

Educators and educational designers can build and provide students with established avatars. Or they can provide learners with more autonomy and agency by allowing students to customize their own avatars. Avatars, whether customized by students or provided by educators, become sentient beings with in the virtual space. Avatars are malleable and fluid representations of student or learner identity. Students constantly reflect on who they are in the real world, how they are represented in the virtual world, and who they hope to become in the future. In this way, the virtual environment also remains fluid and the students occupying the virtual environment cocreate experiences through their expression of self and projected self through their avatars' [8, 9].

When designing characters for immersive virtual environments and setting parameters for customization of avatars it is very important to be in tune with social and cultural norms and mores while avoiding the risk of projecting stereotypes. Whenever possible interactions among characters represented within the virtual world should take place so that they truthfully as possible represent relevant social and cultural mores. These representations should be guided by expert and vetted consultation.

CONCLUSION

The representation of self and the activities available to students in virtual immersive environments must quickly engage learners, be well-designed, and be intrinsically motivating. Intrinsically motivating activity promotes agency and autonomy, competence, and connectedness or affinity to others [26, 27]. Intrinsically motivating experiences provide reward through mastery, where goals are clear, situated, and meaningful. Progress within the intrinsic paradigm is intuitive and immediate so that it endorses or reinforces behavior that the learner is already committed to or hopes to adopt in the future. Intrinsically motivating experiences reinforce the goals required to gain entrance into a profession, in this case a clinical profession. Students must be able to see themselves and their future roles as clinicians through the lens of the immersive learning environments that they are occupying for educational purposes.

This chapter has reinforced the importance of pattern recognition as powerful and key skill that leads to development of expertise [12]. Pattern recognition need not be acquired in the real world, rather pattern recognition occurring through game play, or within virtual learning spaces may be sufficient to prepare students for actual future practice [3, 8, 9, 28]. Pattern recognition is more than a litany of visible variables. Students must learn to understand variables within the context of clinical practice and the role that they will play in recognizing patterns and using them as cues to make informed decisions.

Novices are capable of outperforming or performing on par with experts during task analysis using checklists. However, during clinical encounters taking place via simulation-based learning exercises or in actual practice, experts decisions are often more efficient and accurate than novices [29]. Contemporary theory argues that this occurs because experts have more situated experience reading the totality of clinical encounters, which occurs in an inherently social context and includes both an array of technical and nontechnical patterns. Acculturation of students into clinical professions can in part take place in immersive virtual environments. The process of acculturation is fluid and reflective and can be represented and negotiated through interaction and representation of self in virtual environments.

REFERENCES

1   Sokolowaski, JA and CM Banks. A proposed approach to modeling and simulation education for the medical and health sciences. In *Proceedings of the 2010 Summer Simulation Conference*. Ottawa, Ontario, Canada. San Diego, CA: Society for Computer Simulation International, 2010, July 11–14, (pp. 284–289).

2   Petrakou, A. Interacting through avatars: virtual worlds as a context for online education. *Computers & Education* 54(4) (2010): 1020–1027.

3   Bauman, EB. High Fidelity Simulation in Healthcare. Ann Arbor, MI: Proquest, 2007.

4   Maran, NJ and Glavin, RJ. Low- to high-fidelity simulation – a continuum of medical education? *Medical Education* 37(Suppl 1) (2003): 22–8.

5   Kolb, DA. Experiential Learning: Experience as the Source of Learning and Development. Englewood Cliffs, NJ: Prentice-Hall, 1984.

6   Merriam, SB, Caffarella, RS, and Baumgartner, LM. Learning in Adulthood: A Comprehensive Guide. San Francisco, CA: John Wiley & Sons, 2012.

7   Schön, DA. The Reflective Practitioner: How Professionals Think in Action. New York: Basic Books, 1983.

8   Games, AI and Bauman EB. Virtual worlds: an environment for cultural sensitivity education in the health sciences. *International Journal of Web Based Communities* 7(2) (2011): 189.

9   Bauman, EB and Games, IA. Contemporary theory for immersive worlds: addressing engagement, culture, and diversity. Teaching and Learning in 3D Immersive Worlds: Pedagogical Models and Constructivist Approaches. Cheney, A and Sanders, R. (eds). Hershey, PA: IGI Global, 2011.

10 Benner, P. From Expert to Novice: Excellence and Power in Clinical Nursing Practice. Menlo Park, CA: Addison-Wesley, 1984.

11 Bauman, EB and Wolfenstein, M. The evolving field of virtual reality environments and game-based learning in education. Game-Based Teaching and Simulation in Nursing & Healthcare. New York: Springer, 2012.

12 Gee, JP. What Video Games Have to Teach Us about Literacy and Learning. New York: Palgrave Macmillan, 2003.

13 Bruckman, A. Designing for virtual communities in the service of learning. Designing for Virtual Communities in the Service of Learning. Cambridge, UK: Cambridge University Press, 2004.

14 Bartle, RR. Designing Virtual Worlds. Indianapolis, IA: New Riders, 2003.

15 Squire, K. From content to context: videogames as designed experience. *Educational Researcher* 35(8) (2006): 19–29.

16 Bauman, EB. Virtual reality and game-based clinical education.Clinical Teaching Strategies in Nursing Education (3rd ed). Eds Gaberson, KB & Oermann, MH. New York: Springer, 2010.

17 Buring, SM et al. Interprofessional education: definitions, student competencies, and guidelines for implementation. *American Journal of Pharmaceutical Education* 73(4) (2009): 59.

18 Leape, L et al. Perspective: a culture of respect. Part 1: The nature and causes of disrespectful behavior by physicians. *Academic Medicine: Journal of the Association of American Medical Colleges* 87(7) (2012): 845–52.

19 Rosenstein, AH, Russell, H, and Lauve, R. Disruptive physician behavior contributes to nursing shortage. Study links bad behavior by doctors to nurses leaving the profession. *Physician Executive* 28.6: 8–11.

20 Leape, LL. Errors in medicine. *Clinica Chimica Acta: International Journal of Clinical Chemistry* 404(1) (2009): 2–5.

21 Bauman, EB and Ralston-Berg, P. Serious gaming using simulations. Clinical Simulations in Nursing Education: Advanced Concepts, Trends, and Opportunities. PR Jefferies and National League of Nursing (eds). Philadelphia, PA: Wolters Kluwer Health/Lippincott Williams & Wilkins, 2014.

22 Gisondi, MA et al. Assessment of resident professionalism using high-fidelity simulation of ethical dilemmas. *Academic Emergency Medicine: Official Journal of the Society for Academic Emergency Medicine* 11(9) (2004): 931–7.

23 Wayne, DB et al. Mastery learning of advanced cardiac life support skills by internal medicine residents using simulation technology and deliberate practice. *Journal of General Internal Medicine* 21.3 (2006): 251–6.

24 Bruner, J. The narrative construction of reality. *Critical Inquiry* 18(1) (1991): 1–21.

25 Gee, JP. A linguistic approach to narrative. *Journal of Narrative and Life History* 1.1 (1991): 15–39.

26 Deterding, S. The lens of intrinsic skill atoms: a method for gameful design. *Human-Computer Interaction* 30.3–4 (2014): 294–335.

27 Deterding, S. et al. From game design elements to gamefulness: defining gamification. In *Proceedings of the 15th International Academic MindTrek Conference on Envisioning Future Media Environments*. New York: ACM Press, 2011, September 28–30, (pp. 9–15).

28 Gaba, DM. The future vision of simulation in health care. *Quality & Safety in Health Care* 13(Suppl 1) (2004): i2–10.

29 Murray, D et al. An acute care skills evaluation for graduating medical students: a pilot study using clinical simulation. *Medical Education* 36(9) (2002): 833–41.

PART 3

CHALLENGES: ASSIMILATING THE COMPREHENSIVE DIGITAL PATIENT

15

A ROADMAP FOR BUILDING A DIGITAL PATIENT SYSTEM

SAIKOU Y. DIALLO AND CHRISTOPHER J. LYNCH

Virginia Modeling, Analysis and Simulation Center, Old Dominion University, Suffolk, VA, USA

INTRODUCTION

In the military, it is now common to use interoperability standards to connect existing simulations in order to achieve a goal that none of the simulations can achieve by itself. A similar approach might be possible to achieve a digital patient if we interoperate existing simulations of the human body and mind into a cohesive whole. While the military domain has worked on interoperability since the early nineties, the medical/healthcare domain is at the beginning of its exploration on this topic. In order to achieve a digital patient through interoperability, we need a roadmap that can help guide us as a community and as individuals.

In this chapter, we attempt to identify a roadmap to achieve a digital patient through interoperability by looking at what has been done in the military domain and explore how it can be applied to building a digital patient. In order to study what has been done in the military domain, we analyze the contents of conference and workshop publications of the Simulation Interoperability Standards Organization (SISO) between 2000 and 2010. We chose SISO because it has spent the past 15 years publishing interoperability standards and reporting on their use around the world. This analysis shows that while the focus of interoperability is always on simulations, the intended use and the end user are also very important. Similarly, simulations have to be developed with interoperability in mind, for a given purpose and an appropriate level of detail.

Based on the findings of the content analysis, we propose a roadmap that focuses on developing a digital patient system that (i) is built based on requirements, (ii) has a community of users, (iii) possesses a set of standards rules and practice, and (iv) has a management system and a lifecycle. The proposed digital patient is an interoperability system that serves the medical/healthcare community and has mechanisms to grow, improve, and change and, most importantly, has a responsive flow of communication with its user community.

The Digital Patient: Advancing Healthcare, Research, and Education, First Edition.
Edited by C. Donald Combs, John A. Sokolowski, and Catherine M. Banks.
© 2016 John Wiley & Sons, Inc. Published 2016 by John Wiley & Sons, Inc.

The vision of a digital patient that can be used to train future health professionals, run scientific experiments on the effects of diseases, or test the effect of new cures has the potential to have a tremendous impact in healthcare. One approach to achieve this goal is to unify all the theories and practices of healthcare and medicine; merge them into a new single theory and then construct a unified model that reflects the new theory. The advantage of this approach is that we have a clear and consistent starting point from which to construct a digital patient. While feasible, this approach is time consuming and requires an agreement amongst scientists on the veracity and plausibility of the theory after it has been empirically tested over time. Once the theory is established, it would undergo a simplification process to turn it into a computable form. As our understanding of the human body and how it is affected by external entities and processes increases, the related theory would evolve and that evolution would be reflected in the model.

Another approach is to use existing models that capture years of research in the physical, mechanical, biological, mental, and physiological aspects of human beings and their environment. The advantage is that we leverage existing knowledge borne out of solid research, and we can incrementally create a digital patient by carefully selecting and combining models. The challenge is that the combination of models must have at least the following properties:

- *Consistency*: The digital patient must not have contradicting models. In other words, the models that are merged must form a single, coherent model or be derived from a single model. It also means that the same set of inputs must always produce the same sets of outputs in a consistently repeatable way.
- *"Simulateability"*: The digital patient must be implementable on a digital computer. This means that all of the models used to construct the digital patient must run on a digital computer individually and collectively. It also means that theories that cannot be simplified into a computable form cannot be part of the digital patient.
- *Validity*: The digital patient must consist of valid representations of a real patient and the medical attributes that coincide with that patient (i.e., treatment processes and effects of medicine). Findings from Ref. [1] show that a combination of valid models is not necessarily valid which means that validation has to be performed every time a new model is added to the digital patient.

Achieving a model that has any one of these three properties, let alone all three, is very challenging. Meeting this challenge requires that experts in simulation work closely with medical/healthcare experts. Achieving consistency and validity requires experts who understand how to select appropriate models and how to combine them in a manner that produces a model that is both valid and consistent. Simulateability is typically the domain of the simulation expert who can help further simplify the model into a computable form. With either approach, simulateability is an essential component in achieving the digital patient.

There is no single accepted method for constructing models or simulations. This results in a wide range of models and simulation implementations across all domains. These simulations have different purposes, uses, intended users, and requirements, and they produce different outputs even when they are designed to model similar phenomena. The simulations can differ in the realms of software (i.e., data types), hardware (i.e., the ability to physically connect to a simulation), and the level of abstraction (i.e., whether there conflicting assumptions between the models with respect to the reference system). As a result, pulling different simulations together to try and address a problem that was not the original intent of the individual simulations leads to problems in composability, interoperability, and integratability.

Composability deals with the ability to assemble simulations into a single simulation system [2]. Simulations that already exist within a community are used to compose a new simulation that satisfies the requirements of the user [3]. The composition of a simulation is driven by the intended use of the simulation combined with all of the features contained within the component models. It is likely that the simulations selected to compose a new simulation contain additional features than the minimum features required to comprise the new simulation. Therefore, it is important to determine whether these extra features will cause any unexpected problems in the simulation that will unintentionally invalidate the simulation.

Interoperability deals with the ability of one or more systems (i.e., simulations) to exchange useful information between each other [4]. Interoperability occurs at the system level and focuses on the technical components of data exchange between systems. The two main components of interoperability are (i) the ability to exchange information (interoperation) and (ii) the usability of the information being exchanged (interoperability) [5]. In order for two or more systems to be considered interoperable, there must exist a method for the systems to transmit information to each other. The usefulness of the data refers to not only the ability of a simulation to receive data from another simulation, but to have the ability to know which of the incoming information can and cannot be used by the simulation [3].

Integratability deals with the ability of the simulation infrastructures to talk to each other [6]. This specifically deals with the physical connections between the simulations that permit and facilitate the transferal of data between the simulations [3]. The hardware utilized by the simulation systems is of interest for integratability. Is there a network available for the simulation systems to communicate? Is there a secure network router that will block access to the simulation system? What protocols are available for allowing each simulation to transfer its information across a network? With these questions in mind, it is necessary to determine if the simulation infrastructures are designed in a manner that allows them to be successfully integrated. We refer the interested readers to Refs. [7–9] for more information on composability, integratabilty, and interoperability.

The Levels of Cconceptual Iinteroperability Mmodel (LCIM) defines seven layers of interoperation that differentiate between the integratability, interoperability, and composability components and can be used for determining which layer a model belongs [8]. The seven levels of the LCIM are no interoperability (level 0), technical interoperability (level 1), syntactic interoperability (level 2), semantic interoperability (level 3), pragmatic interoperability (level 4), dynamic interoperability (level 5), and conceptual interoperability (level 6). The first two levels, no interoperability and technical interoperability, deal with the areas of network and infrastructure and fall under the governing concept of integratability. No interoperability means that no network or other infrastructure elements are established to allow for information to be exchanged between systems. Achieving technical interoperability means that network or infrastructure elements that allow for information to be exchanged between systems do exist.

The next three levels deal with the areas of simulation and implementation and fall under the governing concept of interoperability. The level of syntactic interoperability means that the systems are able to use protocols to form common symbols that interpret and structure the information within the systems. These common symbols can then be exchanged. Semantic interoperability introduces common terminology that is used to tag the syntactical structures within the systems and produces a common understanding of the information being exchanged. Pragmatic interoperability allows for common relations between the tagged structures to be captured. The relationships of the tagged structures are then provided with respect to the input and output parameters of the systems.

The final two categories deal with the areas of modeling and conceptualization and fall under the governing concept of composability. Dynamic interoperability means that the systems can account for the various system states and response options that can occur within each system. Conceptual interoperability involves capturing the background information of the systems including the assumptions, constraints, and simplifications that were used in building each system. If the systems are conceptually interoperable, then they share a common view of the problem. According to the LCIM, the ability of the systems to interoperate increases as they increase in level on the LCIM [8, 10].

In this chapter, we focus on the identification of requirements and challenges of creating a simulateable patient. The rest of the chapter is organized as follows: the following section presents our approach for identifying the requirements and challenges associated with combining simulations to build a digital patient; this is followed by a presentation of the results, recommendations, and conclusions.

APPROACH

To identify the challenges inherent to building a simulateable version of the digital patient, we look to the military domain where decreasing budgets and increasing training demands forced the Department of Defense (DoD) to consider combining models in the mid-1990s. Standards such as the distributed interactive simulation (DIS) [11] and the high-level architecture (HLA) [12] were enacted to help foster interoperability. In addition, the DoD promoted and supported the SISO as an organization that brings together people from government, industry, and academia to create, use, and report on standards. SISO holds three annual workshops and conferences on interoperability where peer-reviewed papers are published and presented. Over the past decade, SISO has endeavored to create simulation standards in support of interoperability and composability. Embedded within the collective publications of SISO are years of experience in creating environments for existing models to work together. One way of extracting this knowledge is through content analysis [13].

Content analysis is the process of making valid inferences from text about the content of its uses [14] and [15]. This can be applied to any form of communication that can be transcribed into a textual format. The application of content analysis to a set of text produces the main themes and concepts that comprise the text in a manner that is replicable. Applying content analysis to SISO publications provides a means for identifying the major themes associated with interoperability, composabilitiy, and integratability, along with their main corresponding concepts. The use of content analysis has been previously applied to the healthcare domain in order to identify the main Modeling and Simulation techniques that are identified within the literature [16] and [17]. The interested reader is encouraged to read Refs. [18–20] for additional information on the purpose and uses of content analysis.

As a result, our approach consists of analyzing the content of SISO publications in order to (i) identify the concepts, topics, and themes of interoperability in the past decade and (ii) to discuss how they can be used to build a simulateable digital patient. We use Leximancer to perform automated content analysis. Leximancer uses the frequency of words and the relative co-occurrence of the words to extract the concepts that are most associated with a group of text and provide a visual representation of the connections between them [21]. The interested reader is encouraged to read Refs. [22] and [23] on Leximancer.

TABLE 15.1   Total Number
of SISO Documents per Year

Year	Total
2000	248
2001	278
2002	275
2003	472
2004	378
2005	247
2006	244
2007	253
2008	246
2009	123
2010	132
Total	*2896*

We use a dataset consisting of all SISO conference papers from 2000 to 2010. This resulted in a total of 2825 documents from the 11-year period. A list of the SISO conference papers and presentations per year can be found and viewed at the SISO Digital Library at Ref. [24]. The papers and presentations are divided by year and then further subdivided by each of the three conferences. The number of documents obtained per year are shown in Table 15.1.

We first analyze the overall SISO dataset to identify the focus of SISO as a whole, and we use that focus as the basis to determine the requirements for the digital patient. Second, we analyze each year independently in order to establish a progression of topics in SISO over time. The year-by-year analysis accounts for the papers taken from all three SISO conferences for the corresponding year. We use this progression as a proposed research agenda for the digital patient.

BUILDING THE DIGITAL PATIENT THROUGH INTEROPERABILITY

To support the creation of a digital patient through interoperability, we must identify the main concepts that are associated with the interoperability of simulations within the literature. SISO was selected as the source from which to make this identification. Therefore, content analysis was applied to the publications that occurred during that decade to identify the main themes and concepts that were dominant across the decade. Figure 15.1 shows a concept map of the main themes and concepts over that decade along with the main contributions of each year to the body of knowledge. For instance, in the years 2001, 2005, and 2009 the main theme was "Used." This theme is the biggest bubble shown within the figure. Within each theme in Figure 15.1, the main concepts for that theme are listed and lines are drawn between the concepts that commonly occur together. The folder tags for the folders that contained all of the documents for each year (a total of 11 folders for the years 2000–2010) are also shown in Figure 15.1. The link between each folder tag and that corresponding concept shows the main concept that was identified for that year. Similarly, the theme that the concept is contained within is correspondingly the main theme for that year [21].

Within this section, we explore each theme in detail and draw some recommendations for the digital patient.

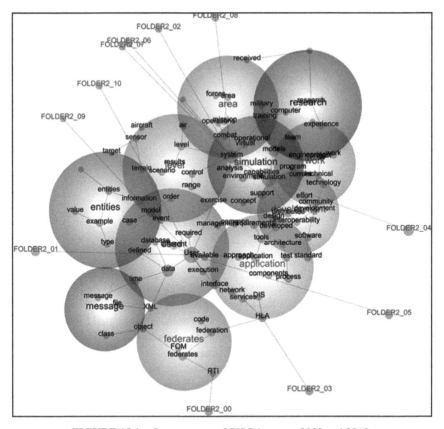

FIGURE 15.1 Concept map of SISO between 2000 and 2010.

For each theme, we provide the percentage relevance. This percentage indicates how closely connected the theme is to the body of knowledge under study. The results for the top five themes are as follows:

1. *Simulation (100% connectivity)*: The main theme is simulation as a system or simulation as a model. This includes what the simulation is used for and how it helps support training and analysis. For the digital patient, the main focus is to identify the simulations that will be integrated and establish a set of selection criteria for including or excluding a model. We discuss this further when we talk about requirements. Simulateability, consistency, and validity are good starting points, but other factors such as cost (i.e., time and labor) can also be included.

2. *Used (98% connectivity)*: The second most prominent theme is used which encompasses both the user and what was used. On the side of the user, the focus is the requirements and the management aspects of running an interoperability model. From the viewpoint of what was used, the focus is on describing the data, the interfaces, and the use cases that were considered. The creators of the digital patient need to define who the end users are and what use cases they intend to support. For existing models, the focus on the user indicates that for each model it is important to understand who the user community is and how the models under consideration are being currently used, managed, and supported (i.e., how

often are they updated and by whom). The focus on what was used is showing that even with standards in place, several implementations of those standards are possible. Therefore, we have to define an accreditation process that vendors can use to determine if their implementations abide by a standard without violating their intellectual property.

3. *Application (78% connectivity)*: The application theme covers the standards (HLA, DIS) and the environment (network and services), components, tools, and process used for testing the simulations individually or collectively. This means that for the digital patient to be successful, a series of tools and services have to be developed or adopted to support the testing, verification, and validation processes. This will help the adoption and growth of the digital patient and provide a standardized set of tools for the user community.

4. *Development (46% connectivity)*: The development theme covers the aspect of designing and developing models for use in a distributed environment as a community. For the digital patient, we have to start thinking about the architecture that we need to adopt and create a mindset of developing for interoperability or for reuse. The idea is that scientists and engineers start thinking about how to build a model that others would use instead of only worrying about what they need from the model. It would mean (i) developing interfaces to access the model parameters, instead of limiting exposure to the parameters, (ii) providing detailed descriptions of the functions and distributions within the model, and (iii) providing a simple user-friendly interface to execute the model.

5. *Level (32% connectivity)*: This theme covers the level of detail or rigor included in testing a simulation and the level of information that a model or the results from a model run provides. In terms of the digital patient, each model could potentially have a different level of scope and resolution in their specification and results. This is potentially a big problem that has to be solved by either mandating a scope and resolution floor (i.e., molecular level and above and millimeters and above) and enforcing very strict validation rules to avoid inconsistency in the federation.

All of these themes strongly overlap with several interconnections between them. While the rest of the themes are around 20% percent connectivity, they reveal several interesting properties. There is a strong overlap between the research theme (9% connectivity) and the simulation theme, which is an indication of the number of researchers working in the area of simulation interoperability as well as the amount of research that goes into making standards. It means that the digital patient must reflect current research from the medical, healthcare, and simulation communities. The digital patient must be an ongoing effort, and therefore must be managed and developed as such.

Having discussed the themes that must be taken into account to build a digital patient through interoperability, we will now focus on creating a set of focus areas that are sequential in theory and concurrent in practice.

Toward an Approach to Building the Digital Patient

Building and maintaining a digital patient is an iterative process that evolves and adapts over time. However, as with everything, it must have a starting point and a direction for proceeding forward. We identified a starting point within the previous section as we now know that both the simulation and the user must be the main focus of the digital patient. However, the five identified themes do not constitute a plan for building the digital patient. Instead, they provide an indication of the lessons that we must learn from a community that has been dealing with the interoperability and composability of simulations for years. Having access to all the papers from each year allows us to examine in greater detail the main concepts for each year and trace these concepts over time. Therefore, we seek to use these publications to establish a path for proceeding forward.

From this year-by-year analysis, we hope to identify the concepts that have stayed relatively permanent during this time period. The goal is to establish a starting point for the digital patient and use the identified concepts to derive a recommendation on the path forward. Concepts that are found to contain a relatively high relevance throughout the decade will be interpreted as being key concepts that the digital patient effort should focus on. For this analysis, we group the SISO publications by year starting with the year 2000 and ending in the year 2010. Then we perform concept analysis to identify the main concepts for that particular year. Table 15.2 shows the top ten concepts for each year.

From Table 15.2, we identify the concepts that repeat more than once and rank them by their average from highest to lowest. Table 15.3 shows the results of the ranking with concepts that are semantically similar ("user" and "used," for instance) grouped together.

Figure 15.2 shows the ranking of the concepts and their prevalence over time. For the digital patient, it means that the user and the use of the simulation must always be at the forefront, followed closely by the simulation itself. This is very important. It implies that for the digital patient to be successful, the digital patient must engage in a permanent conversation with the user community and the digital patient must reflect the data and information needs of the user community in a timely fashion. The concepts also show that the digital patient must be treated as a system, and therefore it must follow Systems Engineering principles that require providing requirements and use cases, as well as creating architecture and performance benchmarks. Additionally, it is essential to provide support in terms of tools, metadata, and man-hours to ensure that the digital patient is useful to the community and that it remains useful over time.

From the list of concepts shown in Figure 15.3, we propose six focus areas for developing and sustaining a digital patient. These focus areas include requirements, modeling and simulation, standards, tools and technology, support, and Systems Engineering. These focus areas are shown in Figure 15.3. While the other concepts shown in Figure 15.3 are not provided their own focus areas, these concepts are incorporated within the six focus areas. Each focus area is discussed in detail in the following sections.

Requirements

For the digital patient to be successful, it is essential to first understand the modeling questions that we want to answer and how we want to answer them. This implies a rigorous data collection effort to gather, classify, and prioritize the requirements for the digital patient. This will create an understanding of the needs and the expectations of the user community. In terms of requirements we distinguish between the following:

- *Data requirements*: A description of the data that is necessary to ensure a functioning digital patient is required. This includes the identification of all relevant inputs, outputs, and functions that will be needed to create the digital patient. Data requirements also include all relevant metadata such as source, format, pedigree, range, and units.

TABLE 15.2   SISO Ranking of Concepts by Relevance Between 2000 and 2010

2000		2001		2002		2003	
Used	16%	Used	100%	User	100%	Used	100%
Data	10%	Simulation	100%	Data	60%	Data	74%
Federation	9%	System	81%	Model	59%	Model	65%
FOM	6%	Model	72%	Federation	38%	Support	44%
HLA	7%	Data	66%	Requirements	42%	Requirements	51%
Model	11%	Requirements	55%	Simulation	83%	Simulation	96%
Requirements	8%	Provide	53%	Provide	47%	Federation	57%
RTI	6%	Support	44%	Support	39%	Provide	51%
System	10%	Process	42%	System	66%	System	75%
Time	6%	Time	40%	Operational	32%	Process	41%

2004		2005		2006		2007	
Used	100%	Used	100%	Used	100%	Used	100%
Model	69%	System	64%	Data	64%	Systems	71%
Data	62%	Model	64%	Systems	62%	Data	53%
Support	40%	Information	40%	Process	38%	Process	36%
Requirements	44%	Requirements	49%	Required	46%	Requirements	44%
Simulation	94%	Simulation	81%	Simulation	89%	Simulation	93%
Provide	53%	Provide	51%	Provide	48%	Provide	51%
Federate	40%	Support	41%	Support	40%	Support	38%
System	70%	Data	78%	Model	70%	Model	81%
Process	38%	Federate	38%	Information	37%	Federation	36%

2008		2009		2010	
Used	100%	Used	100%	Data	100%
Model	70%	Model	67%	Model	55%
Data	57%	Data	61%	Use	53%
Support	36%	Information	45%	Process	40%
Information	44%	Requirements	48%	System	49%
Simulation	92%	Simulation	79%	Simulation	79%
Provide	49%	Provide	51%	Systems	51%
Requirements	44%	Support	47%	Information	45%
Systems	76%	Systems	68%	Used	60%
Process	34%	Federation	39%	Support	37%

TABLE 15.3   Concept Relevance Ranked by Average in Percentages

	2000	2001	2002	2003	2004	2005	2006	2007	2008	2009	2010	Avg.
User/Used	16	100	100	100	100	100	100	100	100	100	53	88.1
Simulation	0	100	83	96	94	81	89	93	92	79	79	80.5
System(s)	10	81	66	75	70	64	62	71	76	68	51	63.1
Model	11	72	59	65	69	64	70	81	70	67	55	62.1
Data	10	66	60	74	62	78	64	53	57	61	100	62.3
Provide	0	53	47	51	53	51	48	51	49	51	0	41.3
Requirements	8	55	42	51	44	49	46	44	44	48	0	39.2
Support	0	44	39	44	40	41	40	38	36	47	37	36.9
Federation/ Federate	9	0	38	57	40	38	0	36	0	39	0	23.4
Information	0	0	0	0	0	40	37	0	44	45	45	19.2
Process	0	42	0	41	38	0	38	0	0	0	40	18.1
Time	6	40	0	0	0	0	0	0	0	0	0	4.2

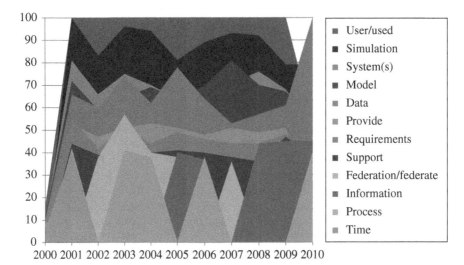

FIGURE 15.2 Percent concept relevance per year.

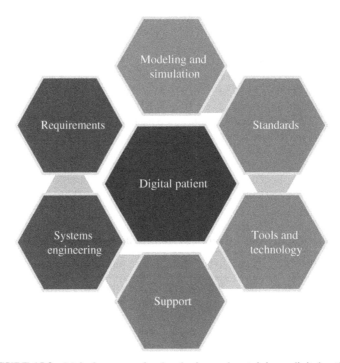

FIGURE 15.3 Main focus area for developing and sustaining a digital patient.

• *System requirements*: A description of the software, hardware, and tools that are needed to effectively run the digital patient is required. This includes not only identifying the operating system, memory size, add-ins, plug-ins, and other environment variables needed for the digital patient but also a description of the desired performance of the digital patient simulation.

- *User requirements*: A description of how the target users desire to use the digital patient should be captured from the view of the functions, interfaces, and use cases that comprise the digital patient. The user requirements should include a description of the interface requirements of the digital patient, a set of modeling questions that they expect the digital patient to be able to answer, and a description of the feedback or outputs they would like the digital patient to provide.
- *Interoperability requirements*: A description of the tools needed to integrate, test, and verify a new simulation model into the digital patient is required. This includes a list of capabilities and functions for each tool.

An important concept that spans across all four of the aforementioned requirement categories is that of time. Note the early prevalence of the concept time in 2000 and 2001, as shown in Table 15.2. The metadata of time is necessary as part of the process of capturing data requirements. This ties directly into the system requirements for determining the software, hardware, and tools that are needed to run the digital patient. Additionally, where it is applicable to use cases, feedback, or simulation outputs for the digital patient, time needs to be incorporated into the user requirements. As part of interoperability requirements, time requirements for the digital patient need to be accounted for when examining the capabilities and functions of the tools that will potentially be used in integrating, testing, and verifying the applicability of new simulations to add to the digital patient.

This is an important issue for the digital patient because it is very likely that models will have different representations of time. Some will contain continuous representations of time, while others will contain discrete representations of time. Similarly, some models will be event based (where change in the simulation is based on event) and some will be state based (where change in the simulation is based on the current state). Other variations are possible but regardless, the time representations have to be resolved very early for the digital patient to work. This also includes resolving potential deadlock situations, including mechanisms for detection and recovery and addressing time management issues such as synchronization and rollback. All of these issues are well known and studied within the domain of parallel and distributed computing [25], and we refer the interested readers to Refs. [10] and [26–28].

There is a possibility that each community of users have differing and sometimes competing requirements. However, a prioritization process should help in organizing a timeline for executing the digital patient. Once these requirements are gathered, we can use them to define the interoperability model. The interoperability model is the final model that we wish to construct by assembling together several candidate models. In addition to providing us with a blueprint and design architecture, the requirements can also be used to derive metrics by which we can evaluate whether a candidate model should be included within the digital patient.

Modeling and Simulation

After the initial requirement gathering, the focus switches to gathering and collecting candidate simulation models. For each candidate model that is under consideration for inclusion into the digital patient, we need (i) a description of the conceptual model, (ii) a description of the data needs for both the model inputs and the outputs produced by the model, (iii) a specification of the assumptions and constraints associated with the model, (iv) a description of the intended purpose of the model, and (v) a description of the means by which the model was validated. The set of models are then vetted against the metrics derived from the requirements and catalogued into a registry of models using either an existing taxonomy or creating a new taxonomy of medical models. This taxonomy of models is critical for determining how models should be connected and the order in which they should be connected. It should also help to identify dependencies and potential contradictions between the models.

The digital patient simulation model catalogue should be open and accessible to the community to allow competing models to be added and evaluated for inclusion within the digital patient. After creating a reasonably stable registry, we can use the metrics and the taxonomy to begin connecting the simulations. For instance, we could decide that models with the same scope, resolution, and time requirements will be integrated first in order to avoid dealing with the obvious problems of multiresolution and scope [5]. This would mean taking all of the equation-based models of the mechanics of the skeleton and putting them together to form a mathematical model of the human skeleton (or parts thereof). While this is a challenging task, it does not require the innovation of software engineering tools to translate time, resolution, and scope. Therefore, it can be attained as a community effort without soliciting specific expertise in computer science.

On the other hand, decisions on how to integrate algorithmic models (models that depend on a finite set of steps) do require that we have tools and standards to deal with the amount and complexity of computer code. It also requires that we have tools and standards for handling the disparity in platforms, operating systems, and environments. As a consequence, the next area of focus is the creation, maintenance, and enforcement of standards.

Standards

Standards promote uniformity and reduce variance in the expected behavior of a system, if standards are followed properly and consistently. In the case of the digital patient, we distinguish between the following:

- *Standard format and language*: This includes the data, metadata, standard, or set of standards that will be followed by the digital patient and are necessary for models to be included into the digital patient. These standards enforce a consistent description of the models and facilitate the creation of gateways and translators to navigate from one standard to another.
- *Standard tools*: It is not recommended to standardize tools. Instead, it is better to let the best tools emerge. However, it is still essential to promote the use of tool sets that are maintained and updated based on the input of the community. The criteria for selecting or developing tools should be obtained during the requirement gathering phase. The use of standardized tool sets reduces integration time and increases cooperation and reuse.
- *Standard practices*: This includes the set of procedures that must be followed in order to submit a model for consideration, the set of procedures that will be used for evaluation, and the set of procedures that must be followed for a model to accepted and incorporated into the digital patient. The object of these standard procedures is to produce and enforce a set of rules for the community in terms of expectations on both sides. This promotes confidence and fairness for everybody involved.

The creation of standards is a social activity that involves technical challenges and is largely successful based on the ability to create consensus. Several standards organizations and applicable standards already exist and can be reused or adapted to fit the requirements of the digital patient. After the creation and implementation of successful standards, an ecosystem of tools and technologies should begin to form around the digital patient. This ecosystem of tools and technology is our next focus area.

Tools and Technology

Even though our intent is to integrate existing models into a digital patient, science continually evolves, and we must account for the continuous creation of new models. The ideal setup for the digital patient would be to allow the community to develop models for the purpose of integrating them into a digital patient. In order to accomplish that goal at least two types of tools are required:

1. *Development and integration tools*: These tools help users create, share, and integrate simulations in a given environment. They should be tailored to fit the user requirements and follow the standards promoted by the digital patient. Several development tools and environments already exist and can be evaluated for reuse. Integration tools are very important and they should conform to a standard.
2. *Testing and evaluation tools*: These tools allow the consistent testing of simulation models to see if they meet an established standard and if the simulation model should be incorporated into the digital patient. Test tools should be automated as much as possible to streamline the process and eliminate human error.

Tool can be created by vendors or can follow a more open track that allows individual users to propose and create new tools and technology. In both cases, the combination of standards and the community should be the driving force behind the tools and technology. The availability of tools is an essential component in the success of a digital patient.

Support

The ecosystem of tools and technology implies the existence of a support system dedicated to maintaining the tools and technology, standards, and an environment for the users. The support system consists of scientists and engineers committed to maintaining these components of the digital patient over time. Standards need to be updated over time dependent upon changes in the state of the art for the digital patient and for the inevitable changes to the uses and requirements for the digital patient. The scientists and engineers will be largely responsible for incorporating new tools that merge simulations together to form the digital patient and for advancing the technology supporting the ability of new and existing simulations to communicate. Additionally, the scientists and engineers are responsible for pushing standards that allow for simulations to become more readily interoperable.

The user environment provides an access point from which the community of users can express emerging requirements and comment on their perception of the effectiveness of current standards. Through the user environment, the community members can comment on if they find current standards desirable, reasonable, or valuable. The value of a standard deals with the whether the standard makes the digital patient faster, cheaper, or better overall. The desirability deals with the ability of the standard to become a significant part of the digital patient's community. The standard is reasonable if it is aligned with current research and is technically sound [29]. Ideally, a standard should be desirable, reasonable, and valuable.

The digital patient could have a large user base that consists of many diverging modeling questions and competing requirements. The user community might also require the inclusion of new practices, technologies, and scientific advancements. The ability to support these requirements from the users will drive the speed and success of the digital patient. This is one of the main reasons for creating SISO and organizing a community of users and volunteers that can create and maintain tools and standards. Changing requirements, tools and technology, and standards suggests that the digital patient has a lifetime that needs to be properly managed. The ability to support the lifetime of the digital patient can be addressed through the application of Systems Engineering principles.

Systems Engineering

The digital patient as described here is a system that has a lifetime and should be managed as such. The system is made up of the digital patient, its user community, its support system, and the tools and technology that are used for testing and evaluating the digital patient. Each of these components has the ability to change and affect the digital patient at any point in time. Therefore, the digital patient should have an architectural blueprint, planned update cycles, a management plan, and a set of rules and guidelines on how it should be used. Systems Engineering handles these types of issues through the design and management of systems over their lifetimes and can be applied to the lifetime of the digital patient.

Integrating and architecting systems, within the Systems Engineering perspective, entails combining multiple systems into a single, functioning whole through the application of process, knowledge, and enterprise integration [30]. The lifecycle of a Systems Engineering project is dependent upon changing technology bases, changing organizational needs, and changing user needs. System architectures include the logical design of the system, the internal and external interfaces of the system (i.e., the physical interface of the system), and functional architectures focus on the requirements of the system. The processes of the systems that Systems Engineering is concerned with are the behaviors of the simulated entities and the effect that the behaviors have on their attributes [9].

The management team also plays an important role in Systems Engineering as they set a direction for advancing the project and dictate the conditions under which the product can be used. Therefore, the management team can be viewed as an additional user for the digital patient. Standards are connected to the management team as the management team maintains a view of the economic incentives associated with the product and can push for developments of standards that make the digital patient faster or cheaper to keep pace with the community. Successful integration of simulation systems can be driven by a management team that balances the perspectives of the simulation integrations with the requirements of the digital patient.

All of these practices connect Systems Engineering with the previous five focus areas that we have discussed up to this point: requirements, modeling and simulation, standards, tools and technology, and support. The concepts that are found in Systems Engineering provide a connection between the requirements for the digital patient, the need for establishing standards that make the digital patient faster and cheaper, and maintaining focus on both the tool and the users throughout the life span of the digital patient.

CONCLUSION

The creation of a digital patient is possible through the development of six focus areas: requirements, modeling and simulation, standards, tools and technology, support, and Systems Engineering. The focus on requirements highlights the importance of data, system, user, and interoperability requirements in building a digital patient out of a collection of simulations. The focus on modeling and simulation highlights the importance of obtaining information about the specific simulations that are being merged into the digital patient.

The focus on standards provides a platform for success by establishing a standard format, language, tool set, and practice for merging simulations and forming the digital patient. The focus on tools and technology allows for emerging technologies to be integrated into the digital patient in the future. The focus on support provides environment through which the users can express their needs and requirements over time. The focus on Systems Engineering highlights that the digital patient needs to have guidelines for how it can be improved upon or updated over time in order to remain useful to the community.

Content analysis of publications pertaining to combining simulations obtained from SISO highlights that the digital patient design needs to maintain focus on the users of the simulation as well as the simulation itself. The focus on the simulation and the simulations' users pertains to the initial creation of the digital patient as well as the process of maintaining the digital patient over time. All of these aspects will allow the digital patient to evolve and remain up to date with current technologies, practices, and needs from the user communities. The ability to evolve simultaneously with advancements in the healthcare domain and by keeping in touch with changing requirements from the users will ensure that the digital patient remains a contribution to the user community into the future.

ACKNOWLEDGMENT

We would like to thank all of our colleagues at the Virginia Modeling, Analysis and Simulation Center (VMASC) for their help and support.

REFERENCES

1 M. D. Petty and E. W. Weisel, "A composability lexicon," in *Proceedings of the Spring 2003 Simulation Interoperability Workshop*, Kissimmee, FL, March 30–April 4, 2003. Orlando, FL: SCS, 2003, pp. 181–187.

2 E. W. Weisel, M. D. Petty, and R. R. Mielke, "Validity of models and classes of models in semantic composability," in *Proceedings of the Fall 2003 Simulation Interoperability Workshop*, Orlando, FL, September 14–19, 2003. Orlando, FL: SISO, 2003, pp. 14–19.

3 A. Tolk, "Interoperability and composability," in Modeling and Simulation Fundamentals: Theoretical Underpinnings and Practical Domains, J. A. Sokolowski and C. M. Banks, Eds., Hoboken, NJ: John Wiley & Sons, Inc., 2010, pp. 403–434.

4 S. Y. Diallo, H. Herencia-Zapana, J. J. Padilla, and A. Tolk, "Understanding interoperability," in *Proceedings of the 2011 Emerging M&S Applications in Industry and Academia Symposium*, Boston, MA, April 3–7, 2011. San Diego, CA: SCS, 2011, pp. 84–91.

5 S. Y. Diallo, "Towards a formal theory of interoperability," Ph.D. dissertation, Department of Modeling, Simulation, and Visualization Engineering, Old Dominion University, Norfolk, VA: UMI Dissertations Publishing, 2010.

6 A. Tolk, Ed. Engineering Principles of Combat Modeling and Distributed Simulation. Hoboken, NJ: John Wiley & Sons, Inc., 2012.

7 S. Y. Diallo and J. J. Padilla, "Military interoperability challenges," in Handbook of Real-World Applications in Modeling and Simulation, J. A. Sokolowski and C. M. Banks, Eds., Hoboken, NJ: John Wiley & Sons, Inc., 2012, pp. 298–328.

8 A. Tolk, S. Y. Diallo, and C. D. Turnitsa, "Applying the levels of conceptual interoperability model in support of integratability, interoperability, and composability for system-of-systems engineering," *Journal of Systemics, Cybernetics and Informatics*, vol. 5, no. 5, pp. 65–74, 2007.

9 W. Wang, A. Tolk, and W. Wang, "The levels of conceptual interoperability model: applying systems engineering principles to M&S," in *Proceedings of the 2009 Spring Simulation*

Multiconference, San Diego, CA, March 22–27, 2009. a: Society for Modeling and Simulation International, 2009, pp. 168–176.

10 A. Tolk, "Challenges in distributed simulation," in Engineering Principles of Combat Modeling and Distributed Simulation, A. Tolk, Ed., Hoboken, NJ: John Wiley & Sons, Inc., 2012, pp. 187–208.

11 *IEEE Standard for Information Technology – Protocols for Distributed Interactive Simulation Applications: Entity information and interaction, IEEE Standard 1278–1993*, pp. 1–64, 2002.

12 *IEEE Standard for Modeling and Simulation (M&S) High Level Architecture (HLA) – Framework and Rules, IEEE Standard 1516–2010*, pp. 1–41, 2010.

13 K. Katsaliaki and N. Mustafee, "Applications of simulation within the healthcare context," *Journal of the Operational Research Society*, vol. 62, no. 8, pp. 1431–1451, 2011.

14 K. Krippendorff, Content Analysis: An Introduction to its Methodology. Thousand Oaks, CA: Sage, 2012.

15 H. H. Kassarjian, "Content analysis in consumer research," *Journal of Consumer Research*, vol. 4, no. 1, pp. 8–18, 1977.

16 S. C. Brailsford, P. R. Harper, B. Patel, and M. Pitt, "An analysis of the academic literature on simulation and modelling in health care," *Journal of Simulation*, vol. 3, no. 3, pp. 130–140, 2009.

17 N. Mustafee, K. Katsaliaki, and S. J. Taylor, "Profiling literature in healthcare simulation," *Simulation*, vol. 86, no. 8–9, pp. 543–558, 2010.

18 B. Berelson, Content Analysis in Communication Research. Glencoe, IL: The Free Press, 1952.

19 S. Stemler, "An overview of content analysis," *Practical Assessment, Research & Evaluation*, vol. 7, no. 17, pp. 137–146, 2001.

20 R. P. Weber, Basic Content Analysis. Sage University Paper Series on Quantitative Applications in the Social Sciences, series no. 07-049. Newbury Park, CA: Sage, 1990.

21 Leximancer (2011). *Leximancer Manual: Version 4 [Online resource document]*. Available at: https://www.leximancer.com/site-media/lm/science/Leximancer_Manual_Version_4_0.pdf. Accessed October 15, 2014.

22 C. Poser, E. Guenther, and M. Orlitzky, "Shades of green: using computer-aided qualitative data analysis to explore different aspects of corporate environmental performance," *Journal of Management Control*, vol. 22, no. 4, pp. 413–450, 2012.

23 A. E. Smith and M. S. Humphreys, "Evaluation of unsupervised semantic mapping of natural language with Leximancer concept mapping," *Behavior Research Methods*, vol. 38, no. 2, pp. 262–279, 2006.

24 Simulation Interoperability Standards Organization. (2014). *Digital Library* [Online]. Available at: http://www.sisostds.org/DigitalLibrary.aspx?EntryId=19116&showSearch=true. Accessed August 7, 2015.

25 R. M. Fujimoto, "Parallel and distributed simulation," in *Proceedings of the 31st Conference on Winter Simulation*, Phoenix, AZ, December 5–8, 1999. New York: Association for Computing Machinery, 1999, pp. 122–131.

26 P. A. Fishwick, Simulation Model Design and Execution: Building Digital Worlds, Upper Saddle River, NJ: Prentice-Hall, Inc., 1995.

27 R. M. Fujimoto, Parallel and Distributed Simulation Systems, Vol. 300, New York: John Wiley & Sons, Inc., 2000.

28 G. A. Wainer and K. Al-Zoubi, "An introduction to distributed simulation," in Modeling and Simulation Fundamentals: Theoretical Underpinnings and Practical Domains, J. A. Sokolowski and C. M. Banks, Eds., Hoboken, NJ: John Wiley & Sons, Inc., 2010, pp. 373–402.

29 A. Tolk, O. Balci, S. Y. Diallo, P. A. Fishwick, X. Hu, M. Loper, M. D. Petty, P. F. Reynolds Jr., H. Sarjoughian, and B. P. Zeigler, "Towards a methodological approach to identify future M&S standard needs," in *Proceedings of the 2011 Winter Simulation Conference*, Phoenix, AZ: IEEE, 2011, pp. 2975–2992.

30 A. P. Sage and C. L. Lynch, "Systems integration and architecting: An overview of principles, practices, and perspectives," *Systems Engineering*, vol. 1, no. 3, pp. 176–227, 1998.

16

MULTIDISCIPLINARY, INTERDISCIPLINARY, AND TRANSDISCIPLINARY RESEARCH: CONTEXTUALIZATION AND RELIABILITY OF THE COMPOSITE

ANDREAS TOLK

Simulation Engineering Department, The MITRE Corporation, Hampton, VA, USA

INTRODUCTION

Medical Research comprises many disciplines. During his research on the support of constructing a concise medical taxonomy, McGregor [1] identified 53 general topics derived from established specialties, recognized diseases, therapies, and general topics. His subdivisions resulted in 374 topics and subtopics. When he compared his results with MEDLINE's Medical Subject Headings used to categorize research topics in medical journals, he was able to show that straightforward mapping is possible. This insight is important for the contextualization and reliability of modeling and simulation (M&S) composites supporting medical research: as each medical specialty comes with its own terms and methods, the simulation systems support the needs of these researchers and their way of conducting their research. They display the characteristics of disciplines, representing branches of knowledge in their field of study and profession.

Within this chapter, we are using a systems engineering viewpoint and understand modeling as a task-driven activity, resulting in a purposeful simplification and abstraction of a perception of reality [2]. The task initiates the modeling process. Each model is generated for a task, such as answering a question within the domain of analysis or providing a certain functionality to support training, etc. Modeling is a creative act during which the various activities are driven by the task and are done knowingly and purposefully to fully reach the goal. Within this process, researchers usually eliminate elements that are not important and distract from the main task (simplification). They also aggregate components that may have an effect, but they consider them secondary or less important. Finally, their discipline or specialty significantly shapes their perception and their problem solving skills in addition to other physical-cognitive aspects and constraints. The resulting conceptualization is the foundation of the following simulation. For the simulation, this conceptualization becomes the representation of the real-world reference. *The model becomes the reality of the simulation.*

With this insight of the variety of specialties and the pivotal role of specialty domain knowledge and methods when conceptualizing and modeling, it becomes obvious that contextualization and reliability of M&S composites supporting medical research needs to be understood in the context of multiple disciplines. This chapter will address various ways of interdisciplinarity as well as, techniques and methods to support collaboration. We assume that a composite works reliable within its own discipline, so the challenges to be addressed are the following: How do I prepare an M&S composite to be used in M&S-based research involving more than one discipline? How do I ensure that an M&S composite, which components are reliable in their own disciplines, is also reliable in the broader context of M&S-based research, involving more than one discipline? What can I do about reliability in the first place?

INTERDISCIPLINARITY AND INTERDISCIPLINARY RESEARCH

In order to answer the question of contextualization, we first have to understand in more detail how various disciplines collaborate. Klein [3] contributed to a taxonomy of interdisciplinarity that looks at the way different disciplines are working together. She observed that since the late nineteenth century, taxonomies of knowledge in the Western intellectual tradition have been dominated by a system of disciplinarity. Experts in a discipline or specialty agreed on a comprehensive and concise representation of concepts, terms, and activities needed to explain their professional domain by representing the common understanding of relevant professionals and professional organization, also known as a common body of knowledge. However, in recent years, this partition of knowledge into more or less independent expert domains fell short in providing the required insights into complex problems. Even today, more and more problems are discovered that require a common effort of experts from more than one expert domain, which is the object of interdisciplinarity.

Klein [3] observed that whenever more than one discipline works together, there are three different ways to accomplish this: multidisciplinarity, interdisciplinarity, and transdisciplinarity. The following sections will describe these main categories in more detail and show the application in the context of M&S-based medical research.

Multidisciplinarity, Interdisciplinarity, and Transdisciplinarity

Multidisciplinarity describes the loosest coupling of disciplines to solve a common problem. In a multidisciplinary effort, each discipline remains sovereign. This approach juxtaposes disciplines and their methods. The multidisciplinary team coordinates and sequences the contributions of various disciplines. The methods are complementing each other, but have no real overlap. Once the problem is solved, each discipline continuous their work as before. The definition of terms may have been aligned in support of this collaborative effort; but in general, there is no persistent contribution to the overall body of knowledge beside—hopefully—the proposed solution to the common problem. The information exchange is an *ad hoc* established by the team.

Interdisciplinarity creates a closer linkage between participating disciplines. Although the disciplines remain sovereign as a whole, interdisciplinary teams focus on identifying overlapping domains of knowledge. By identifying knowledge components that are able to interact with each other, domains are identified that can actually be blended into a new common domain subset that uses integrated solutions from all participating disciplines. Interdisciplinary teams are building permanent bridges that link domains together into something bigger. These bridges are still focused on common problems; but besides the proposed solution, a new quality of linked knowledge is supported as well. As a rule, common information exchange models—in other words, common semantics—are established that describe the common problem space.

Transdisciplinarity represents the strongest coupling of disciplines. Within transdisciplinary teams, new disciplines are created by transcending, transgressing, and transforming the contributing disciplines and specialties. Concepts, terms, and activities are not only described in common terms, but they are systematically integrated and new interactions are defined across the sectors of original contributions. While knowledge components are used to complement each other in multidisciplinary teams, transdisciplinarity hybridizes the knowledge. New theory needs to be created to explain the resulting body of knowledge, and restructuring is the rule. As the integration is systematic and transparent, all disciplines do not only agree on the information to be shared but also on the common use of this information—in other words, common pragmatics are established.

Integratability, Interoperability, and Composability

The terms *integratability*, *interoperability*, and *composability* were coined by Page, Briggs, and Tufarolo [4] with the objective to provide a categorization of challenges that have to be addressed when teams of different specialties are composing simulation solutions to provide new solutions. They define the three governing concepts of challenges that have to be addressed to support such teams as follows, as extended in Ref. [2]:

1. *Integratability* contends with the physical/technical realms of connections between systems, which include hardware and firmware, protocols, networks, etc. A common syntax allows exchanging data. As a rule, the sending and receiving systems use different data models, so that data mediation between the system interpretations is necessary.

2. *Interoperability* contends with the software and implementation details of interoperations; this includes exchange of data elements via interfaces, the use of middleware, mapping to common information exchange models, etc. Common protocols use common information exchange data models. The sending systems map their data to these exchange models, and the receiving systems are able to map the exchange models to their data. This establishes a common semantics.

3. *Composability* contends with the alignment of issues on the modeling level. The underlying models are task-driven, purposeful simplifications, and abstractions of a perception of reality used for the conceptualization being implemented by the resulting systems. These conceptualizations describe the entities, their attributes and relations, and processes, allowing for common pragmatics.

Successful interoperation of M&S-based solutions of different disciplines or specialties requires integratability of applied infrastructures on the technical level, interoperability of

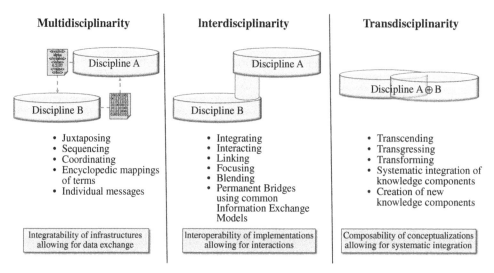

FIGURE 16.1   Multidisciplinarity, interdisciplinarity, and transdisciplinarity.

simulation systems on the implementation level, and composability of models—which are conceptualizations on the cognitive level captured in an agreed formats to contribute to the body of knowledge—on the conceptual level.

Figure 16.1 shows the relation between multidisciplinary and integratability, interdisciplinarity and interoperability, and transdisciplinarity and composability.

If we want to support M&S-based medical research in the multidisciplinary context, we need integratable infrastructures. In some cases, we may be able to simply sequence and coordinate the supporting simulation systems by using the output data of one system as input data for the next system. In the interdisciplinary context, we likely need a more integrative and interactive approach, which requires integrated and interactive simulation system solutions as well. As a rule, we will use a common protocol to exchange information structured in a common information exchange data model. As disciplines and specialties merge in transcending and transgressing manner, resulting in a transformation of knowledge, we will likely have to transform our simulation systems as well, in order to support the systematic integration characteristic for transdisciplinarity. The next section will present various techniques and methods that can be applied to adapt simulation systems to support these various degrees of collaboration between specialties or disciplines.

DATA ENGINEERING TO SUPPORT INTERDISCIPLINARITY AND INTEROPERABILITY

In multidisciplinary teams, the disciplines, specialties, and their tools remain untouched. As long as there is a way to use data provided by one tool by sequencing and coordinating the use of simulation systems within the team, there is no problem. Mapping of data is conducted based on encyclopedic mappings that are done by team members.

When moving into the realm of interdisciplinarity, common information exchange models are needed. As described in more detail in Ref. [5], a structured and systematic effort can lead to the construction of a common reference model that captures the conceptual

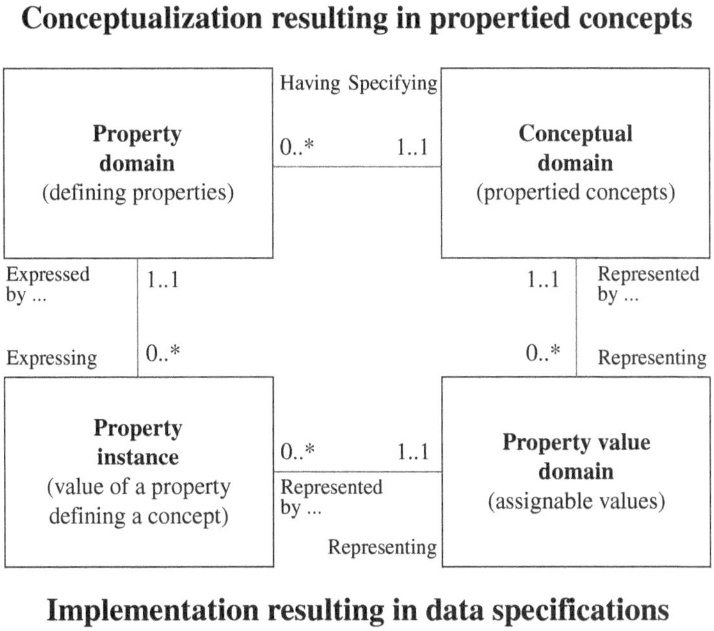

Conceptualization resulting in propertied concepts

Implementation resulting in data specifications

FIGURE 16.2   Domains of information exchange in ISO/IEC 11179 [6].

meaning of data elements, as well as the implementation thereof. For an improved understanding of the principles, the ISO/IEC 11179 [6] defines the domains of information exchange as shown in Figure 16.2.

The conceptual domain describes the concepts that are derived in the conceptualization phase of the modeling process. This domain comprises all the concepts that are needed to describe the referent or referents relevant to the information exchange. For example, the concept of *time* can be identified as an important one.

The property domain describes the properties that are used to describe the concept. Concepts are characterized by the defining properties. ISO/IEC 11179 refers to this domain as the data element concept. In the example of time, the data elements needed to describe *time* may be *year, month, day, hour, minute,* and *second*.

The property value domain comprises the value ranges, enumeration, or other appropriate definition of values that can be assigned to a property. ISO/IEC 11179 refers to this domain as the value domain. To address the property *month* describing the concept *time*, we can use the enumeration of the 12 months (*January, February, March, …, December*). Alternatively, we can use three-letter codes (*Jan, Feb, Mar, …, Dec*), or we can use numerals (1, 2, 3, …, 12). All these are possible and valid value ranges. These ranges need to be captured for each property for each concept.

Finally, property instances capture the pieces of information that can be exchanged. They minimally comprise the value of one property, which can be interpreted as updating just one value. They can also become an n-tuple of n properties describing a group of associated concepts, which represents complex messages or updates for several objects. ISO/IEC 11179 calls these property instances data elements. The property instance is the datum captured at a given moment. In case of databases, the property instance is what we assign to a table entry; in case of XML-tagged information, this is the value assigned to a tagged data field, etc.

Multiscope, Multiresolution, and Multistructure Challenges

When two disciplines get together to conduct interdisciplinary research, they normally have a clear understanding of their information exchange needs (what input data they need for their systems), as well as their information exchange capabilities (what output data they can produce with their systems). If they both structure their information exchange and capabilities according to the ISO/IEC 11179 standard, it becomes easier to find out if all information exchange requirements between the systems can be satisfied or if data gaps, that have to be addressed, exist.

If two disciplines use the same concept in their conceptual domain, they can exchange information, as they are interested in the same real-world referent. However, it is possible that the number and type of properties they use to capture the concept differ. Worldwide organization may include the property *time zone* in their description of *time*, as they may have to orchestrate worldwide operations. Other specialties may need to address various cultures and have to capture a reference point for the calendar, like BC/AD, BCE/CE, the year of the hegira, and other options. If the same concept is represented by different properties that only overlap partly, we have a difference in the scope. Whenever we face such multiscope challenges, we need to find a way to populate the properties missing in the source system from an alternative source. Often, we can also use default values based on application and domain-specific constraints.

Similarly, we may encounter multiresolution problems. If the same concept is represented using higher resolution properties, or if the same property is modeled using property value domains with different resolutions, we encounter such challenges. For many applications, the ABO blood types as discovered by Karl Landsteiner with A, B, AB, and 0 blood types is sufficient, while several specialties are interested in additional subtypes (A1, A2, B1) and the presence or absence of the Rhesus D antigen, etc. It is often possible to aggregate higher resolution data fields to provide for lower resolution fields; but in order to generate higher resolution data from lower resolution data, additional information is needed. In the blood-type example, the AB blood type on the one hand is represented by (A1B −ve), A1B Positive (A1B +ve), (A2B −ve), and (A2B +ve) on the other hand.

The last challenge group, multistructure challenges, arises often in different disciplines. While the same properties are observed, these properties may be used to characterize different concepts for each discipline. The logistics group of a hospital that is responsible for storing and purchasing may look at the same medicaments like the nurses, but both expert groups look at the medicaments differently, as nurses look at them from the perspective on how to use them to treat patients. The resulting concepts for logistic experts and nursing experts may be very different, and both viewpoints are justified.

Another example is the categorization of vessels: typical properties are that vessels are arteries or veins and that they are systemic or pulmonary. Specialties interested in blood flow from or to the heart will talk about veins and arteries, while specialties interested in blood flow from and to the lungs are interested in systemic or pulmonary vessels. It is important to understand that, in both cases, both structures are valid within the specialty. Having different viewpoints resulting in different groupings and structures may make it difficult to identify elements that can be exchanged, as the identification of common ideas normally starts with the conceptual domain; and if the resulting concepts are different, although the same properties are used, a mapping possibility may easily be overlooked.

Multiscope, multiresolution, and multistructure challenges can be observed in any imaginable combination, and encyclopedic challenges like homonyms and synonyms contribute to the complexity of the problems, but the structured approach of ISO/IEC

11179 allows identifying many of them based on set theoretic mappings. As an example, the different sets used for the representation of months, in the concept of *time* as *(January, February, ..., December)* versus *(Jan, Feb, ..., Dec)* or (1, 2, ..., 12), are all equivalent and can easily be mapped without loss of information. It also helps to understand that lung and heart specialties both share ideas about systemic arteries, systemic veins, pulmonary arteries, and pulmonary veins, and that they do this in a systematic manner.

Standards Supporting Contextualization

For the medical community, these observations are not new. Schuyler et al. [7] give examples and possible solutions using the Unified Medical Language System (UMLS [8]) in their work. Many of these lessons learned can be applied in this context as well. Another current initiative with significant potential for future applications is the National Information Exchange Model (NIEM [9]). NIEM is a community-driven, government-wide, standards-based approach to exchanging information. It defines in concepts, properties, and relations as they are agreed upon within different communities of interests or practices. NIEM originates from the need of local and state governments to exchange information across governance borders to exchange juristic data. The original model was successfully applied and soon extended to support not only justice departments but also homeland security efforts. NIEM was formally initiated in April 2005, by the chief information officers of the US Department of Homeland Security and the US Department of Justice. In October 2010, the US Department of Health and Human Services joined as the third steward of NIEM, which implies applicability for the topic of this section as well. At the time this chapter is written, NIEM is released as version 3.0 and all 50 states and 19 federal agencies are committed to using NIEM at varying levels of maturity. NIEM distinguishes between the NIEM Core, NIEM Domains, and Future Domains, as shown in Figure 16.3.

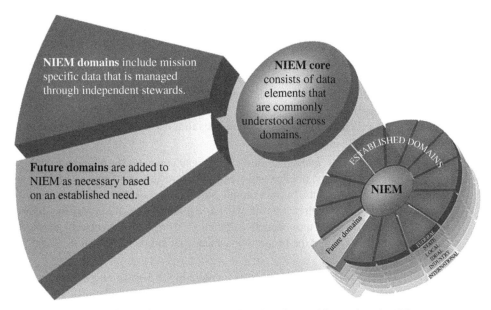

FIGURE 16.3   NIEM core, NIEM domains, and future domains [9].

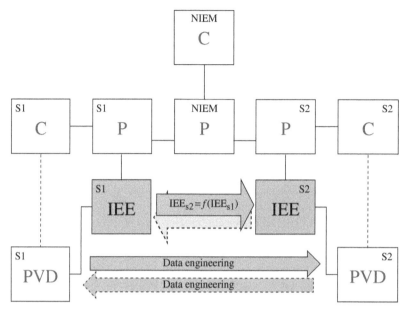

FIGURE 16.4   NIEM-based information exchange contextualization.

The concepts and properties defined in the NIEM can be extended, following the common rules to reflect the information exchange need of each discipline or specialty—hence supporting simulation systems of this domain as well. As such, NIEM and its domain (healthcare) and specialty specific extensions provide the common vocabulary needed to communicate with this specialty. Following the technical detailed principles described in Ref. [5], NIEM concepts and properties can be used to identify specialty specific data components that can be mapped to each other. Only property instances are data that flow over the infrastructure; all other information captured in the ISO/IEC 11179 are metadata allowing the correct interpretation.

Figure 16.4 illustrates the steps that result in data transformation allowing for valid information exchange under the contextualization of information under NIEM (or any other applicable common reference model capturing agreed concepts and properties) resulting from data engineering.

Data engineering as described in Ref. [5] comprises four necessary domains as follows:

1. *Data administration* is managing information exchange needs including source, format, context of validity, fidelity, and credibility. It results in awareness of the data sources and their constraints. In our example, this includes capturing the information exchange needs and requirements of the participating specialties—in the figure indexed S1 and S2—using the conceptual domain (C), property domains (P), property value domains (PVD), and the property instances that are the information exchange elements (IEEs).

2. *Data management* comprises all processes for planning and organizing data including definition and standardization of the meaning of data as of their relations. The availability of NIEM with its core elements and domain elements is a reasonable start.

The interdisciplinary team should extend these initial concepts and properties to allow for all information exchange requirements. In Figure 16.4, NIEM concepts and NIEM properties represent these identified common elements.

3. *Data alignment* processes ensure that information exchange requirements can be fulfilled, which means information exchange capabilities of source systems can be mapped to information exchange needs on the target system side. This is depicted by the connection of the property of the source specialty via the property of the NIEM to the property of the target specialty system. This connection, however, only ensures that we have a conceptual consensus. In addition, data engineering must also map the property value domain of the source system IEE to the target system.

4. *Data transformation* is the technical process of mapping data elements from the source to the target system. To this end, the data alignment process results in a function that takes the source IEE and produces the target IEE. This function needs to be injective. If the property value domains of source and target are equivalent sets, this function is surjective and an inverse function exist, which allows for bijective informative exchange.

Data engineering ensures that possible information exchange requirements are established and potential gaps are identified. Model-based data engineering processes using the NIEM as their model allow for the contextualization of information exchange requirements in a clear, common semantic context. NIEM is the common vocabulary that holds the various data representations conceptually together.

BASE OBJECT MODELS TO SUPPORT TRANSDISCIPLINARITY AND COMPOSABILITY

Model-based data engineering is a powerful method to identify if information exchange capabilities and needs are aligned with information exchange requirements in support of interdisciplinary research needs. Transdisciplinarity results in systematic integration of knowledge and creation of new knowledge. While integratable infrastructures and interoperable implementations are satisfied by common symbols and their interpretation, also known as syntax and semantics, transdisciplinarity requires understanding how this information is used as well, which requires common pragmatics. We need to understand how data are coded, what they mean, and how they are applied within the system.

This high degree of transparency is often an issue for solution providers, as they want to protect their intellectual property (IP). To address this dichotomy of required transparency of solutions and the protection of implementation details to address IP issues, the Simulation Interoperability Standards Organization (SISO) developed the Base Object Model (BOM) standard [10, 11]. This standard uses diagrams utilizing the Unified Modeling Language (UML) to describe what events occur that influence BOM, in what order or pattern such events occur, and how the state of the BOM changes.

For the medical simulation community, the use of UML in support of their efforts is not a new approach. Kumarapeli et al. [12] describe how they are using UML as a process-modeling technique for clinical-research process improvement. They use the same diagrams applied to describe events and event flows for the BOM approach. Vasilakis, Lecnzarowicz, and Lee [13] give a broader view on related research, in their literature and application overview of UML in health care. Both of these contributions make a strong case for the general applicability of UML to describe composites used to capture certain viewpoints of interest to the digital human efforts.

BOM uses standardized structures to capture the context of its applicability. It captures the conceptual model definition using the UML artifacts, describes a model interface to a simulation interoperability standards, and maps from the conceptual model to the model interface. This allows supporting several interoperability standards with the same conceptual model. As this conceptual model provides for the contextualization of the composite, this will be our focus.

The conceptual model definition uses four structures:

1. The *pattern of interplay* that defines how two or more composites interact with each other.
2. The *state machine* that describes how the state of an entity changes depending on events it receives within these patterns.
3. An enumeration of *entity types* that are used to describe the composite.
4. An enumeration of *event types* that are used to describe the interactions and events.

This conceptual model documents entities, events, and behavior patterns that take place among one or more entities, while the state machines describe the behavior of individual entities. This provides the required transparency of the composites, while at the same time protecting the IP for the provided detailed solutions. Implementation focused characteristics—such as data distribution management, transportation types, update rates, and synchronization—are not part of the conceptual model, but of the simulation interoperability standard-specific structures.

Figure 16.5 is an example of the well-known interplay of insulin and glucose in the human body. When we eat, our stomach digests the food and the glucose level in our blood rises. This high level triggers the pancreas to produce insulin and release it into the blood. The blood flow brings insulin and glucose to the body cells. The insulin ensures that the cells become receptive for the glucose and receive it to produce energy or store it for later use. This decreases the glucose level in the blood, and no more insulin is produced until it is needed again.

The model shown in Figure 16.5 has three entities: pancreas, blood, and body cells. Everything else has been deleted in the simplification process. Also, we aggregated all different main recipients, such as muscle and liver, into body cells. The pancreas entity has two states: "produces insulin" and "produces no insulin." The state change is triggered by the events "glucose high" and "glucose low." The pancreas entity furthermore creates the event "insulin" to trigger a state change in the blood. Similarly, body cells can be receptive or nonreceptive. They need insulin to become receptive; and once they receive enough glucose, they become unreceptive again. Finally, the blood is modeled using three states to address glucose and insulin level. The whole series of events between blood, pancreas, and body cells establish the pattern of interplay that is expected to be supported by simulation systems representing these entities as well.

Gustavson and Chase [14] show how this approach can bridge the gaps between conceptualization and implementation. Another viewpoint on simulation interoperability and how standards can be used to support this objective is given in Ref. [15].

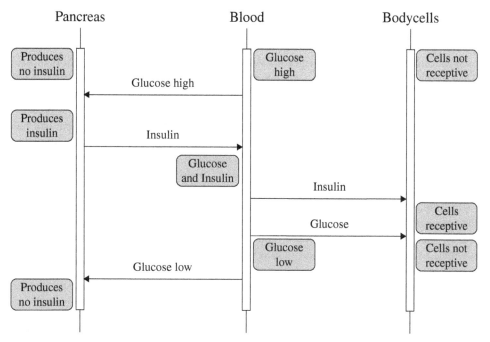

FIGURE 16.5   BOM example.

OPEN CHALLENGES ON RELIABILITY

Up to this section, our focus was the contextualization of M&S composites. This last section looks closer at reliability. There are many related terms that have to be taken into account when we address reliability: credibility, trustworthiness, validity, accuracy, soundness, authenticity, and more. Brade addressed this challenge in his dissertation [16] as follows:

> The credibility of a model is based on the perceived suitability and the perceived correctness of all intermediate products created during model development. The correctness and suitability of simulation results require correctness and suitability of the model and its embedded data, but also suitable and correct runtime input data and use or operation of the model. Verification and validation aim to increase the credibility of models and simulation results by providing evidence and indication of correctness and suitability. [16, p. 13]

In the simulation community, we usually apply validation and verification (V&V) to address the concept of reliability of M&S composites. The standard literature on V&V is summarized by Balci [17] and Sargent [18], who both contributed significantly to this field themselves. Validation ensures that we build the right composite, while verification ensures that we build the composite right! In other words, validation determines the degree to which a composite is an accurate representation of the real-world problem entity in the context of the intended use. It deals with behavioral or representational accuracy of representing the system. Verification focuses on the accuracy of all transformation processes: Does our model represent all concepts, relations, and requirements the user asks for? Does the computer model represent the conceptual model? Is the simulation providing all the functionality asked for in the right context?

The US Department of Defense (DoD) requires that all simulation solutions that are used to train soldiers undergo a rigorous V&V process to become accredited for their use. They compiled the Verification, Validation, and Accreditation (VV&A) Recommended Practice Guide (RPG) to support simulation professionals with guidelines and best practices [19]. The compilation takes several roles and viewpoints into account and presents documents to deal with them. The VV&A RPG is a living, web-based document that has been influenced by contributions from V&V experts all over the world and is not limited to the DoD. It can be downloaded for free and is a good starting point for every simulation expert or manager to deepen their understanding of processes and procedures that are applied in the biggest simulation application domain to this day.

In summary, validation is generally being applied to increase the reliability. However, the very recent observations in Ref. [20] show that validation is never conducted against reality, but at best against a reference model: an explicit model of a real—or imaginary— referent, its attributes, capabilities, and relations, as well as governing assumptions and constraints under all relevant perceptions and interpretations. The reference model captures what is known and assumed about a problem situation of interest. It captures requirements and theories and allows the identification of inconsistencies. It is complete in the sense that it captures what is known and lends itself to multiple and even competing interpretations. But it is still a model of one or several perceptions of reality. As such, we can only validate against currently known theories, and science has shown again and again that theories continuously change, improve, or are replaced themselves.

Another aspect often underestimated by those interested in the epistemology of simulation is that computer simulations obey the same limits and constraints as all computer programs: decidability, computability, and computational complexity.

- In 1931, Kurt Gödel presented his incompleteness theorem and shocked the academic world. Mathematical logic was considered the key for unambiguous, consistent, and complete description of knowledge and theories. Gödel proved that this was not the case: as soon as one devises a system that is powerful enough and that supports mathematical reasoning, the same system will necessarily contain statements that we could never prove to be true, even though it is true. Similarly, only a few years later Alan Turing showed that some problems never can be solved with a computer. He used the halting problem as an example, and by extending his argument showed that no algorithm can ever exist to answer questions like: "Will the system terminate?", "Are two modeled actions order independent or do I have to orchestrate them?", "Is the system specification complete?", "Is the system specification minimal?", or "Are two specifications functionally equivalent, in other words, do they deliver the same functionality?" There can be no algorithm to decide these problems; therefore, no computer simulation program can decide them either. They are undecidable problems!

- Computability addresses that only computable functions can be used on computers. Lambda calculus, the Turing machine, and recursive function theory explain what computable functions are. In simple terms, computable functions have a limited and discrete range and domain. If range and domain are not limited, they cannot be handled in the finite space of the computer. If they are not discrete, they cannot be mapped to the digital space. We can approximate other functions, but that always encompasses numerical errors. Again, this is a systemic challenge that cannot be solved. They are not computable problems!

- Finally, not everything that can be computed in theory can also be computed in practice: solving some problems simply takes too long, even on fast supercomputers. Computational complexity studies the use of resources, in particular computer memory needs and computing time. Computational complexity, as a discipline, is interested in the order of magnitude of functions to describe their general behavior. As a rule, only problems that require polynomial growth of resources with the size of the problem are generally solvable. Many additional problems can be solved based on good heuristics, but a huge number of computational complex problems cannot be solved with a computer anyhow, and this holds for simulations as well. These problems are computationally too complex to be solved in practice!

The interested reader is pointed to Huber L. Dreyfus books on the limits and constraints of computers: "What Computers Can't Do: The Limits of Artificial Intelligence" [21] and "What Computers Still Can't Do: A Critique of Artificial Reason" [22].

A final limitation of reliability of composites is based on the earlier insight that simulations and composites are based on models, which in turn are based on theories. While it is technically possible to combine simulation using handshake protocols and loose coupling methods, such as service-oriented architectures, the result of such a composition must be conceptually meaningful as well. Winsberg [23, pp. 72–92] uses nanosciences as an illustration. In his example, scientists are interested in how cracks evolve and move through material in order to predict, for example, the stability of a bridge or a building. To address this problem, three different levels of resolution are necessary. In order to understand how cracks begin, sets of atoms governed by quantum mechanics are modeled in small regions. These regions are embedded into medium-scale regions that are governed by molecular dynamics. Finally, most of the material is neither cracking nor close to a developing crack and can be modeled using continuum mechanics based on linear-elastic theory. The challenge is that these three theories—quantum mechanics, molecular dynamics, and linear-elastic theory—cannot all be valid at the same time, each exists with excluding principles. When composing contributing simulations to the digital human, such problems on the conceptual level need to be addressed in order to avoid *conceptual chimeras* as a result.

SUMMARY AND CONCLUSION

Computer simulation has become a powerful tool. New integration methods and paradigms are supporting the construction of composites of various disciplines to support multidisciplinarity, interdisciplinarity, and transdisciplinarity. This chapter addressed several supporting methods that allow the contextualization of components. In order to better understand what metadata is needed to allow for composition of independently developed solutions into a valid and reliable component, the levels of conceptual interoperability model (LCIM) was developed and successfully applied in many domains. Figure 16.6 shows the levels as explained in Ref. [15].

The LCIM exposes a base layer and six layers of interoperation:

- The base layer represents the stand-alone systems; they are not connected and therefore expose no interoperability.
- The *technical layer* deals with infrastructure and network challenges, enabling systems to exchange carriers of information. We define common protocols allowing exchanging signals.

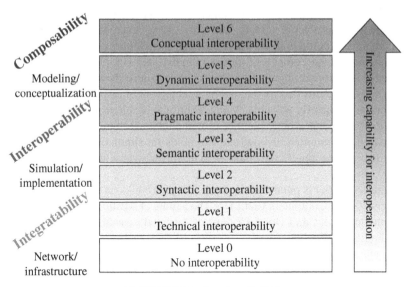

FIGURE 16.6   Levels of LCIM.

- The *syntactic layer* deals with challenges to interpret and structure the information to form symbols within protocols. We introduce a common way to interpret the signals.

- The *semantic layer* provides a common understanding of the information exchange. On this level, the syntactical structures are interpreted as objects, messages, and other higher structures. The symbols get a common semantic interpretation.

- The *pragmatic layer* recognizes the patterns in which data are organized for the information exchange, which are in particular the inputs and outputs of procedures and methods to be called. This is the context in which data are exchanged as applicable information. These groups are often referred to as (business) objects. We know not only what the data mean but also how the data is used.

- The *dynamic layer* recognizes various system states, including the possibility for agile and adaptive systems. The same business object exchanged with different systems can trigger very different state changes. It is also possible that the same information sent to the same system at different times can trigger different responses. The conceptual models of BOMs explained earlier in this chapter are an example of how this can be done.

- Finally, assumptions, constraints, and simplifications need to be captured. This happens in the *conceptual layer*. The conceptual challenges of contradicting theories discussed in the previous section are examples of challenges that have to be addressed.

Reliable composites require integratable infrastructures, interoperable simulation, and composable models. The LCIM allows identifying the necessary metadata allowing for meaningful contextualization. As discussed in more detail in Ref. [2], interoperability standards allow exchanging information between the systems and using the information in the receiving system. Composability ensures the consistent representation of truth in all participating components of the composites. The necessary mathematical foundations have been identified [20] and their practical application demonstrated [5]. Methods and tools for contextualization and reliability of composites, in support of the Digital Human, are identified and are ready to be applied.

It should be pointed out that these technical challenges described in this chapter may not be the major challenge that the Digital Patient will encounter. As described by Dunn and colleagues [24], the integration into the organizational complexity may be the bigger issue. Internally, engineering, culture, execution, and infrastructure have to be addressed as inter-related fields of concerns, while externally in addition challenges of media, accreditation, certification, industry, government, malpractice, public, and advocacy have to be addressed. A purely technology-driven view is not sufficient to address the resulting issues. Gheorge and Masera [25] identified infranomics as a crucial discipline for this century. They define infranomics as the body of disciplines supporting the analysis and decision-making, regarding the metasystem. The metasystem is defined by the totality of the technical components, stakeholders, mindframes, legal constraints, etc. It is the set of theories, assumptions, models, methods, and associated scientific and technical tools required for studying the conception, design, development, implementation, operation, administration, maintenance, service supply, and resilience of the metasystem. As such, infranomics will be the discipline-of-disciplines grouping all needed knowledge. Technical approaches as described in this chapter have to be embedded into such an overarching approach in order to be successful.

REFERENCES

1 McGregor B. Constructing a Concise Medical Taxonomy. *J Med Libr Assoc.* Jan 2005; 93(1): 121–123.

2 Tolk A. Interoperability, Composability, and Their Implications for Distributed Simulation: Towards Mathematical Foundations of Simulation Interoperability. In *Proceedings of the IEEE/ ACM 17th International Symposium on Distributed Simulation and Real Time Applications (DS-RT)*, October 30–November 1, 2013, Delft, the Netherlands, pp. 3–9.

3 Klein JT. A taxonomy of interdisciplinarity. In The Oxford Handbook of Interdisciplinarity, edited by Frodeman R, Klein JT, Mitcham C. 2010. Oxford University Press, Oxford, pp. 15–30.

4 Page EH, Briggs R, Tufarolo JA. Toward a Family of Maturity Models for the Simulation Interconnection Problem. In *Proceedings of the Simulation Interoperability Workshop*, April 18–23, 2004, Arlington, VA.

5 Tolk A, Diallo SY, King RD, Turnitsa CD, Padilla JJ. Conceptual modeling for composition of model-based complex systems. In Conceptual Modeling for Discrete-Event Simulation, edited by Robinson S, Brooks R, Kotiadis K, van der Zee DJ. 2010. Baco Raton, FL: CRC Taylor & Francis Press, pp. 355–381.

6 International Organization for Standardization (ISO)/International Electrotechnical Commission (IEC). Information Technology Metadata Registries Part 3: Registry Metamodel and Basic Attributes. ISO, Geneva. ISO/IEC 11179-3; 2003.

7 Schuyler PL, Hole WT, Tuttle MS, Sherertz DD. The UMLS Metathesaurus: representing different views of biomedical concepts. *Bull Med Libr Assoc.* 1993; 81(2):217–22.

8 Campbell KE, Oliver DE, Shortliffe EH. The Unified Medical Language System: toward a collaborative approach for solving terminologic problems. *J Am Med Inform Assoc.* 1998; 5(1):12–6.

9 United States Government. *National Information Exchange Model.* Available at: http://www. niem.gov (accessed on August 13, 2015).

10 Simulation Interoperability Standards Organization. SISO-STD-003-2006: Base Object Model (BOM) Template Specification. SISO, Orlando, FL.

11 Simulation Interoperability Standards Organization. SISO-STD-003.1-2006: Guide for Base Object Model (BOM) Use and Implementation. SISO, Orlando, FL.

12 Kumarapeli P, De Lusignan S, Ellis T, Jones B. Using Unified Modelling Language (UML) as a process-modelling technique for clinical-research process improvement. *Informatics for Health and Social Care*, 2007; 32(1), 51–64.

13 Vasilakis C, Lecnzarowicz D, Lee C. Application of Unified Modelling Language (UML) to the modelling of health care systems: an introduction and literature survey. *International Journal of Healthcare Information Systems and Informatics*, 2008; 3(4), 39–52.

14 Gustavson P, Chase T. Building Composable Bridges between the Conceptual Space and the Implementation Space. In *Proceedings of the Winter Simulation Conference*, December 9–12, 2007, J.W. Marriott Hotel, Washington, DC. IEEE CS Press, pp. 840–814.

15 Tolk A. Interoperability and composability. In Modeling and Simulation Fundamentals: Theoretical Underpinnings and Practical Domains, edited by Sokolowski JA, Banks CM. Wiley, Hoboken, NJ 2010, pp. 403–433.

16 Brade D. *A Generalized Process for the Verification and Validation of Models and Simulation Results*. Ph.D. Thesis, University of the Federal Armed Forces of Germany, Munich. 2004.

17 Balci O. Verification, validation, and Testing. In: The Handbook of Simulation, edited by Banks J, John Wiley & Sons, New York, 1998; pp. 335–393.

18 Sargent RG. Verification and validation of simulation models. *Journal of Simulation*, 2013; 7(1), 12–24.

19 US Modeling and Simulation Coordination Office. Verification, Validation, and Accreditation (VV&A) Recommended Practices Guide (RPG). US Modeling and Simulation Coordination Office, Alexandria, VA; 2006. Available at: http://www.acq.osd.mil/se/pg/guidance.html (accessed on August 13, 2015).

20 Tolk A, Diallo SY, Padilla JJ, Herencia-Zapana H. Reference Modeling in support of M&S—Foundations and Applications. *Journal of Simulation*, 2013; 7(2): 69–82.

21 Dreyfus HL. What Computers Can't do: The Limits of Artificial Intelligence. New York: Harper & Row; 1972.

22 Dreyfus HL. What Computers Still Can't Do: A Critique of Artificial Reason. Boston, MA: MIT Press, 1992.

23 Winsberg E. Science in the Age of Computer Simulation. The University of Chicago Press, Chicago, IL, 2010.

24 Dunn W, Deutsch E, Maxworthy J, Gallo K, Dong Y, Manos J, Pendergrass T, Brazil V. Systems integration. In: The Comprehensive Textbook of Healthcare Simulation, edited by Levine AI, DeMaria Jr S, Schwartz AD. Sim AJ, Springer, New York, 2013; pp. 121–133.

25 Gheorghe AV, Masera M. Infranomics. *International Journal of Critical Infrastructures*, 2010; 6(4), 421–427.

17

BAYES NET MODELING: THE MEANS TO CRAFT THE DIGITAL PATIENT

Joseph A. Tatman[1] and Barry C. Ezell[2]

[1] Innovative Decisions, Inc., Vienna, VA, USA

[2] Virginia Modeling, Analysis and Simulation Center, Old Dominion University, Suffolk, VA, USA

INTRODUCTION

Judea Pearl and other researchers introduced the concept of Bayesian networks in the mid-1980s [1, 2]. Many of the earliest applications were in the field of medicine.

Figure 17.1 shows a standard introductory example of a Bayesian network (BN). A BN consists of nodes and arcs. The nodes represent random variables or uncertain events. The arcs represent probabilistic dependencies between the nodes. In each node is a conditional probability table (CPT) that represents the knowledge of the relationship between that node and its parent nodes (its predecessor nodes in the network). The CPT is shown for the Dyspnea node in the figure. Importantly, each BN corresponds to a specific expansion of a joint probability distribution. The BN is mathematically precise. All constructs and operations in the BN correspond to constructs and operations in probability theory. The unique feature of BNs is the propagation algorithm, developed from Bayes' theorem, which provides efficient analysis of the BN, even those containing hundreds or thousands of nodes.

BNs have many unique advantages for diagnostic and other problems in medicine. These will be pointed out as each application area is covered and summarized at the end of the chapter. We cover four application areas: automation of patient aids, clinical diagnosis and treatment, medical image interpretation, and public health.

The Digital Patient: Advancing Healthcare, Research, and Education, First Edition.
Edited by C. Donald Combs, John A. Sokolowski, and Catherine M. Banks.
© 2016 John Wiley & Sons, Inc. Published 2016 by John Wiley & Sons, Inc.

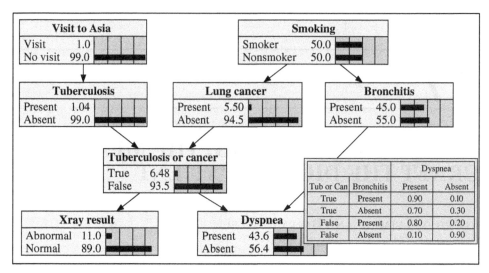

FIGURE 17.1   Bayesian network example [1].

Automation of Patient Aids

A small but important application of BNs in medicine has been to automation of patient aids. We provide two examples. The first is the application of a BN to tune the 150 parameters of a cochlear implant to improve patient hearing ability. The second is an application that recommends an insulin dose to control the serum glucose level of a patient.

Cochlear Implants   First, we will discuss the cochlear implant application. The purpose of a cochlear implant (CI) is to treat hearing loss [3]. In some cases, a CI restores a sense of hearing to a person who is deaf. The CI is an electronic device consisting of a speech processor and an array of electrodes implanted in the cochlea of the ear. The electrodes directly stimulate the auditory nerve to provide the sense of hearing. This particular application uses a unique algorithm to solve the network for an optimal strategy instead of the typical propagation algorithm used to solve BNs. The authors use the more general term "probabilistic graphical models" (PGMs) instead of "networks." We consider this a BN application, but use the term PGM throughout our summary to be consistent with the authors.

Problem. The CI has up to 150 tunable parameters. These can be associated with individual electrodes or with the implant as a whole. The role of the PGM is in the tuning process. It takes as input the current settings of the control parameters and the results of audiological tests, and tries to find a change to the set of parameters that will provide maximum improvement to the patient's hearing ability.

Approach. The researchers develop the concept of a "tuning network" which is a special PGM that contains not only chance nodes but also decision and utility nodes. Like an influence diagram, the tuning network contains decision nodes, used to model a tunable parameter such as the sensitivity of the microphone. It also contains chance nodes to model variables representing the effect of a change in a tunable parameter. Evidence nodes update the chance nodes. The evidence nodes might represent the result of a test, such as an audiometric, phoneme discrimination, or speech recognition test. Finally, the tuning network contains utility nodes to assign a value representing a change in hearing performance due to changes in some subset of the tuning parameters. The set of utility nodes in the tuning network represent the value function associated with the patient's hearing capability that is to be optimized.

In addition to the tuning network, the researchers develop a new type of "independence of causal interaction (ICI)" node. The most popular example of these kinds of nodes is the commonly used nisy-or. Their ICI node or "tuning model" implements a type of majority voting function. To facilitate this, they assume that every variable involved in the tuning model has exactly one of three values: increased, decreased, or "not changed."

Bayesian Network Development. Their model contains 202 nodes and 664 links. To facilitate building of the large PGM, they use an object-oriented paradigm for PGMs [4]. Elicitations from experts provide the probabilities required.

Inference. Using the utility nodes as described earlier, the researchers computed a global expected utility given the strategy using an inference algorithm. Because of the large number of variables and the high connectivity of the model, they used a likelihood weighting method [5] adapted to be used for networks containing utility nodes.

Results and Verification. Initial results were promising. Formal verification not being performed, the results from applying the PGM to a set of cases from real CI users were compared with the FOX model, an experts system based on deterministic rules. In addition, the expert who developed FOX reviewed the results. This expert judged results on cases in which the PGM CI tool diverged from FOX reasonable. In one notable case, a set of audiologists using FOX could not improve a patient's ability to understand spoken words, but this tool increased her performance to that of normality.

Current State. Current work involves learning the conditional probabilities from data, instead of relying wholly on expert elicitation. Discretization of nodes into three states now seems too coarse. Increasing the number of states would allow sensitivity to smaller changes. Finally, a partially observable Markov decision process approach is under consideration.

Discussion. The researchers chose a PGM because they provide a structured way to combine knowledge elicitation from experts with learning from data, and they provide a powerful probabilistic reasoning capability.

Insulin Regulation   In the Intensive Care Unit (ICU), patients who are critically ill frequently experience hyperglycemia [6]. This may be due to a preexisting diabetic condition or due to stress-response mechanisms. Such patients must maintain their serum glucose level within tolerances. Intensive insulin therapy performs this control function.

Problem. Intensive insulin therapy requires that the intravenous glucose drip be monitored and adjusted every 2 h or less. This control could be performed without human intervention; however, the risk of death demands a clinician in the loop. This research attempts to provide the clinician with a tool that allows them to do this job effectively and safely. This is a two-part problem. First, the system must accurately predict the serum glucose level accurately. Second, the system must be able to recommend insulin doses to control the serum glucose of the patient within the appropriate bounds.

Approach. The researchers chose dynamic BNs (DBNs) to model the evolution of a set of state variables in time. The DBN provides a way to model changing situations in which evidence is gathered over time. A set of nodes is defined as the state for the model. The values of these state nodes depend only upon the previous state, that is, the Markov property. Typically, the DBN is defined by modeling the relationship between two time steps. Therefore, the user needs only to define the relationship between two time steps to specify completely the DBN. These models rapidly become intractable with the addition of more complexity (increased number of arcs) or more time steps or both.

The researchers modeled all nodes as discrete. The time between states was 2 h. An exact inference algorithm was used. The primary tool was Bayes Net Toolbox, which is an open-source package in MATLAB [7].

Bayesian Network Development. The structure of the model, shown in Figure 17.2, was formulated based on information from the medical literature. The gray-shaded nodes are those that are directly observable. The unshaded nodes are those that are not directly observable (but can be estimated by the observable nodes). Figure 17.2 shows two time periods of the dynamic model for times $t-1$ and t. Nodes marked with the same circled number will have the same CPT. Comparing the $t-1$ stage to the stage at time t, shows that only Serum Glucose will have a different CPT across the stages. The Serum Glucose node at time $t=2$ will have the same CPT as this node at time $t=1$, but at $t=1$ it will not have the same CPT at time $t=0$, simply because $t=0$ is the first stage.

Anonymized data from 796 patients was used to learn the 11 unique CPTS indicated in the model pictured above. The model was learned with two-thirds of the data, and tested with the remaining one-third.

The researchers realized the importance of discretization in obtaining accurate results with a discrete BN model. They tried a combination of domain-based and equal interval discretization, and compared this to k-means clustering. Interestingly in this application, even though standard values for very low, low, normal, high, very high for physiological variables were taken from the clinical literature, the results for the domain-based approach were not nearly as accurate as with k-means clustering.

Results and Verification. The key component of their verification of the model was to randomly remove some fraction of the observed values of serum glucose and insulin drip rate, have the DBN algorithm estimate these removed values, and then compare the actual values (that were removed) to the values estimated by the algorithm. The results, when compared to what is considered the gold standard (eProtocol-Insulin), showed the model to be highly accurate even though the patient's nutrition and severity of illness were not included in the data set used in the machine learning of the model.

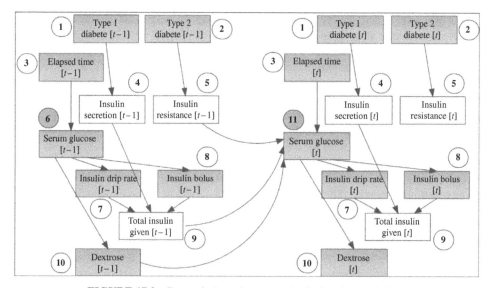

FIGURE 17.2 Dynamic Bayesian networks for insulin regulation.

Discussion. "Dynamic Bayesian Networks (DBN) support modeling changes in patients' condition over time due to both diseases and treatments, using probabilistic relationships between different clinical variables, both within and across different points in time" [6]. This leads to several important advantages for this application. For example, nodes that are not directly observable can be estimated from the values of observed nodes. In fact, at any point in time, whatever nodes have not been observed will be estimated by the nodes have been observed at that point in time. "This is an advantage of the DBN model over models such as regression and neural networks that have preset input and output variables" [6].

Clinical Diagnosis and Treatment

Selecting Treatment for Lung Cancer   "A prime example of a clinical setting, in which uncertainty is ubiquitous, is treatment selection in cancer care, where the diverse nature of the patient and disease characteristics and the rapidly expanding range of treatment options often present dilemmas regarding optimum treatment decisions" [8]. This leads to multidisciplinary teams playing a large role in treatment decisions. BNs offer an effective framework for discussion among the members of these teams.

Problem. There are two tasks. First, survival must be predicted as a basis for comparing treatments and making other decisions regarding the patient. Second, a method for selecting the optimal treatment option must be defined. These tasks must be done in an environment containing a high degree of uncertainty. This uncertainty is unavoidable in patient care processes—medicine is inherently uncertain. This uncertainty has many impacts including a distortion in the understanding of causal relationships. Other aspects of the problem environment are datasets having many blank entries, inconsistent formatting, and incorrect entries. A high degree of uncertainty and missing data are problems for which BNs are uniquely suited.

Approach. The ability of the BN to account for causal interventions allows calculation of the probability of survival for each treatment. Therefore, the doctor using this research will be able to select a treatment that maximizes the probability of survival.

Bayesian Network Development. The researchers used a broad variety of techniques for building the model: BN models elicited solely from human experts, BN models using machine-learning techniques, BN models using a hybrid approach that folds expert judgment into the machine learning process, and finally non-Bayesian statistical approaches. Across these four approaches, they used 12 different algorithms. The MATLAB BNT toolbox and the Weka 3 machine learning software tools were used. In addition, for the hybrid modeling approach, they used Causal Minimum Message Length (CaMML), a causal discovery algorithm. CaMML incorporates limited expert knowledge into the automated structure learning in the form of relationships between pairs of nodes in terms of time, direct causality or undirected influence between the two nodes.

An anonymized subset of the Lung Cancer Database (LUCADA) lung cancer database from England provides the basis for the machine learning in the various approaches and for measuring the quality of the resulting models. They used 4 years of anonymized data collected during diagnoses from 2006 to 2010. This data, obtained from LUCADA, contained more than 1,26,000 patient records. Over 30% of the fields in LUCADA were missing data, and so a key part of the knowledge engineering was addressing this problem. These researchers considered missing data for a field value to be a meaningful value for that field, and so the text value "Unknown/Missing" replaces the missing value. Therefore, the model makes inferences based on the node value "Unknown/Missing."

Verification and Validation. The models (nine BN models and three statistical models) were used to predict the 1-year survival outcome. The results are mixed across the 12 algorithms used and show no dominant winner. On the other hand, the BN built by eliciting both structure and probabilities from human experts, a purely manual built model, performs noticeably worse than all the algorithmically built models. The authors believe that "this low predictive performance of the manual DAG structure may be explained by implicit dependencies in the data that the clinically elicited network is unable to capture" [8].

The ability of the BN to recommend a treatment by finding the treatment that maximized the probability of one-year survival given that treatment was not overwhelming. The BN recommendation only matched the recorded treatment 29% of the time. This rose to 76% when partial matches were considered. It is important that the comparison of treatment recommended by the models was to the treatment selected by the patients' doctors, not to ground truth.

Discussion. The results show that BNs score about the same as non-BN approaches for this problem. In particular, BNs build with careful consideration of causal structure do not perform significantly better than the TAN BNs that give absolutely no consideration to causal structure. Even given this, however, BNs are still valuable in this problem. They can provide answers even when some variables are not observed (by doing inference from the variables that are observed to those that are not). Also, the CPTs in the nodes of the BN, which model the relationship of a node to its parent nodes, can be updated as additional information (in the form of cases) becomes available. The need to predict survival probabilities given different treatment options requires causal reasoning, which is supported by BNs with causal structures but not with "discriminative machine learning methodologies such as regression models" [8].

On the one hand, there is much research and applications work on BNs hoping to identify the underlying causal structure of a BN from data, while at the same time comparison of causal BNs to Naïve Bayes and Tree augmented Naïve Bayes show little or no advantage. However, even given this mediocre performance by the BN solutions, there are still strong advantages for using BNs when their structure is causal. The section "Conclusions" discusses the advantage of this causal structure.

There are many other interesting applications of BNks in the general category of clinical diagnosis and treatment. Three examples are given in the following text.

OTHER INTERESTING APPLICATIONS

The current technique for predicting the pathological stage for prostate cancer relies on a logistic regression-based approach. Predicting the pathological stage is important for determining the patient's treatment. The authors have compared a range of classifiers for improving performance against this problem. Though a Naïve Bayes classifier did the best using the four variables in the current approach, BNs generally outperform the other methods as additional variables were added to the model [9].

The prognosis of cancer patients treated with intensity-modulated radiation-therapy (IMRT) is complex due to uncertainty, the number of decision variables, and the need to balance objectives of maximum tumor control and minimal treatment complications. A BN was developed to predict outcomes of IMRT such as tumor control and regional spread [10].

DBNs were applied to modeling the Sequential Organ Failure Assessment (SOFA) severity score for critically ill patients admitted to the ICU. The SOFA score is based on individual system scores for the respiratory, cardiovascular, hepatic, coagulation, and renal and neurological systems. The purpose was to identify probable sequences of organ failures, a major cause of death in the ICU. DBNs were shown to be a promising tool for prognosis and supporting physician decision making in this case [11].

Medical Image Interpretation

Images are extremely important in medicine allowing insight into a patient otherwise would not be known [12, 13]. Since 1895, imaging methods have improved in parallel with the advancements of the computer. Image interpretation and processing have improved over time as well but still remain a very complex problem. To that end, BNs have been used in hopes of improving mammographic analysis, breast cancer detection, and specifically in interpreting results. Velikova *et al.* [12] developed an approach where they compared medical interpretation of results from a breast cancer screening practice that included the mammographic examinations of 795 patients of which 344 were cancerous. The study purpose was to determine whether data discretization and structure learning can be used to scrutinize the modeling assumptions to improve the quality of a manually developed BN model. The results showed that discretization could improve the representation and the accuracy of the models in comparison to the model with continuous variables. First, the discrete data better captures the way radiologists analyze mammograms and evaluate abnormalities. This allows for easier interpretation and usability of the BN model. Second, appropriate discretization provides better approximation of the true probability distribution of the data used and avoids the strong Gaussian assumption imposed on the continuous variables, leading to better accuracy and data fitting capabilities of the models, as shown in this study.

Public Health

Biosurveillance   There are many important and substantial problems in the field of public health [14]. One problem is in detecting the emergence of an outbreak of disease in the human population as quickly as possible. The key factor in reducing the casualties of such outbreaks is early detection. The goal of DTRA's Biosurveillance Ecosystem (BSVE) program is to significantly reduce the time required to identify threats to human health, whether of malicious or natural origin, and respond appropriately. Rapid and thorough information access will benefit US government analysts, local public health authorities, and individual citizens attempting to mitigate such outbreaks.

Problem. A BN anomaly detector (BNAD) contributes to early detection of outbreaks by being able to detect anomalous conditions. The BNAD does not require knowing the signature of the outbreak. It finds anomalies and provides a capability for the user to look into the nature of the detected anomaly and determine if it is an outbreak of interest or not. The BNAD's success requires having a model of normality. It provides a capability for analysis of the current situation with respect to this model of normality. Then the current situation can be judged to be anomalous or not compared to the BNAD's model of normality.

Approach. In building the BNAD, the approach used machine-learning techniques to learn the probabilities of the BN model that describes "normality." Ideally, the BN probabilities should be learned from data that was collected when conditions were normal—in this case, a non-outbreak situation. The BN is dynamic and models day-to-day transitions; looking for unusual day-to-day transitions across approximately 90 syndromes and 68 counties. The structure is shown in Figure 17.2. The database used to learn the probabilities was furnished by DTRA and included several datasets that recorded clinic visits by individual patients. From this data, we were able to build a data table that gave syndrome counts for each of 68 counties over a given set of days (about 100–200). This data table was used to learn the probabilities of the BN.

To use the BNAD, the analyst enters a case into the BN. Each case typically consists of a county, a season of the year, and the standardized syndrome count data for 2 sequential days. A standard function in Netica calculates the probability of this case. An anomaly is defined as a case with a relatively low probability of occurrence. Since the BN model represents what is normal, a low probability of the case given the model indicates an anomaly. An anomaly score was defined to be the negative log of the probability of the case given the model. Higher scores are more anomalous. If the user identifies an anomalous case, they can look at specifically what syndromes are resulting in this anomaly and compare with other information in and out of the BNAD to make a decision about an alert.

Bayesian Network Development. The raw dataset was very large, about 3–5 million records. It consisted of records of individual patient visits to clinics across counties in a specific state. The data had been carefully anonymized. Standard tools such as Excel or R were unable to process the dataset because of its size. A unique combination of various data tools had to be used to reduce the raw data to array data objects that could be handled by R. Excel and R and other software were then used to prepare a data table formatted appropriately for the Netica BN software to ingest and learn the model (Fig. 17.3).

This learning was only for the probabilities in the BN model. The structure of the model was developed manually. This structure is shown in Figure 17.4.

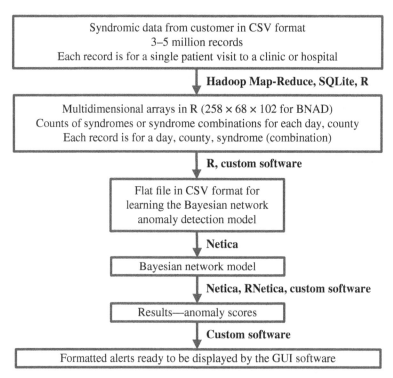

FIGURE 17.3   Steps in development of the Bayesian network model.

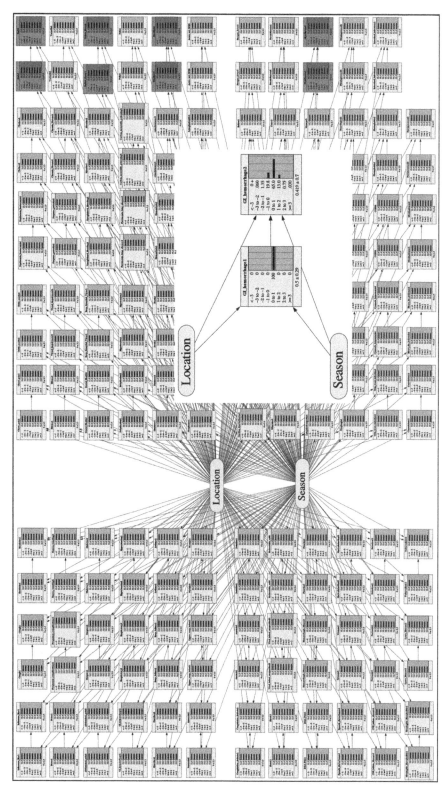

FIGURE 17.4 The Bayesian network structure is modeled with uniform probabilities. Inset shows the day 1 and day 2 nodes for a single syndrome after learning.

The inset in Figure 17.4 shows the nodes representing the standardized syndrome count data for 2 consecutive days for GI Hemorrhage. When data is entered for this node for a specific county and 2 sequential days of a specific season, Netica calculates the probability of this case. With this process performed for all 90 syndromes, Netica calculates the probability of this entire case. This probability of case given model is then used to calculate the anomaly score.

Verification and Validation. To facilitate the Biosurveillance Ecosystem contractors verifying their models, data representing a shigellosis outbreak was injected into a syndromic data set for a specific county. All of the data had been heavily "anonymized." In the initial testing scenario, analysts knew there was a shigellosis outbreak in the given county, but they did not know when the outbreak began or ended.

The BNAD was applied to the data set containing the injected shigellosis data. Using a simple alert rule of looking for 1 day with a high anomaly score resulted in too many false alarms. By trying different alert rules, one was found that provided an adequate probability of detection of the outbreak with a small false-alarm probability. This was considered acceptable for this initial prototype.

Discussion. There are many advantages to using the BN for this problem. First, the BN allows information from other sources to contribute to the analysis. For example, during the BSVE project, techniques for mining twitter data were also developed. This information source could be easily integrated with the BNof the BNAD to produce improved results [15]. Also, BNs provide a causal model that a human user can more easily understand, interact with, and explore. Causal relations are represented directly. In addition, trend effects can be easily modeled by including a node representing a context variable in the BN. Dynamic variables like syndrome counts at each time period and static variables like county, season, mitigation strategies, and weather are all easily incorporated into the BN. Case data and expert knowledge can be easily synthesized in the BN machine learning algorithms. Finally, complex dependencies are straightforward to represent in the BN.

A key disadvantage of BNs is that in nearly all BN software all variables must be discretized. Also, BNs can be awkward for modeling dynamics. These issues did not pose a problem in this case, because the model had only two stages.

Future Work. Immediate needs include analysis tools to help the analyst better understand the underlying causes when an alert is given. The probabilities of detection and false alarm depend strongly on the definition of an alert. This requires working with the analyst community to explore the impact of different ways to define the alert. The BNAD must be more thoroughly tested in diverse scenarios and refined accordingly.

Less immediate needs include increasing the scope of the BNAD to account for seasonal flu variation and other context variables. In addition, one of the key advantages of BNs is the ability to model dependencies between nodes, for example in our case, between nodes representing the standardized syndrome counts. Taking advantage of this and accounting for dependencies could improve performance. Finally, the capability of BNs to synthesize data with knowledge from human experts should be explored.

Other Interesting Applications There is a broad and diverse literature of the application of BNs in the public health arena. Samplings of those applications are summarized here.

Researchers applied BNs to modeling the risk of diarrhea infection in children in Cameroon to understand the cause of the disease and to quantify its effects [16]. They illustrate the capability of BNs to model the causal relationships between risk factors and to model hierarchical and other complex interrelationships between factors. The paper shows advantages of BNs over the more standard logistic regression approaches. This includes the ability to infer unknown values of some risk factors given other risk factors with known values.

A diverse team of researchers applied BNs "to develop a method for the optimization of epidemic alerts and the spatial and temporal targeting of immunizations and other interventions for the management of meningitis in the Niger, with the ultimate goal of preventing meningitis epidemics in the country" [17]. A key problem was to extract clinically meaningful information from an epidemiological database. Unfortunately, the size and quality of the dataset used in the Niger is not available for other areas. Simulation and resampling are being considered to address this problem. Validating their BN model (built from 2004–2006 results) against 2006–2008 data showed promise.

Researchers [18] used BNs to discover relations between genes, environment, and disease. They applied their approach to a study of bladder cancer in the United States. A key model building issue was missing data. The authors used the Expectation Maximization (EM) algorithm to provide "a practical means for estimating model parameters without disregarding observations with missing values. In our example, this greatly increased our sample size and allowed for the discovery of toenail arsenic levels as a significant predictor of bladder cancer" [18]. It is interesting that complex associations of variables (i.e., gene environment interaction) were only found when looking for other than causal interpretations of BN structure. Usually, attention to causality contributes to the insight and usefulness provided by the BN model.

CONCLUSION

Table 17.1 summarizes the five applications discussed in some detail in this chapter. Each column corresponds to an application. Each row corresponds to a different summary topic including the following:

- Role of the BN in the application
- knowledge was acquired to build the structure of the BN and determine its probabilities
- How knowledge was represented in the model
- Anything the researchers did that was unique compared to similar applications
- Software used to build and exercise the BNs
- Status of the work focusing especially on verification

As in all modeling approaches, there are disadvantages in modeling with BNs. For example, in almost all BN software all variables must be discretized. In addition, BNs can be awkward for modeling dynamics. However, the publications discussed in this chapter have shown many advantages to applying the BN modeling approach in the medical environment. These include the followi ng:

- Complex dependencies are straightforward to represent in the BN.
- BNs provide a structured way to combine knowledge elicitation from experts with learning from data.

TABLE 17.1 Summary of the Five Applications Described in Detail in this Chapter

	Cochlear Implant	Insulin Regulation	Clinical Diagnosis and Treatment	Image Interpretation	Bio-surveillance
Role of BN	To find optimal setting of 150 tuning parameters for a cochlear implant	Recommend insulin doses to control serum glucose level of patient in ICU	Predict probability of survival; select optimal treatment to maximize this probability	Cancer detection in the interpretation of mammograms	Identify anomalous conditions across a region of clinics and issue alert to public health analysts
Knowledge acquisition	Elicitation of structure and probabilities from experts	Structure knowledge from the medical literature	Machine learning from LUCADA database (>126,000 records); expert elicitation	Data from screening mammographic exams of 795 patients, of whom 344 were cancerous.	Used standard structure and machine learning of probabilities
Knowledge representation	Contains chance, decision, and utility nodes; used object oriented paradigm to facilitate structuring	Used dynamic Bayesian networks (DBNs); probabilities from anonymized 796 patient database	Standard BN structures	Experimented with machine learned structures versus expert-elicited structures	Two-stage DBN
Uniqueness	Developed a new *independence of causal interaction* node as a tuning model	Careful treatment of discretization to maximize accuracy	Compared 12 algorithms (9 BN-based); treatment of missing data; technique to input expert knowledge	Compared expert-elicited BN structure using continuous Gaussian nodes to machine-learned structure using discretization	Use of DBNs to base anomaly score on day-to-day transitions of syndrome counts
Software used	Adapted a likelihood weighting method due to model complexity	Primarily open-source Bayes Net Toolbox in MATLAB	Bayes Net Toolbox in MATLAB, Weka 3, in-house package CaMML	Bayes Net Toolbox in MATLAB, Weka	R, Netica, Excel, various software to process large datasets
Status	Performed expert-based verification along with a few actual cases	Detailed verification to a gold standard model	Verified to doctor's treatment selection in LUCADA database	Verified in detail against actual data	Verified against dataset with constructed outbreak

- The CPTs in the nodes of the BN, which model the relationship of a node to its parent nodes, can be updated as additional information (in the form of cases) becomes available.

- In most real-world datasets, much information is lost when only complete observations are considered in statistical analysis. An important benefit of BNs is their ability to handle missing information.

- An advantage of BNs over the more standard logistic regression approaches includes the ability to infer unknown values of some nodes given other nodes with known values.

- The need to predict survival probabilities given different treatment options requires causal reasoning, which is supported by BNs with causal structures but not with "discriminative machine learning methodologies such as regression models."[8]

- BNks facilitate causal models that a human user can more easily understand, interact with and explore [1].

REFERENCES

1   Pearl J. Probabilistic Reasoning in Intelligent Systems: Networks of Plausible Inference. 1988. Morgan Kauffmann, San Francisco, CA.

2   Gold V. Judea Pearl Wins ACM A.M. Turing Award for Contributions that Transformed Artificial Intelligence. Press Release from Association for Computing Machinery, March 15, 2012.

3   Bermejol I, Diez FJ, Govaerts P, and Vaerenberg, BA Probabilistic graphical model for tuning cochlear implants. In Artificial Intelligence in Medicine Lecture Notes in Computer Science, Volume 7885. *Proceedings of the 14th Conference on Artificial Intelligence in Medicine*, AIME 2013, Murcia, Spain, May 29–June 1, 2013. Springer Berlin/Heidelberg.

4   Koller D, Pfeffer A. Object-oriented Bayesian networks. In *Proceedings of the 13th Conference on Uncertainty in Artificial Intelligence (UAI-97)*. August 1–3, 1997, San Francisco, CA.

5   Shachter R, Peot M. Simulation approaches to general probabilistic inference on belief networks. In Henrion M, Shachter RD, Kanal LN, Lemmer JF, eds. Uncertainty in Artificial Intelligence 5. 1990. Elsevier Science Publishers, Amsterdam.

6   Nachimuthu SK. Temporal Reasoning in Medicine Using Dynamic Bayesian Networks. May 2012. PhD Dissertation, The University of Utah, Utah.

7   Murphy K. The Bayes net toolbox for MATLAB. *Computing Science and Statistics*. 2001; 33(2):1024–1034.

8   Sesen MB, Nicholson AE, Banares-Alcantara R, Kadir T, Brady M. Bayesian networks for clinical decision support in lung cancer care. *PLoS One*. 2013; 8(12): e82349. Doi:10.1371/journal.pone.0082349 (accessed October 20, 2015).

9   Regnier-Coudert O, McCall J, Lothian R, Lam T, McClinton S, N'dow J. Machine learning for improved pathological staging of prostate cancer: A performance comparison on a range of classifiers. *Artificial Intelligence in Medicine*. 2011; 55(1): 25–35.

10 Smith WP, Doctor J, Meyer J, Kalet IJ, Phillips MH. A decision aid for intensity-modulated radiation-therapy plan selection in prostate cancer based on a prognostic Bayesian network and a Markov model. *Artificial Intelligence in Medicine*. 2009; 46(2): 119–130.

11 Sandri M, Berchialla P, Baldi I, Gregori D, De Blasi RA. Dynamic Bayesian Networks to predict sequences of organ failures in patients admitted to ICU. *Journal of Biomedical Informatics*. 2014; 48: 106–113.

12 Velikova M, Luca P, Samulskic M, Karssemeijer N. On the interplay of machine learning and background knowledge in image interpretation by Bayesian networks. *Artificial Intelligence in Medicine*. 2013; 57 (2013): 73–86.

13 Newell, J. Medical images and automated interpretation. *Journal of Biomedical Engineering.* 1988; 10(6): 555–561.

14 Tatman J, Ciminera C, Smith G, Guikema S, Tatman S. Bayesian Network Anomaly Detector for Biosurveillance. 2014. Innovative Decisions, Inc., Vienna, VA.

15 Mahoney S, Comstock E, deBlois B, Darcy S. "Aggregating forecasts using a learned Bayesian network." 2011. In McCarthy PM, Charles Murray R. Twenty-Fourth International FLAIRS Conference, May 18–20, 2011, The Colony Hotel, Palm Beach, FL. AAAI Publications.

16 Nguefack-Tsague G. Using Bayesian networks to model hierarchical relationships in epidemiological studies. *Epidemiology and Health.* 2011; 33.

17 Beresniak A, Bertherat E, Perea W, Soga G, Souley R, Dupont D, Hugonnet S. A Bayesian network approach to the study of historical epidemiological databases: modelling meningitis outbreaks in the Niger. *Bulletin of the World Health Organization.* 2012; 90: 412A–417A.

18 Chengwei Su, Andrew A, Karagas MR, Borsuk ME. Using Bayesian networks to discover relations between genes, environment, and disease, *BioData Mining.* 2013; 6: 6.

PART 4
POTENTIAL IMPACT: ENGAGING THE DIGITAL PATIENT

18

VIRTUAL REALITY STANDARDIZED PATIENTS FOR CLINICAL TRAINING

ALBERT RIZZO AND THOMAS TALBOT

Institute for Creative Technologies, University of Southern California, Los Angeles, CA, USA

INTRODUCTION

A virtual revolution is ongoing in the use of simulation technology for clinical purposes. When discussion of the potential use of virtual reality (VR) applications for human research and clinical intervention first emerged in the early 1990s, the technology needed to deliver on this "vision" was not in place. Consequently, during these early years VR suffered from a somewhat imbalanced "expectation-to-delivery" ratio, as most users trying systems during that time will attest. Yet it was during the "computer revolution" in the 1990s that emerging technologically driven innovations in behavioral healthcare had begun to be considered and prototyped. Primordial efforts from this period can be seen in early research and development (R&D) that aimed to use computer technology to enhance productivity in patient documentation and record-keeping, to deliver cognitive training and rehabilitation, to improve access to clinical care via internet-based teletherapy, and in the use of VR simulations to deliver exposure therapy for treating specific phobias. Over the past 20 years, the technology required to deliver behavioral health and medical training applications has significantly matured. This has been especially so for the core technologies needed to create VR systems where advancements in the underlying enabling technologies (e.g., computational speed, 3D graphics rendering, audio/visual/haptic displays, user interfaces/tracking, voice recognition, artificial intelligence, and authoring software) have supported the creation of low-cost, yet sophisticated VR systems capable of running on commodity-level personal computers. In part driven by digital gaming and entertainment sectors, and a near insatiable global demand for mobile and networked consumer products, such advancements in technological "prowess" and accessibility have provided the hardware and software platforms needed to produce more usable and high-fidelity VR scenarios for the conduct of human research and clinical

The Digital Patient: Advancing Healthcare, Research, and Education, First Edition.
Edited by C. Donald Combs, John A. Sokolowski, and Catherine M. Banks.
© 2016 John Wiley & Sons, Inc. Published 2016 by John Wiley & Sons, Inc.

intervention. Thus, evolving behavioral health applications can now usefully leverage the interactive and immersive assets that VR affords as the technology continues to get faster, better, and cheaper moving into the twenty-first century.

While such advancements have now allowed for the design and creation of ever more believable context-relevant "structural" VR environments (e.g., combat scenes, homes, classrooms, offices, and markets), the next stage in the evolution of Clinical VR will involve populating these environments with Virtual Human (VH) representations that can engage real human users in believable and/or useful interactions. This emerging technological capability has now set the stage for the next major movement in the use of VR for clinical purposes with the "birth" of intelligent VH agents that can serve the role of virtual standardized patients (VSPs) for clinical training. One problem in trying to understand VSPs is that there are several quite distinct educational approaches that are all called a "virtual patient." Such approaches include case presentations, interactive patient scenarios, virtual patient games, human standardized patients (HSPs), high-fidelity software simulations, high-fidelity manikins, and VH conversational agents. This chapter emphasizes on VH conversational agents, and the reader is referred to Talbot et al. [1] for a very clear detailing of the salient features of the wide variety of approaches that are commonly referred to as virtual patients.

THE RATIONALE FOR VIRTUAL STANDARDIZED PATIENTS

An integral part of medical and psychological clinical education involves training in interviewing skills, symptom/ability assessment, diagnosis, and interpersonal communication. In the medical field, students initially learn these skills through a mixture of classroom lectures, observation, and role-playing practice with standardized patients—persons recruited and trained to take on the characteristics of a real patient, thereby affording medical students a realistic opportunity to practice and be evaluated in a simulated clinical environment. This method of clinical training was first attempted in 1963, when Dr. Howard Barrows at the University of Southern California trained the first HSPs [2]. Since that time, the use of live actors has long been considered as the gold standard medical education experience for both learning and evaluation purposes [3, 4]. HSPs are paid actors who pretend to be patients for educational interviews and provide the most realistic and challenging experience for those learning the practice of medicine because they most closely approximate a genuine patient encounter. HSPs are also a key component in medical licensing examinations. For example, the United States Medical Licensing Examination (USMLE) Step 2 Clinical Skills exam uses SPs and is mandatory for obtaining medical licensure in the United States (cf. http://www.usmle.org/). HSP encounters engage a number of clinical skill domains such as social skills, communication skills, judgment, and diagnostic acumen in a real-time setting. All other kinds of practice encounters fall short of this because they either do not force the learner to combine clinical skill domains, or they spoon feed data to the student with the practice case that turns the learning more into a pattern recognition exercise, rather than a realistic clinical problem-solving experience. The HSP is the only type of encounter where it is up to the learner to naturalistically pose questions to obtain data and information about the case that then needs to be integrated for the formulation of a diagnostic hypothesis and/or treatment plan.

Despite the well-known superiority of HSPs to other instructional methods [5, 6], they are employed sparingly. The reason for this limited use is primarily due to the very high costs to hire, train, and maintain a diverse group of patient actors. Moreover, despite the expense of standardized patient programs, the standardized patients themselves are typically low-skilled actors and administrators face constant turnover resulting in considerable challenges for maintaining the consistency of diverse patient portrayals for training students. This limits the value of this approach for producing realistic and valid interactions needed for the reliable evaluation and training of novice clinicians. Thus, the diversity of clinical conditions that HSPs can characterize is limited by the availability of human actors and their skills. HSPs that are hired may provide suboptimal variation control and are typically limited to healthy-appearing adult encounters. This is even a greater problem when the actor needs to be a child, adolescent, elder, person with a disability, or in the portrayal of nuanced or complex symptom presentations.

The situation is even more challenging in the training of students in clinical psychology, social work, and other allied health professions. Rarely are live standardized patients used in such clinical training. Most direct patient interaction skills are acquired via role-playing with supervising clinicians and fellow graduate students, with closely supervised "on-the-job" training providing the brunt of experiential training. While one-way mirrors provide a window for the direct observation of trainees, audio and video recordings of clinical sessions is the most common method of providing supervisors with information on the clinical skills of trainees. However, the imposition of recording has been reported to have demonstrable effects on the therapeutic process that may confound the end goal of clinical training [7] and the supervisor review of raw recordings is a time consuming process that imposes a significant drain on resources.

In this regard, VSPs can fulfill the role of HSPs by simulating diverse varieties of clinical presentations with a high degree of consistency, and sufficient realism [8, 9], as well as being always available for anytime–anywhere training. Similar to the compelling case made over the years for Clinical VR generally, VSP applications can likewise enable the precise stimulus presentation and control (dynamic behavior, conversational dialog, and interaction) needed for rigorous laboratory research, yet embedded within the context of an ecologically relevant simulated environment. Toward this end, there is a growing literature on the use of VSPs in the testing and training of bioethics, basic patient communication, interactive conversations, history taking, clinical assessment, and clinical decision-making and initial results suggest that VSPs can provide valid and reliable representations of live patients [1, 9–16].

CONVERSATIONAL VIRTUAL HUMAN AGENTS

Clinical interest in artificially intelligent agents designed for interaction with humans can trace its roots to the work of MIT AI researcher, Joe Weizenbaum. In 1966, he wrote a language analysis program called "ELIZA" that was designed to imitate a Rogerian therapist. The system allowed a computer user to interact with a virtual therapist by typing simple sentence responses to the computerized therapist's questions. Weizenbaum reasoned that simulating a nondirective "Rogerian" psychotherapist was one of the easiest ways of simulating human verbal interactions, and it was a compelling simulation that worked well on teletype computers (and is even instantiated on the Internet today: http://www.manifestation. com/neurotoys/eliza.php3). Despite the fact that the illusion of Eliza's intelligence soon disappears due to its inability to handle complexity or nuance, Weizenbaum [17] was reportedly shocked upon learning how seriously people took the ELIZA program [18].

Moreover, this led him to conclude that it would be immoral to substitute a computer for human functions that "…involves interpersonal respect, understanding, and love."

More recently, seminal research and development has appeared in the creation of highly interactive, artificially intelligent (AI) and natural language capable VH agents. No longer at the level of a prop to add context or minimal faux interaction in a virtual world, these VH agents are designed to perceive and act in a three-dimensional (3D) virtual world, engage in face-to-face spoken dialogues with real users (and other VHs); and in some cases, they are capable of exhibiting human-like emotional reactions. Previous classic work on VHs in the computer graphics community focused on perception and action in 3D worlds, but largely ignored dialogue and emotions. This has now changed. Artificially intelligent VH agents can now be created that control computer generated bodies and can interact with users through speech and gesture in virtual environments [19]. Advanced VHs can engage in rich conversations [20], recognize nonverbal cues [21, 22], reason about social and emotional factors [23], and synthesize human communication and nonverbal expressions [24]. Such fully embodied conversational characters have been around since the early 1990s [25], and there has been much work on full systems to be used for training [26–29], intelligent kiosks [30], and virtual receptionists [31]. Both in appearance and behavior, VHs have now passed through "infancy" and are ready for service in a variety of clinical and research applications.

USC EFFORTS TO CREATE VIRTUAL STANDARDIZED PATIENTS

Early Work in Psychiatry

The USC Institute for Creative Technologies began work in this area in 2007 with an initial project that involved the creation of a virtual patient, named "Justin" (see Figure 18.1). Justin portrayed a 16-year-old male with a conduct disorder who was being

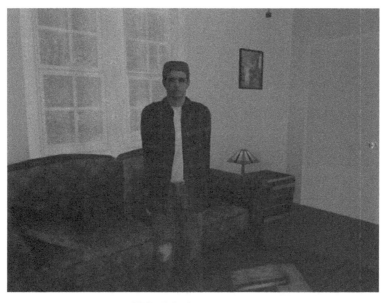

FIGURE 18.1   "Justin."

forced to participate in therapy by his family. The system was designed for novice clinicians to practice asking interview questions, to attempt to create a positive therapeutic alliance and to gather clinical information from this very challenging VSP. Justin was designed as a first step in our research. At the time, the project was unfunded and thus required our lab to take the economically inspired route of recycling a virtual character from a military negotiation-training scenario to play the part of Justin. The research group agreed that this sort of patient was one that could be convincingly created within the limits of the technology (and funding) available to us at the time. For example, such resistant patients typically respond slowly to therapist questions and often use a limited and highly stereotyped vocabulary. This allowed us to create a believable VSP within limited resources for dialog development. As well, novice clinicians have been typically observed to have a difficult time learning the value of "waiting out" periods of silence and nonparticipation with these patients. The system used voice recognition technology to translate speech to text, upon which the system would match questions to a limited bank of VSP responses. We initially collected user interaction and dialog data from a small sample of psychiatric residents and psychology graduate students as part of our iterative design process to evolve this application area. The project produced a successful proof-of-concept demonstrator and generated interest in the local medical community at Keck School of Medicine at USC that subsequently led to the acquisition of funding that supported the development of our next VSP.

Following the Justin proof of concept, our second VSP project involved the creation of a teenage female sexual assault victim, "Justina" to more formally assess student views toward interacting with a VSP in a training context (see Figure 18.2). We also aimed to explore the potential for creating a clinical interview trainer that could evaluate students in terms of their ability to ask questions relevant for assessing whether Justina met the criteria for the DSM-4r diagnosis of PTSD based on symptoms reported during the clinical interview. The interaction were also informally reviewed to get a sense as to whether students

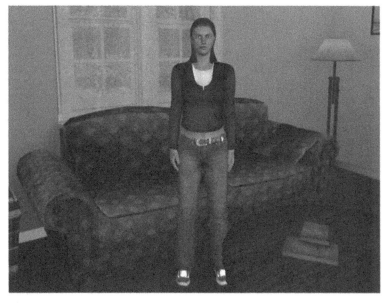

FIGURE 18.2 "Justina."

would interact with the VSP in a "sensitive" fashion as one would expect with a real-life clinical interaction with someone who had experienced significant personal trauma.

For the PTSD content domain, 459 questions were created that mapped roughly 4 to 1 to a set of 116 responses. The aim was to build an initial language domain corpus generated from subject matter experts and then capture novel questions from a pilot group of users (psychiatry residents) during interviews with Justina. The novel questions that were generated could then be fed into the system in order to iteratively build the language corpus. We also focused on how well subjects asked questions that covered the six major symptom clusters that can characterize PTSD following a traumatic event. While this approach did not give the Justina character a lot of depth, it did provide more breadth for PTSD-related responses, which for initial testing seemed prudent for generating a wide variety of questions for the next Justina iteration.

In the initial test, 15 Psychiatry residents (6 females, 9 males; mean age=29.80, SD 3.67) participated in the study and were asked to perform a 15-min interaction with the VSP to take an initial history and determine a preliminary diagnosis based on this brief interaction with the character. The participants were instructed to speak normally, as they would to a live standardized patient, but they were informed that the system was a research prototype that uses an experimental speech recognition system that would sometimes not understand them. They were instructed that they were free to ask any kind of question relative to a clinical interview and the system would try to respond appropriately, but if it didn't they could ask the same question in a different way.

From postquestionnaire ratings on a 7-point Likert scale, the average subject rating for believability of the system was 4.5. Subjects reported their ability to understand the patient at an average of 5.1, but rated the system at 5.3 as frustrating to talk to due to speech recognition problems, out-of-domain answers, or inappropriate responses. However, most of the participants left favorable comments that they thought this technology will be useful in the future, and that they enjoyed the experience of trying different ways to talk to the character in order to elicit a relevant response to a complex question. When the patient responded back appropriately to a question, test subjects informally reported that the experience was very satisfying. Analysis of concordance between user questions and VSP-response pairs indicated moderate effects sizes for Trauma inquiries ($r=0.45$), re-experiencing symptoms ($r=0.55$), avoidance ($r=0.35$), and in the non-PTSD general communication category ($r=0.56$), but only small effects were found for arousal/hypervigilance ($r=0.13$) and life impact ($r=0.13$). These relationships between questions asked by a novice clinician and concordant replies from the VSP suggest that a fluid interaction was sometimes present in terms of rapport, discussion of the traumatic event, the experience of intrusive recollections, and discussion related to the issue of avoidance. Low concordance rates on the arousal and life impact criteria indicated that a larger domain of possible questions and answers for these areas was not adequately modeled in this pilot effort.

Social Work Standardized Virtual Patients

The next USC VSP project involved collaboration with the USC School of Social Work, Center for Innovation in Research (CIR). This MSW program is novel for its focus on preparing social workers for careers working with military Service Members, Veterans, and their families. This project resulted in the creation of a VSP named "Sgt. Castillo" (see Figure 18.3a and b) designed to help social work trainees gain practical training experiences with VSPs that portray behavior more relevant to military culture and common

(a)

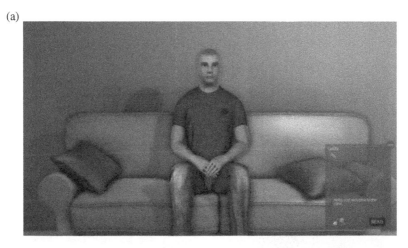

(b)

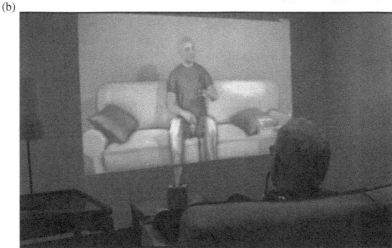

FIGURE 18.3   (a) Sgt. Castillo military virtual standardized patient and (b) in use with trainee using wall projection.

clinical conditions that Service Members and Veterans experience. This work also supported our first effort to create a limited authoring system that would allow for the creation of new VSP dialog that would support the flexible modification of the training goals. The vision was to build an interface that allowed clinical educators to create a virtual patient with the same ease as creating a PowerPoint presentation. If such authoring could be done by clinical educators, it would be possible for subject matter experts (social work educators in this case) to create VSPs that could represent a wide range of clinical conditions with the ability to manipulate the intensity and complexity of the clinical presentation and subsequent training challenge. Unfortunately, the resulting authoring system was somewhat difficult to learn without a deeper understanding of dialog management. Consequently, the authoring system was poorly adopted by our collaborators in social work, and only a few VSP instantiations were created. A sample video of a social work trainee interviewing one of these military VSPs can be found at http://www.youtube.com/watch?v=PPbcl8Z-8Ec.

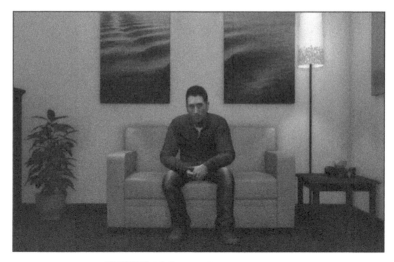

FIGURE 18.4   MILES virtual patient.

In view of these difficulties with authoring, the ICT/CIR project changed direction in order to meet the immediate need to provide clinical training to social work students currently enrolled in the CIR program. Instead of focusing on authoring and modification of the characteristics of the VSP, the emphasis shifted to training a specific psychotherapeutic approach that could involve concurrent individual and group/classroom practice. This resulted in the development of the motivational interviewing learning environment and simulation (MILES) to provide future social workers with the opportunity to practice motivational interviewing (MI) skills in a mixed-reality setting with a VSP. MILES was designed as an instructor-facilitated experience that enables an individual student to practice an MI-oriented interaction with a military veteran VSP while a classroom of students observes real-time video of the student/client interaction. The individual student trainee "speaks" to the VH through a microphone, selecting what he or she says from a multiple-choice list of carefully constructed statements. The MILES VSP (see Figure 18.4) has the ability to understand the spoken dialog and respond to the student in a lifelike, natural manner with realistic voice, body language, gestures, and facial expressions. As the single student progresses through the scenario, a branching dialog system can lead to various successful and unsuccessful outcomes depending on the response options selected by the individual trainee. At the same time, the rest of the class follows along viewing the real time video and selects their choice of the dialog options at each interaction juncture via individual response "clickers." An instructor control station captures performance data, including the answers selected by the lone student and their fellow classmates, to support of instructor awareness of the class's knowledge status to facilitate feedback in the form of an after action review (AAR) following an interaction. This system is currently in classroom use and learning evaluations are ongoing. A sample video of the MILES project can be found at http://www.youtube.com/watch?v=Sg8x1rttBho&feature=youtu.be.

Standardized Virtual Patients for Medical Training

After a number of prototypes and experiments conducted by the authors and elsewhere, it had become clear that a plateau had been reached in VSP applications and technology that left progress short of the threshold required for broader adoption of interactive

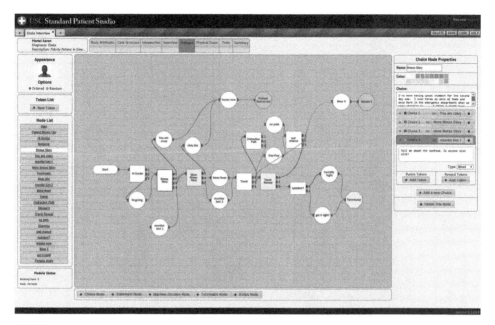

FIGURE 18.5 USC standard patient "select-a-chat" structured virtual human encounter authoring tool.

conversational characters for training. The primary factors limiting further improvement in experimental VSP systems were many, with the primary cause being the considerable effort required to create a single VSP encounter. Generally, it required a team of experts about 6 months to create a VSP, including up to 200 h of expert language training [32]. Additional factors included the low performance of natural language understanding (NLU) systems needed to understand the learner's questions and the effort involved in animating, creating voices, lip syncing, and scheduling motion of a VH avatar. The Justina prototype had a maximum NLU accuracy of 60% [33], with other systems achieving over 75%. That level of performance resulted in frustrating encounters, whereas NLU accuracy nearing 90% is more likely to result in a more positively received interaction that flows well as a clinical interview.

One strategy around the NLU accuracy problem is to avoid NLU altogether. VH conversations are possible that include an avatar that responds to pre-selected choices; such an interview is called a "structured encounter." There are many kinds of structured encounters. They may be linear, branching, unlocking style, and state-machine/logic-based. Structured encounters can be employed for patient interviews, surrogate interviews, counseling sessions, difficult conversations, persuasive conversations, and many other purposes (Figs. 18.5 and 18.6). Learner choices are definite and appropriate responses are guaranteed. Assessments are based on accurate data and have no potential for assessment bias.

The use of structured VHs for training is established; it has been successfully integrated into routine training with the previously mentioned MILES being an example. Another MILES variant, ELITE Lite has been accredited by the US Army for training. According to the accreditation document [34], ELITE Lite survey feedback reported 88.7% of respondents indicated practice exercises provide a sufficient representation of an informal interaction between a counselor and counselee. Subjects (87%) indicated the training experience was

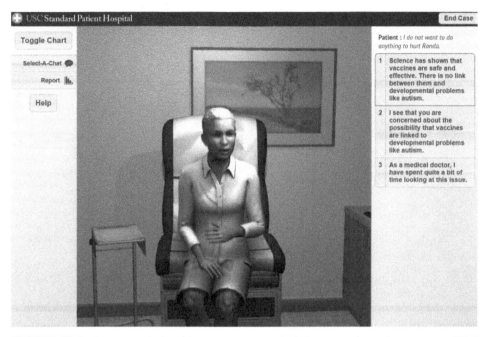

FIGURE 18.6   A structured virtual human encounter depicting a vaccine-resistant parent (USC standard patient).

engaging and effective, while 77% indicated they have a better understanding of the counseling process after using ELITE Lite. Most users indicated they would rather use ELITE Lite vs. lecture and PowerPoint instructional method (85%).

Another compelling structured encounter prototype is Virtual Child Witness (VCW). (See Figure 18.7.) VCW is a structured VH encounter intended to assess forensic interviewing skills. This effort focused on questioning strategy and compared "experts," a group of professionals who completed a forensic interviewing course with novices. The study, designed to see if the VH encounters could be an effective assessment tool, showed significantly higher performance in the expert group compared with novices. Analysis of the study data also revealed a strong training effect with subjects who unexpectedly played the structured encounter multiple times [35]. Of interest, VCW was created with very small budget on the SimCoach VH platform. SimCoach shortened the development time because it handled all the tasks required to create animated VHs and provided an online delivery mechanism [9].

Although structured encounters are a useful tool for many training applications, there is still a desire to simulate the medical interview with a VSP. The expense and limited access to HSPs coupled with the potential for objective assessments and repeatable, low-cost encounters make a compelling case for the success of VSPs. Fortunately, recent technology advancements have succeeded in breaking the VSP plateau to the point where the major problems inhibiting VSP creation and adoption are being addressed.

The USC Standard Patient (USP) project is a freeware open-source VSP community (www.standardpatient.org) that has applied considerable resources to improving natural language random access (NLRA) VSPs—the kind that mimic typical conversations with human patients (Fig. 18.8). The improvements [36] include creation of an automated online

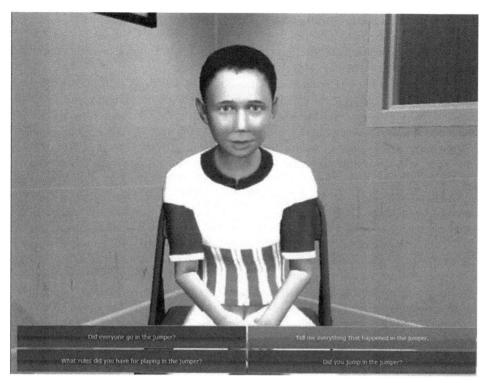

FIGURE 18.7 Virtual Child Witness—a structured encounter.

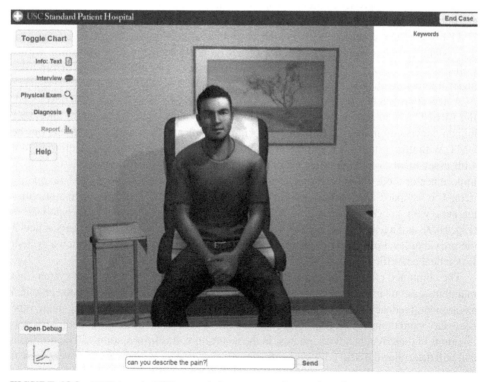

FIGURE 18.8 NLRA-style VSPs permit learners to ask questions in a natural manner through speech or typed input (USC standard patient).

VH tool, an improved medical NLU system, a universal VSP taxonomy, and a new approach to assessing human–computer conversations.

An automated online VH tool, SimCoach, was created first. SimCoach enables the rapid creation of cloud-based online VHs. SimCoach VSPs work on current-generation web browsers and greatly simplify the development burden for VH creation. SimCoach automates speech actions, animation sequencing, lip synching, nonverbal behavior, NLU integration, and AI processing and interaction management. With assets in place, new VHs can be created by providing text content. SimCoach was initially employed for training for VCW and is now the VH technology platform for USP.

The next impediment to be addressed is the fact that most prior NLRA VSPs were authored by creating a language focus around a specific medical problem or diagnosis. Questions would be compiled and answers associated to create a case that receives training data. This labor-intensive process needed for every patient case. Additionally, off-topic questions were poorly handled and caused such VSPs to appear inflexible. The USP project adopted a unified medical taxonomy (UMT) instead. UMT provides a common patient description regardless of actual patient condition. This makes new patient cases much more easily authorable and provides a fixed NLU training domain. Every Standard Patient VSP is represented by the complete unified taxonomy. Baseline and nonauthored case elements are filled in by the UMT system based on age/sex appropriate default responses.

NLU, one main impediment to fluent learner–patient interactions, was addressed through the creation of a new medical NLU system called "LEXI Mark 1." LEXI is a vastly improved NLU system specifically developed for medical interactions. The system is closely tied to the UMT and includes lexical assessment, probabilistic modeling, and content matching approaches. Lexi is capable of improving performance through human-assisted and machine learning. The implication of an approach that trains the NLU for the UMT rather than a specific case is that NLU training affects improvements in all cases on the system. Lexi has demonstrated better than 90% NLU accuracy in early testing with a well-trained taxonomy. Further evaluation will be necessary to assess actual performance under training conditions.

A new approach to conversational assessment, INFERENCE-RTS, was then developed. INFERENCE is an advanced game-based assessment engine that is capable of analyzing human conversations in real-time and associating learner speech acts with effects on the UMT. With this system, case authors annotate patient utterances in the case-authoring tool with assessment tags. Such tags are employed to indicate information that is of critical importance or moderate importance to the diagnosis. Tags exist for every UMT taxonomy item. The feedback intervention system encapsulates diagnostic performance and provides learners with concrete improvement tasks, a mind-map case taxonomy visualization (Fig. 18.9), and a learning-curve tool. INFERENCE was designed for deliberate practice at the proximal level of learner development. Future research will establish if such a system is practical and efficacious.

The combined effect of all these recent improvements results in a practical system that maintains ease of use, allows content creation in a timely manner, and provides practical assessment feedback to learners and educators. Researchers have yet to conduct the necessary validations to determine the educational impact of VSP systems that employ combinations of these recent advancements. In the near future, this information will be available and will determine the next course of action to advance VSPs for medical and psychological education purposes. If these combined technologies prove efficacious, it will be of great interest to see how this influences the milieu of medical and professional training.

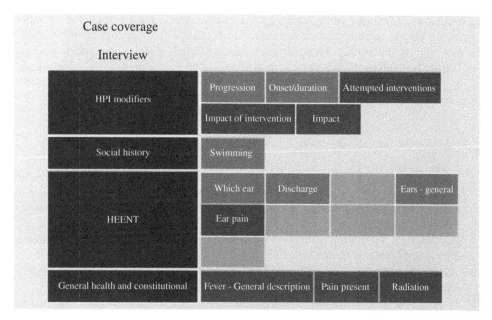

FIGURE 18.9   VSP interview mind-map.

Most VSPs attempted to date have been on traditional computers. With the increased prevalence of mobile devices, it is logical to consider the migration of VSP technology to phones and tablets. Regardless, there are significant usability barriers to adoption of VSPs on mobile platforms. The limitations are more human factors-based rather than caused by technical limitations. For example, how will a person interact with a conversational VSP? Will people talk to their phones? Will people type on tablet screens? Computers have excellent keyboards and when speech recognition is performed, this is usually with the benefit of a headset microphone to isolate speech. Phone and tablet microphones capture surrounding sound, and this may result in too many speech recognition errors. It may also present a more awkward interaction. Structured encounter-style VSPs do not suffer from these limitations and are much more readily adaptable to mobile device adoption.

Another promising idea is to imbue a manikin or task trainer with VSP capabilities. Such a capability could greatly improve the interactive potential of plastic-based physical training systems. The main technical limitation is similar to the mobile device problem: voice recognition. Future distant recognition (DSR) systems will require a high level of individual speaker discrimination and will likely adopt microphone array-based acoustic beamforming technology [37]. Unfortunately, DSR technology is not yet at a sufficient level of maturity for effective use with VSPs.

CONCLUSION

Virtual reality standardized patients have come a long way from faux-interactions on time-sharing mainframes starting half a century ago. Work over the past 15 years, in particular, has produced a wealth of knowledge and practical lessons in both the advancement of VSP technology as well as experience with VSPs in clinical training applications. Despite these advancements, VSPs have yet to see mainstream adoption in clinical training for a number of reasons. Recent work appears to have advanced sufficiently to ameliorate or overcome the most significant barriers. Thus, the age where VSPs may play a major role in training may finally be upon us. Future success may no longer be rate-limited by the pace of technology, but by the creativity and innovation of educators who will create compelling VSP experiences and curricula.

REFERENCES

1   Talbot, T. B., Sagae, K., John, B., & Rizzo, A. A. (2012). Sorting out the Virtual Patient: How to exploit artificial intelligence, game technology and sound educational practices to create engaging role-playing simulations. *International Journal of Gaming and Computer-Mediated Simulations*, 4(3): 1–19.

2   Barrows, H. S. & Abrahamson, S. (1964). The programmed patient: A technique for appraising student performance in clinical neurology. *Journal of Medical Education*, 39: 802–805.

3   Adamo, G. (2004). Simulated and standardised patients in OSCEs: Achievements and challenges 1992–2003. *Medical Teaching*, 25(3): 262–270.

4   Jack, B., Chetty, V., Anthony, D., Greenwald, J., Sanchez, G., Johnson, A., Forsythe, S., O'Donnell, J., Paasche-Orlow, M., Manasseh, C., Martin, & S., Culpepper, L. (2009). A reengineered hospital discharge program to decrease rehospitalization: A randomized trial. *Annals of Internal Medicine*, 150(3): 178–187.

5   Howley, L., Szauter, K., Perkowski, L., Clifton, M., & McNaughton, N. (2008). Quality of standardised patient research reports in the medical education literature: Review and recommendations. *Medical Education*, 42: 350–358.

6   Berkhof, M., Van Rijssen, H. J., Schellart, A. Anema, J., & Van der Beek, A. (2011). Effective training strategies for teaching communication skills to physicians: An overview of systematic reviews. *Patient Education and Counseling*, 84(2): 152–162.

7   Bogolub, E. B. (1986). Tape recorders in clinical sessions: Deliberate and fortuitous effects. *Clinical Social Work Journal*, 14(4): 349–360.

8   Stevens, A., Hernandez, J., Johnsen, K., Dickerson, R., Raij, A., Harrison, C., DiPietro, M., Allen, B., Ferdig, R., Foti, S., Jackson, J., Shin, M., Cendan, J., Watson, R., Duerson, M., Lok, B., Cohen, M., Wagner, P., Lind, D. S., & Lind, D. S. (2006). The use of virtual patients to teach medical students history taking and communication skills. *The American Journal of Surgery* 191(6): 806–811.

9   Rizzo, A. A., Kenny, P. G., & Parsons, T. D., (2011). Intelligent virtual humans for clinical training. *International Journal of Virtual Reality and Broadcasting*, 8(3): 1–16.

10 Beutler, L. E. & Harwood, T. M. (2004). Virtual reality in psychotherapy training. *Journal of Clinical Psychiatry*, 60: 317–330.

11 Bickmore, T. & Giorgino, T. (2006). Health dialog systems for patients and consumers. *Journal of Biomedical Informatics*, 39(5): 556–571.

12 Bickmore, T. W., Pfeifer, L. M., & Paasche-Orlow, M. K. (2007). Health document explanation by virtual agents. *Lecture Notes in Computer Science*. 4722: 183–196.

13 Kenny, P. G., Rizzo, A. A., Parsons, T. D., Gratch, J., & Swartout W. (2007). A virtual human agent for training clinical interviewing skills to novice therapists. *Annual Review of Cybertherapy and Telemedicine*, 5: 81–89.

14 Lok, B., Ferdig, R. E., Raij, A., Johnson, K., Dickerson R., Coutts, J., … Lind, D. S. (2007). Applying virtual reality in medical communication education: Current findings and potential teaching and learning benefits of immersive virtual patients. *Journal of Virtual Reality*, 10(3–4): 185–195.

15 Parsons, T. D., Kenny, P. G., Ntuen, C. A., Pataki, C. S., Pato, M. T., Rizzo, A. A, … Sugar, J. (2008). Objective structured clinical interview training using a virtual human patient. *Studies in Health Technology and Informatics*, 132: 357–362.

16 Triola, M., Feldman, H., Kalet, A. L., Zabar, S. Kachur, E. K., Gillespie, C., … Lipkin, M. (2006). A randomized trial of teaching clinical skills using virtual and live standardized patients. *Journal of General Internal Medicine*, 21: 424–429.

17 Weizenbaum, J. (1976). Computer Power and Human Reason. San Francisco, CA: W. H. Freeman.

18 Howell, S. R. & Muller, R. (2000). Computers in Psychotherapy: A New Prescription. Retrieved from: http://www.psychology.mcmaster.ca/beckerlab/showell/ComputerTherapy.PDF (accessed on August 5, 2015).

19 Gratch, J., Rickel, J., Andre, E., Cassell, J., Petajan, E., & Badler, N. (2002). Creating interactive virtual humans: Some assembly required. *IEEE Intelligent Systems*. 17(4): 54–63.

20 Traum, D., Marsella, S., Gratch, J., Lee, J., & Hartholt, A. (2008). Multi-party, multi-issue, multi-strategy negotiation for multi-modal virtual agents. Proceedings of the Eighth International Conference on Intelligent Virtual Agents. Tokyo, Japan, September 2008. Springer. Retrieved from: http://people.ict.usc.edu/~traum/Papers/multi-neg5.pdf (accessed on August 25, 2015).

21 Morency, L.-P., de Kok, I., & Gratch, J. (2008). Context-based recognition during human interactions: Automatic feature selection and encoding dictionary. Proceedings of the 10th International Conference on Multimodal Interfaces, ICMI 2008, Chania, Crete, Greece, October 20–22, 2008. IEEE.

22 Rizzo, A. A., Scherer, S., DeVault, D., Gratch, J., Artstein, R., Hartholt, A., Lucas, G., Marsella, S., Morbini, F., Nazarian, A., Stratou, G., Traum, D., Wood, R., Boberg, J. & Morency, L-P. (In press). Detection and computational analysis of psychological signals using a virtual human interviewing agent. *International Journal on Disability and Human Development*, 15(3).

23 Gratch, J. & Marsella, S. (2004). A domain independent framework for modeling emotion. *Journal of Cognitive Systems Research*, 5(4): 269–306.

24 Thiebaux, M., Marsella, S., Marshall, A. N., & Kallmann, M. (2008). Smartbody: Behavior realization for embodied conversational agents. In *Proceedings of the Seventh international Joint Conference on Autonomous Agents and multiagent Systems—Volume 1*, May (pp. 151–158). International Foundation for Autonomous Agents and Multiagent Systems.

25 Bickmore, T. & Cassell, J. (2005). Social dialogue with embodied conversational agents. In J. van Kuppevelt, L. Dybkjaer, & N. Bernsen (Eds.), Advances in Natural, Multimodal Dialogue Systems. New York: Kluwer Academic.

26 Evans, D. R., Hern, M. T., Uhlemann, M. R., & Ivey, A. E. (1989). Essential Interviewing: A Programmed Approach to Effective Communication. Pacific Grove, CA: Brooks/Cole Publishing Company.

27 Kenny, P. G., Hartholt, A., Gratch, J., Swartout, W., Traum, Marsella, S., & Piepol, D. (2007). Building interactive virtual humans for training environments. Paper Presented at the Interservice/Industry Training, Simulation and Education Conference (I/ITSEC), November 26–29, Orlando, FL.

28 Prendinger H. & Ishizuka, M. (2004). Life-Like Characters – Tools, Affective Functions, and Applications. Cognitive Technology Series. Heidelberg: Springer.

29 Rickel, J., Gratch, J., Hill, R., Marsella, S., & Swartout, W. (2001). Steve goes to Bosnia: Towards a new generation of virtual humans for interactive experiences. In papers from the 2001 AAAI Spring Symposium on Artificial Intelligence and Interactive Entertainment. Technical Report FS-00-04. Stanford University, Stanford, CA.

30 McCauley, L. & D'Mello, S. (2006). MIKI: A speech enabled intelligent kiosk. In J. Gratch, M. Young, R. Aylett, D. Ballin, & P. Olivier (Eds.). IVA 2006, LNAI 4133. Berlin/Heidelberg: Springer-Verlag, pp. 132–144.

31   Babu, S., Schmugge, S., Barnes, T., & Hodges, L. (2006). What would you like to talk about? An evaluation of social conversations with a virtual receptionist. In J. Gratch M. Young, R. Aylett, D. Ballin, & P. Olivier (Eds.). IVA 2006, LNAI 4133, Springer-Verlag, Berlin/Heidelberg. pp. 169–180.

32   Rossen, B, Lind, S, & Lok, B. Ruttkay, Z., Kipp, M., Nijholt, A., & Högni Vilhjálmsson, H. (2009). Human-centered distributed conversational modeling: Efficient modeling of robust virtual human conversations. Zs. Ruttkay et al. (Eds.). IVA 2009, LNAI 5773, pp. 474–481.

33   Kenny, P. G., Parsons. T. D., Gratch J., & Rizzo, A. A. (2008). Evaluation of Justina: A virtual patient with PTSD. In H. Prendinger, J. Lester, & M. Ishizuka (Eds.). IVA 2008, LNAI 5208, pp. 394–408.

34   Martin, J. M. ATZL-CTN-I, August 8, 2014, subject: *Emergent Leader Immersive Training Environment (ELITE) Lite Accreditation*. US Government Document.

35   John, B. S., Talbot, T. B., Lyon, T., Rizzo, A., & Buckwalter, J. G. (2013). Training effective investigative child interviewing skills through use of a virtual child: A pilot study comparing two different skill-level groups performance with a prototype of the Virtual Child Witness (VCW) program. In Fifth International Pediatric Simulation Symposia and Workshops, April 23–25. New York Academy of Medicine, New York: IPSSW, p. 236.

36   Talbot, T. B., Sagae, K., John, B., & Rizzo, A. A. Designing useful virtual standardized patient encounters. Interservice/Industry Training, Simulation and Education Conference Proceedings, 2012, December 3–6, Orlando, FL USA.

37   Kumatani, K., Arakawa, T., Yamamoto, K., McDonough, J., Raj, B., Singh, R., & Tashev, I. (2012). Microphone array processing for distant speech recognition: Towards real-world deployment. Proceedings of the APSIPA ASC, December 3–6, Hollywood, CA USA.

19

THE DIGITAL PATIENT: CHANGING THE PARADIGM OF HEALTHCARE AND IMPACTING MEDICAL RESEARCH AND EDUCATION

V. Andrea Parodi

Virginia Modeling, Analysis and Simulation Center, Old Dominion University, Suffolk, VA, USA

INTRODUCTION

Not so many years past, the study of anatomy and physiology (A&P) entailed spending long hours in the library "stacks" reading and memorizing details from Guyton's textbook and the beautiful Netter anatomical illustrations. Those drawings were our roadmap, helping to steer our way through the body's curves, connections, contractions, and joints. A strong foundation in A&P was, and is, essential to formulate sound clinical assessment skills. But the road to building these skills in the digital age is quite different.

Today's medical and healthcare students are able to select learning tools that visualize aspects of the anatomy and physiology with far greater fidelity than we would have thought possible. The student can choose from an array of learning tools with methods that appeal to their individual learning style, as well as aspects of their active and mobile life style. Training methods range from being passive to highly interactive, even immersive. Some reinforce eye/hand coordination using task trainers, or systems with embedded haptics. But for all these educational advantages, the medical student of the digital age still faces significant educational and professional hurdles, like the time and cost of their education/ training, as well as the steady influx of new knowledge and technologies creating challenges for the medical instructor and students to remain current. These issues coincide with notable problems in a healthcare delivery system that is struggling to meet unmet societal healthcare needs. Impacting the education of physicians and other healthcare professionals, the students are educated and enter the American healthcare process amid concerns regarding the organization, management, and delivery of healthcare that falls short of

The Digital Patient: Advancing Healthcare, Research, and Education, First Edition.
Edited by C. Donald Combs, John A. Sokolowski, and Catherine M. Banks.
© 2016 John Wiley & Sons, Inc. Published 2016 by John Wiley & Sons, Inc.

delivering quality health care reliably, consistently, and affordably according to the "Roundtable" collaboration between the Institute of Medicine (IOM) and the Nation Academy of Engineering (NAE). They contend that as the scope and complexity of health-care demands increase, so will the challenges to efficiency. What is needed is the development of information about the systems' relative effectiveness of interventions [1].

Their goal for the healthcare system is simply to "deliver the best care every time, and to learn and improve with each care experience" [2]. Consequently, medical and the health-care professional students will train and ultimately enter a metric-driven system that will actively measure, among other things, patient outcomes. These outcomes will be evaluated as part of an extensively utilized process improvement program that impacts all aspects of the care delivery system while generating knowledge as a "natural by-product of patient care delivery" along with the digital records of the data created from that care [3].

As the healthcare system undergoes extensive system-wide overhaul, recommendations specific to medical education and residency training were made by the Carnegie Foundation in 2010, as part of a series of studies of professional education. This report stated that like Flexner, "...medicine has served as the 'model profession,' and most other professions and forms of professional education have been interpreted through the lens of medicine" [4]. But, substantial system-wide changes are being called for in the areas of "curricular integration, as well as the essential tension between standardization of curriculum and indi-vidualization of instructional opportunities, and the critically central role of professional and personal identity in learning to become a physician" [5]. Internally, medical education is reexamining how to best prepare the next generation of physicians, in a manner reflecting a legacy of quality academic and professional preparation, but in less time and in a more cost-effective manner for both the school and the student.

Emerging fields of science, such as systems biology, biomedical engineering, medical informatics, and integrative computational biomedicine using complex modeling and sim-ulation techniques are making significant inroads in medical science. A project like the Virtual Physiological Human (VPH) is collecting massive amounts of anatomical, physiological, and pathological human data internationally across disparate data networks to create an open, transparent, resource for education, research and the development of interventional procedures and therapies. The long-range goal for these programs and others like them is to have sufficient data to create the whole patient digitally from DNA to being fully represented as a human or the Digital Patient (DP). This patient is the "every" patient, young, old, female, or male, representing data from all races and ethnic groups, both healthy and those with significant pathology. Discoveries will no doubt offer incredible opportunities and solutions changing in many ways how and what can be provided for instructional support, and how research is conducted. It is highly likely there will be a rapid increase in research and development. Clinical practice, based on patient specific knowledge from the DP's data, will create a twenty-first-century view of medical practice that may routinely reflect collaboration with an expanded team that includes biomedical engineers, modeling and simulation professionals, and computer scientists. Consequently, physicians-in-training must be prepared to either be an active member of a team working with a com-putationally derived biomedical data set modeling human anatomy, physiology, and pathology, or be conversant enough with this type of data to use and benefit from such a system, or both. Curriculum and pedagogies, while currently all under self-study and trans-formation, will need to integrate the necessary capabilities for a VPH-type medical practice in medical school, and to further develop these skill sets in residency. This chapter looks at today's medical education and recommendations for curricular support of computational medicine and its translation to practice. The following sections will introduce the emergence of computationally based medical support in the United States. Then, the chapter will focus on the grandest of the digital medicine plans from Europe that is generating great interest and speculation. And finally, a presentation of education and training recommendations from panels of subject matter experts are presented and discussed relative to the transformative changes anticipated in the education of America's physicians.

OVERVIEW DIGITAL MEDICINE PROJECTS

Visionary leaders in systems biology, medicine, modeling and simulation, medical informatics, computer science, and engineering recognized the merits of bringing systems science and computational integration to the process of analyzing larges sets of aggregate human anatomical, physiological, and medical data. We are a society using and generating massive amounts of data. With the emergence of supercomputers, and the digitalization of almost every aspect of the world around us, and within us, we are now able to gather anatomical and physiologic measures in real time or near real time that provide great insight into the innermost functions of the human body, providing a valuable educational and clinical support. Through the use of predictive models, it will be possible to control/eradicate the effects of injury and illness through drug and interventional care protocols customized to the needs of an individual patient or tailored to a whole population. Programs like the DP will only increase the opportunities for population-based and health/disease-based models to add to the data that will ultimately support customization of treatments and therapies.

In 2014, researchers at a Conference on Knowledge Discovery and Data Mining in New York City noted that society is better at generating new information than analyzing what it already has. The researchers felt that this leads to inefficiencies in translating research into progress for humanity. They emphasized that we must accelerate our rates of real discovery and gave an example of one solution. This solution was an autonomous supercomputer system that was programmed to conduct a specific scientific literature review, analysis, and synthesis. This computer system, designed through a collaboration with IBM and Baylor College of Medicine, is making discoveries by identifying gaps in the literature, and it suggests areas for further inquiry or validation at rates beyond that of any human [6]. The automated knowledge discovery and data management system is just one example of the digital era's use of the growing data supply. The following information will present the development of early projects that evolved from the use of digital human data.

Visible Human Project®

Prior to the availability of present-day supercomputers, significant advancements were still being made. In 1986, the National Library of Medicine envisioned creating a collection of complete, anatomically detailed three-dimensional (3D) images of a normal male and female human body. The images and data came from a variety of sources such as cadaveric CT and MRI scans. These scans were able to generate a rich dataset from the digitized images producing organ and tissue images and measures of great detail. The ultimate goal of this collection called the Visible Human Project® (VHP) was "...to produce a system of knowledge structures that will transparently link visual knowledge forms to symbolic knowledge formats such as the names of body parts" [7]. These materials form an anatomy instructional and practice guide of great value to the learner and practitioner alike. As this project has grown, it continues to incorporate data from PET scans to microscopy and includes 3D model rendering tools. The accompanying data set continues today to be widely used by students and researches alike. From this project, research methods and hypothesis have emerged that would not have been possible without this rich resource.

Using digitalized data from the Visible Human Project, researchers were able to identify 83 acupuncture points along ascribed meridians, skin surface points, and blood vessels within a three dimensional plane. Point location was achieved through the use of computerized tomography data [8]. This research project exemplifies how access to the VHP data helped begin opening a door within Western medicine and into the medical practices of another culture. In this case, Chinese traditional medicine and acupuncture points were being mapped against other anatomical structures by location. Acupuncture, we are reminded, has a history of efficacious anecdotal reports spanning a history of 5000 years.

The data from VHP or other integrated computational biomedical datasets provide great opportunity and diversity for use, such as the development of a virtual endoscopy. The digital data enables the physician to conduct an invasive body examination using a noninvasive virtual method. Virtual endoscopy (or computed endoscopy) is a method of diagnosis using computer processing of 3D image datasets (i.e., CT or MRI scans) to provide simulated visualizations of patient-specific organs similar or equivalent to those produced by standard endoscopic procedures. Conventional CT and MRI scans produce cross-sectional "slices" of the body that are viewed sequentially by the radiologists who must imagine or extrapolate from these views what the actual 3D anatomy should be. Using sophisticated algorithms and high-performance computing, these cross sections may be rendered as direct 3D representations of human anatomy. Specific anatomic data appropriate for realistic endoscopic simulations can be obtained from 3D MRI digital imaging examination or 3D-acquired spiral CT data [9].

This is a remarkable breakthrough because…thousands of endoscopic procedures are performed each year. They are invasive and sometimes have serious side effects such as perforation, infection and hemorrhage. Virtual endoscopic visualization avoids the risks associated with real endoscopy, and when used prior to performing an actual endoscopic exam can minimize procedural difficulties and decrease the rate of morbidity, especially for endoscopists in training. Additionally, there are many body regions not accessible to or compatible with real endoscopy that can be explored with virtual endoscopy. Eventually, when refined, virtual endoscopy may replace many forms of real endoscopy. Although there has been speculation about virtual endoscopic capabilities since the early 1970's, as dramatized in the science fiction movie *Fantastic Voyage*, the recent availability of the Visible Human Datasets (VHD) from the National Library of Medicine coupled with the development of computer algorithms to accurately and rapidly render high resolution images in 3-D and perform fly-through examinations instead of inserting long instruments (endoscopes of any kind) into a patient, has provided modern realization of these capabilities. The VHD provides a rich opportunity to help advance this important new methodology from theory to practice [10].

And techniques such as this could have the benefit of greatly reducing patient discomfort, fear, and noncompliance with screening plans.

Virtual Soldier Project

In the 1990s, DARPA collaborated with Army medical research and a number of universities, with Stanford as the lead. This collaboration created the Virtual Soldier, a training program that used complex models and simulation, even holographic images to create high fidelity physiologic representations of unique battlefield-type wounds and the cardiac system. Using real-world-based specific patient scenarios and wounding patterns, this program was able to generate predictive outcomes based on patient condition, wounds, and the learner's selected interventional choices. Much of this demonstration project was computationally derived, giving the learner feedback related to the success of management of the virtual patient's trauma. This program would be considered unique and innovative to this day [11, 12].

The Virtual Physiological Human Project and the Digital Patient

We reviewed examples of how the use of digital human data and sophisticated computing capability coupled with complex modeling, simulation, and visualization can enable the modeling of biomedical and anatomical data with high degrees of complexity and holistic data representation. Various levels of simulation capability allow for improved outputs and analysis of discrete and continuous events, and the state-of-the-art visualization allows for graphics that can represent details [13]. With more robust computational methods and technologies available, medicine, biomedical engineering, and allied health disciplines are seeing greater opportunities for the use of computational biomedical science.

In 2001, the International Union of Physiological Societies established objectives "to develop and share separate but integrated computational models of the organs and systems that make up the human body and their structure and function in health and disease, ... eventually integrating them into a 'virtual human'" [14]. Coveney et al. further noted that all projects funded through this initiative would generate computational human organ and systems models representing healthy and disease states, and decision assist tools for the clinicians to project the best course of action for the DP [15].

Europe's way of aggressively progressing along this highly focused research plan was to base the work on the physiome concept. The physiome concept is "...a comprehensive framework for modeling the human body using computational methods which can incorporate the biochemistry, biophysics and anatomy of cells, tissues and organs" [14]. It was thought that the current way of conducting research was highly compartmentalized, lacked transparency, and was inefficient. Consequently, the VPH project came into existence. This new project incorporated an all-embracing philosophy that includes many disciplines, nations, and approaches. Here is a description of the initial vision and function of the teams' work toward a final collaboration:

> Teams integrated their work based on the focused problem at hand, but the means to solving the problems were unconstrained as to scientific disciplines involved, anatomical subsystem studied, temporal or dimensional scales used. They expected the framework to be radical, thus deserving of the nature of the work at hand. They would make observations in laboratories, hospitals, clinics, across nations, collect, catalog, organize, and share observations and findings so that the clinical and non-clinical experts could collaboratively interpret, model, validate, and understand the data. Using this framework, the goal of the VPH, will be to create work that is descriptive; that the scientists and clinicians enable integrative analysis and develop systemic hypothesis that incorporate the knowledge of multiple scientific disciplines; and that the framework should be predictive and facilitate the interconnection of predictive models defined at different scales, with different methods and with different levels of detail, producing systemic networks that breathe the life into systemic hypotheses; simultaneously, the framework should enable their validity to be verified by comparison with other clinical or laboratory observations [16].

This highly ambitious work, as described by Hunter et al., describes the key stages of the VPH model development as follows:

- **Descriptive stage**: This stage includes using refereed journal publications to describe experimental data and to develop the quantitative aspects of the models. Researchers from labs all over the world are willing to help identify key papers for this literature search. Then the papers are placed in a web-accessible database with review comments from experts in the field. Since the ultimate goal of the project is health related, it is important that documentation is such to make it accessible to clinicians and biologists without "particular mathematical expertise."
- **Formulation stage**: Biologic data is transformed into mathematical models containing the variables and parameters of interest.
- **Implementation stage**: Mathematical analysis is conducted to solve systems of equations via computer simulation. A second analysis of the original analysis is often conducted to further reduce the model. This is the stage that forms links between models at different levels, for example, between the cell to the tissue level, to the organ level.
- **Model validation**: When validating the model, it is important to use independent data that has not been used in the original model formulation.
- **Biomedical interpretation**: This is the end process of using the model to gain insight into the biology and pathology, which is the goal of project. This is hypothesis-driven research [14].

It is also Hunter's contention that in time, there will be a union or link of the genomic and proteomic data revolution, with the revolution in medical imaging and the physiome data for an individual. It will take the merging of these revolutions to generate the vast data needed to enable the treatment or diagnosis of diseases. Then the data will span all spatial and temporal scales [17]. When this is all achieved medical practice, healthcare management and clinical research will indeed be radically different and changed forever.

Characteristics of the VPH Program

For any healthcare system to be deemed successful, and the VPH is such a program, four major characteristics should be evident. The system should be *personalized*, reflecting the unique needs of a single person or a unique group, especially related to prognosis, diagnosis, and treatment. The data would support *predictive* capabilities to enable the physician to be more proactive, timely, and specific and the system must be *integrative* for it to function, from the infrastructure to the data acquisition to aggregation or sequestration. And, finally, the system needs to be *affordable*. As escalating costs are anticipated with the increasing numbers of aging in the population as a normal consequence, this situation is likely to be accentuated by presumed extended life expectancy [18].

The VPH program is all about the generation of "actionable" knowledge and the deliverables to support this knowledge. The program is strongly focused on translating research models that are being developed into real, usable clinical applications. For example, a decision assist tool must be specific to the person or situation to have value, predictive to enable the support needed and expected, integrated with current data or near-real-time date to generate the best possible solution, and affordable to provide a cost benefit. But, what will make one clinical application stand apart from another usually comes down to the interface with the actual people who will use the device. The clinicians must be brought in from the beginning to the end of the design for features such as utility, ease of use, durability, and cleaning requirements to be incorporated into the design. This input is invaluable. Coveney et al. also recognized the importance of having ongoing clinical input on the VPH program team. In fact "… all VPH projects are expected to include clinicians and to aim to produce tools and simulations that are (or, at least, that have potential to be) of practical use in the clinic. … Simply stated human biology is a science of complexity. If a computational tool is to be accepted within the clinical community as, for example, an aid to rapid diagnosis or clinical decision making, it must be user-friendly, based on models reflecting community standards of practice and it must be validated to accepted standards of accuracy" [18].

In 2012, Hunter et al. set forth a vision and strategy that relates to the use of the modeling and simulation in VPH creating significant opportunities, the most compelling being the application of this data to tailor models with the unique characteristics and variables of an individual. It is possible to create a diagnosis, or therapeutic intervention, medical or surgical, that uniquely addresses the state of one individual. Likewise, this capability can also be used to "batch" the need characteristics and variables for target groups or populations. However, with the clinical focus being individualized, the physician can anticipate far more personalization of diagnosis, prognosis, treatment plans, and patient monitoring. One may also anticipate improved patient support or compliance as they are intimately involved in the treatment plan. Individualized treatments and interventions can take the form of a device tailor-made for the patient, or a drug that elicits a unique or targeted response. Screening and some interventions may be deemed necessary based on calculated or projected patient risk, not just generalized protocols. The DP is "…a vision of a coherent digital representation of each patient that is used to provide an integrative framework for personalized, predictive, and integrative medicine" [18].

PERSONALIZED PATIENT CARE CLINICAL USE

How do the findings, results, or deliverables stemming from the analysis of the DP data translate to clinical practice? Using a modification of the wholistic and dynamically organized Neuman's Systems Model as a guiding conceptual framework, individualized DP recommendations and deliverables can be associated with an anticipated level of interventional care to estimate likely real-world use. This model has been used internationally to guide both clinical practice and clinical education across a number of disciplines and is predominantly a wellness-oriented view of the continuum of health to illness. Briefly, the patient (pt.) or client is the center of the focus of care. The pt./client can be a unique individual or a group of people sharing some common element. At the core of the model is the basic person structure and resources comprised of inherent characteristics impacting health and wellness (i.e., one's genetic make-up, body strength, structure, and systems functionality). The basic structure has inherent strength and weaknesses and maintains a balance of wellness against stressors that may be from within, external, or environmental. Within the wholistic Neuman System's Model, the organization of the system considers the reaction of the client to stressors as a system taking into consideration the simultaneous effects of the interacting variables: physiological, psychological, socio-cultural, developmental, and spiritual. The concepts of De Chardin and Cornu have influenced Neuman's Model according to Neuman and Fawcett. They suggest that in any dynamically organized systems, the properties of a part are determined to an extent by the whole that contains it. … "This means that no part can be considered in isolation; each must be viewed as part of the whole. The single part influences our perception of the whole, and the patterns or features of the whole influence our awareness of each system part" [19].

The DP, as a unique individual, will promote the individual patient to routinely experience *primary prevention as a healthcare intervention*. The plan of care for primary prevention is to prevent illness, and injury for the patient and those around them. For example, the individual patient's immune system may be engineered to fend off many or most contagious diseases or a particular type of cancer. For another example, the patient may be identified at high risk for colon cancer and will have a plan of virtual colonoscopies created for him/her with their physician. What about using an individual's model of the likelihood of manifesting a genetic disorder? The unique information, specific and used in a timely fashion, could become a decision-assist tool for the patient and physician together, enabling genetic counseling to be far more specific regarding the likelihood of manifestation, if one was contemplating having a child. This informs and empowers the patient. The physician is able to provide a more detailed and informative guide to his or her patients, enabling them to better decide their choices of care.

For the DP as individual, the *secondary prevention as a healthcare intervention* would create or recommend ways to mitigate or largely eliminate acute care requirements such as avoiding preventable illness and injuries, and minimize or correct/cure injury/illness or disease. The plan of care for secondary prevention is about managing actual conditions and symptoms while optimizing repair and function. The DP as individual may have created a medication to kill a virus or bacteria, attack a tumor, or design the approach for a complex surgical procedure and be able to rehearse the operative team. The DP as individual experiences *tertiary prevention as a healthcare intervention* by promoting the patient's re-adaptation, or re-education to prevent future occurrences of illness or injury, in addition to regaining or maintaining their health stability. The plan of care is initially focused on the reduction of pain, if appropriate, along with increased functionality including the activities of daily living, for both physical and cognitive needs, while promoting, teaching, and engineering for safety and function. The DP as individual may be able to benefit from the use of macro- or microprosthetics, such as customized major joint replacements to enable ambulation and steady gait, or increase the fine motor dexterity in one's hands. By reducing chronic discomfort while enabling greater independence for extended periods of time, the patient will reap an improved quality of life, and over all, this growing population of oldest old will likely demonstrate a reduction in the social and financial burdens of dependency. The use of the Neuman System's Model in this context of unique individual person, placed the proposed future capabilities of an evolving, complex, research-based system into a framework that helped generate a plausible view of what personalized clinical practice can be like from primary care to tertiary care levels. Correspondingly, the DP as a unique group or population could also have been demonstrated across the care levels reflecting the unique needs of the group through the specialized care they received, tailored to their needs. The Neuman System's Model helps frame the vision for identifying what is needed to support the educational and experiential preparation of clinicians for this exciting, but challenging new practice paradigm. The patient care plans, interventions, therapies, and medications derived from the individualized or personalized DP processes can be designed, researched, developed, validated, and tested virtually, prior to introduction to the live patient. This process adds to the patient's safety, and that of the clinical team. It enables fine-tuning or rejection of a therapy, device, medication, or procedure prior to doing actual harm.

Consequently, interventions focused toward primary, secondary, or tertiary care interventions will reliably be more efficacious. These positive patient outcomes are good for the health-care system, they are fiscally responsible, and provide valuable additional data to the clinician for follow-on studies.

RECOMMENDED EDUCATION AND TRAINING FOR VPH PROJECT PARTICIPATION

Establishing education and training competencies for team participation in the VPH or a program similar to the VPH comes best from those involved with the work and by looking at the composition of the team. Currently, team members work in the following areas: information technology, big data management and bioinformatics, biomedical modeling/simulation and visualization, genomics and proteomics, and structural and functional imaging. The VPH builds on a broad range of educational backgrounds, and disciplines. The majority of team members are engineers, or they have a physical science, or a computer science background, with few medical experts. Efforts to correct this imbalance focus on outreach, recruitment, as well as through training. But, there is a disconnection between the need for integrative research and the lack of interaction and collaboration between the research disciplines working largely separated from one another according to Lawford et al. "As a consequence, fragmented expertise and differing conceptual and terminological backgrounds have led to a situation where advanced integrative research increasingly depends on the availability of 'translators'" [20]. The literature reflects discussion related to the research *being conducted* in a vertical fashion and urges more of a horizontal approach. Although many disciplines are involved with this work, it does not appear to be conducted in an intraprofessional collaborative manner. These teams are challenged by competing taxonomies and a lack of standardization compounding the difficulties in collaboration. What is being described here is not unique to Europe or the VPH, but is rather common. Not only do the team members not see themselves as one team, but as many teams working on many parts independently with little communication. Hence, it is not surprising that the necessary integration of work to form a unified whole suffers. The teams are also challenged by the need to stay current. They are inundated with constantly emerging new scientific discoveries and technologies.

What has been done in Europe to sustain and grow the science and technology work-force for projects like the VPH and others like the VPH was to established the "Bologna process." "This is a collaboration between 46 European countries. It aims at building an integrated 'European higher education area,' where increased modularity of educational contents supports mobility of students and graduates" [20]. Overall, what is needed for proper preparation for VPH team membership is experience in the practical application of problem solving, interdisciplinary work experience, and a strong background in the sciences, especially engineering, biomedicine, and computer science.

It is also advisable to have experience and a demonstrated ability in dealing with technology and information handling, as well as the ability to communicate across subject boundaries, with a focus on the acquisition of common terminology to foster understanding, and a broad background of successful research. There are also system wide efforts to improve both undergraduate- and graduate-level education across Europe. The VPH also established a network of excellence (NoE). With 14 partners from the top academic institutions across Europe, the NoE comprises clinical and industrial advisory boards. Their aim is to support the VPH community, and promote success by training future specialists [21]. The design or identification of a curriculum supporting a physician workforce and support team able to participate in integrative computational biomedical research, design, or development, must incorporate both concepts of interdisciplinary team process and communication training supporting collaboration and safety. In addition to a strong science background, engineering, visual analytics, and the study specifically of modeling and simulation are core components of the VPH. Computer science and familiarity with technology in general is recommended.

Currently at the VPH lab, the data is annotated to support the clinician. Techs prepare data and models. They are reviewed and analyzed with the clinician to extract maximum advantage from the information. To support the analysis, heavy emphasis is placed on the visual analytics [22, 23]. Putting the clinician in the center of the process helps their understanding of the process as well as the cross learning and checking that are natural consequences.

Recommendations from the Institute of Medicine and National Academy of Engineering

The Carnegie Foundation issued a call to reform and transform the education of two of the largest healthcare professions: medicine and nursing [22–24]. Medicine is called to engage in new curriculum and pedagogies, as is nursing. But, nursing was found to be unprepared for the use of new technologies in our digital era. In fact, all aspects of our healthcare system is stressed, stretched, and all too often, unreliable. It is also clear that each group acting on their own will only confound an already burdened and flawed system. A strong, integrated and united system is possible only with programmatic transparency and open collaboration.

When trying to identify a resource for innovative ideas supporting academic reform, physicians and other healthcare clinicians in the United States sought council from the Institute of Medicine (IOM). In the United States, the National Academies of Sciences is the pre-eminent private society representing distinguished scholarship in science and engineering research. In 1863, the National Academy of Sciences was granted a charter by the Congress that mandates they advise the federal government on scientific and technical matters. In 1964, the National Academy of Engineering (NAE) was established under the National Academy of Sciences charter. The NAE sponsors engineering programs aimed at meeting national needs, encourages education and research, and recognizes the superior achievements of engineers. In 1970, the IOM was established. The IOM advises the federal government on issues related to medical care, research, and education.

In 2006, the Roundtable on Value & Science-Driven Health Care convened. The membership comprises a group of renown physicians, pharmacists, a nurse, a professor of public health and a lawyer, to be joined by a team of engineers. They established a goal that "… by the year 2020, 90% of clinical decisions will be supported by accurate, timely, and up-to-date clinical information, and will reflect the best available evidence" [25]. Over years of meetings, it was clear to the Roundtable that there was a need for cross-disciplinary collaboration and they identified engineering, with their system design science, as being able to make very positive contributions to the development of a learning healthcare system. They felt the goal of a learning healthcare system was to deliver the "best care every time, and to learn and improve with each care experience" [26]. The Roundtable established a series of workshops to develop the learning healthcare system by identifying learning opportunities from healthcare disciplines and teaching opportunities from engineering, particularly systems, industrial, and operations engineering.

Specific common themes were identified with the 2011 Roundtable report [27]. The following themes, observations, and recommendations reflect on approaches to creating a learning healthcare system in the United States:

- The healthcare system's processes must be centered on the right target—the patient.
- System excellence is created by the reliable allowance for tailored adjustments.
- Learning is a nonlinear process. There is a need to bridge the gap between formal clinical research trials and the use of process improvement for rapid cycle lessons learned. The goal is to constantly improve.
- Emphasize interdependence and tend to the process interfaces. Patients and information/data transfer are most vulnerable to error during periods of turnover. This clearly reflects and supports improved collaboration and the establishment of interprofessional education that promotes the knowledge of and respect for the disciplines one works with. There is also reference to the dangers of patient or patient information hand-offs. The use of a structured process to help organize, formalize, and safeguard the turnover process is becoming more commonly used (e.g., SBAR).
- Teamwork and cross-checks trump command and control. Establish a system of parity among all responsible parties. Foster teamwork principles of communication and work. Formalized training, such as TeamSTEPPS®, a patient safety and communication program based on crew resource management research, is strongly recommended as it deals with these issues, as well as the observations that follow.
- Performance transparency and feedback serve as the engine for improvement. Capture feedback and make adjustments.
- Expect errors in the performance of individuals, but perfection in the performance of systems. Safeguards and redundancies can deliver perfection in system performance. Use process mapping, embed prompts, cross-checks, and information loops.
- Align institutional rewards on the key elements of continuous improvement. Incentives can come from Human Resources (HR): rewards for improving efficiency, effectiveness, and safety of the system and patient outcomes.
- Education and research can facilitate understanding and partnerships between engineering and the health professions. Develop common vocabulary, concepts, and ongoing joint education and research activities that help generate stronger questions and solutions.
- Foster a leadership culture, language, and style that reinforce teamwork and results. Provide supportive and integrated leadership.

Areas for Innovation and Collaboration [28]

- Clarify terms and terminology
- Identify best practices
- Explore health professions education changes
- Advance the science of payment for value
- Explore fostering the development of a science of waste assessment and engagement
- Support the development of a robust health IT system

The Roundtable is an important group as their work targets practicing clinicians, but this group is also mindful of the issues and challenges of today's healthcare system. As we look to a future with data-driven practice, research and development, we must put the care delivery into context. For data-driven systems derived from the DP to provide the best possible outcomes, live patients must be assured that their interventions and medications are reliably safe. Hence, team process for communication and safety are requisite components of any clinical curriculum. It enhances not only safety and communication but also improves efficiency, with less waste creating less cost.

The observations and themes of the Roundtable also relate to issues within the VHP team as well. The recommendations based on themes and the way ahead for innovation and collaboration reflect areas for identifying capabilities for the emerging medical curriculum of the future.

FROM FLEXNER TO THE 2010 CARNEGIE REPORT

In 2010, an in-depth analysis of American medical schools and residency programs were conducted by the Carnegie Foundation as part of a series of professional preparation studies of five major disciplines (medicine, nursing, law, chaplaincy, and engineering). Interestingly, this was one hundred years after the original Carnegie-funded landmark study conducted by Abraham Flexner [29]. Unlike the medical school programs scrutinized by Flexner, the medical education of today is characterized by a great deal of creativity and innovation, yet changes still must be made. The 2010 report entitled "Educating Physicians: A Call For Reform of Medical School and Residency," notes that fundamental changes are needed to support the rising challenges to medical education. These changes include adopting new curricula, new pedagogies, and new forms of assessment [30]. In 1997, during the first meeting with the Board of Directors of the Foundation, Dr. Lee Shulman, President Emeritus of the Carnegie Foundation for the Advancement of Teaching, informed the group that he intended to "undo the unintended consequences of some of the Foundation's most successful historical contributions to the field of education including the Flexner Report… the very act of resolving one era's problems often contributed to the dilemmas of the next generation" [31]. Specifically, the Flexner Study made a clear distinction between "legitimizing a metric" that determined the rigor of a program or course in terms of the length of time and intensity of the course… Unfortunately, in doing so it reified the value of 'seat time' as a measure of academic rigor instead of looking to students' actual learning as the real gold standard. In fact, what Flexner advocated was: Standardization in rigorous education; Integration—This means physicians should train in university teaching hospitals and integrate laboratory advances with the practice at the bedside; Habits of inquiry and improvement—Formally, excessive use of rote memorization was used, Recommended that physicians are trained to "think like a scientist" and require medical education to be taught by scientifically trained faculty; Professional formation—This means that the school must facilitate close and sustained contact between learners and scientifically based faculty role models [32].

Over the century, as patient needs increased and the sciences grew, so too did schools of medicine, but not by absorbing, synthesizing and then simplifying the curriculum. Rather, the schools would grow "…through division and multiplication… New domains are added, new topics are identified, and new specializations are added to the canon. For each addition, there must be a new course, a new rotation, and a new set of journals. Yet medical students are expected to learn all these domains and somehow to connect, combine, and integrate them within their own understandings and their own professional identities…Medical schools need to foster more of these integrations rather than leave the work entirely to the students" [5]. In every discipline, there is the development of the professional identity. It is this identity that links the discipline with values such as integrity, ethical conduct, professionalism, and responsibility to name just a few. Cooke et al. contends that professional preparation and the formation of the professional identity, moral and ethical core of service was the most overlooked aspect of the students professional development. Consequently, one of the cardinal recommendations for curriculum reform is to incorporate the foundations of forming the physician's professional integrity so that the physician-in-training will have studies aimed at forming… "a deeply internalized moral responsibility" [5] in addition to the expected programs developing critical thinking, the sciences and complex technical competence. This is where standardization of content can be integrated into a curriculum fostering a more individual approach to the guided development of professionalism. It is at this point that one would anticipate Flexner cringing from the digression from standardization. This leads to the final recommendations (2010) made for curricular reform for medical schools and residency programs in the United States.

Recommendations for Medical Education and Residency Reform fom the 2010 Carnegie Foundation Report: Educating Physicians

In 2010, the Carnegie Foundation Report on medical education and residency programs identified four goals for medical education. These goals are largely an extension of and consistent with the work of Flexner. These goals are (1) standardization and individualization; (2) integration of core content, concepts, and skills; (3) insistence on excellence; and (4) formation of the professional identity [33].

Cooke et al. identified the educational goals along with those from Flexner's report and put the recommendations into the context of today. It is from this breakout that one can envision where the curriculum design would thread competencies for computational biomedical practice, and to a somewhat lesser degree, provide the ability to understand the process, benefits and concerns that may be raised with using DP data-based research, decision assists, or procedure/device development. At the core of the DP process is the use of complex modeling and simulation. It is reasonable to anticipate foundational-level knowledge be acquired in modeling and simulation for physicians in practice or in research science.

The following presentation of the educational goals for today's physicians helps align curriculum content. For example: (1) standardization and individualization reflects the need to standardize learning outcomes through assessment of competencies. This also brings up considerations related to setting the grade criteria and standards as well as alternative approaches to grading. Guskey makes a case against percentage grades stating they distort accuracy, objectivity and reliability [34]. McGaghie et al. favor the use of mastery-level performance based on the use of deliberate practice [35]. (2) Integration refers to connecting formal knowledge to clinical experiences. It also identifies where immersive opportunities should be given to advanced learners while engaging all learners at all levels with more comprehensive patient experiences. This might be where an immersive humanitarian mission experience might be conceptually linked. After being conceptually linked, there exists an opportunity for inserting interprofessional education and essential concepts and techniques of teamwork into the curriculum. These are not spectator events; they must be practiced. This conceptual slot is linked with the learner experiencing the broader professional roles of physician including educator, advocate, investigator, or VPH-like team member. (3) Habits of inquiry and quality improvement enable the learner to engage in addressing problems and learn the process of improvement through inquiry, innovation, and evaluation of the quality of the care. Orient the learner to initiatives based on population health, quality improvement, and patient safety. Identify and teach clinical education topics outside of a teaching hospital environment in a setting of quality patient care. (4) Professional formation denotes the promotion of ethics, through various means, like stories or cere-monies. Learners should be given opportunities to reflect on professionalism in the context of monitoring and advising. Offer and allow feedback. Promote faculty relationships that support learners and hold them to high standards [36]. The role of the physician in a VPH-like team should include the ethical oversight of the DP process. Concerns have been raised regarding rights of intellectual property, and liability if a predictive model or designed therapy generates a negative patient outcome [37]. The final curriculum recommendation gives ample opportunity to use interesting and innovative pedagogies (simulation, serious games, virtual reality, augmented reality) to inspire, engage, and clarify students under-standing and commit to excellence and continuous improvement in all things.

SUMMARY STATEMENTS

The near future poses great challenges from new technologies, and the use of DPs as part of the physician's future practice. This novel practice influences treatment modalities, therapeutics, and even surgical interventions. Of significance, the recommendations made by the IOM and the NAE reflect recommended solutions for our nation's healthcare system, but also reflect recommendations for similar problems in both the VPH team and targeted goals and objectives for American medical education. However, there is not a single targeted or prescribed academic degree, or specific course of study that best prepares the physician-in-training or resident for integration into the practice of medicine in a computa-tional biomedicine team. But, general recommendations do include acquiring a strong foundation in the sciences, familiarity with computers and principles of biomedical engineering and mathematics. Modeling and simulation is an important course of study for those interested in VPH-like team membership, as are competencies in team communica-tion and patient safety. These capabilities need not be a fixed course, but integrated into every course as the "way to do business." This approach helps simplify the number of courses offered, yet promotes the content, facilitating collaboration and respectful, but firm negotiation. Experience in an interprofessional working team will prepare the learner for interdisciplinary discussions and valuable learning about the shared roles and responsibil-ities of other professions as well as heighten one's awareness of their own disciplinary responsibilities to the patient, science, and the discipline. The team communication and safety program components of the curriculum should be considered graded content; otherwise, the likelihood of behavior adoption across the enterprise would be low. Like Flexner's input, the four goals for the curriculum development threads have stood the test of time, with some modifications. The development of new and evolving medical education programs supporting the DP will bring medical practice to new scientific heights. But, while remaining grounded in the four educational goals with twenty-first-century objectives, educators must be mindful and clarify to their students that we owe respect, dignity, and security to our to our human patients, always.

REFERENCES

1 IOM (Institute of Medicine). 2011. Engineering a learning healthcare system: A look at the future. Workshop summary. Washington, DC: The National Academies Press.

2 IOM (Institute of Medicine). 2011. Engineering a learning healthcare system: A look at the future. Workshop summary. Washington, DC: The National Academies Press, p. 1.

3 IOM (Institute of Medicine). 2011. Engineering a learning healthcare system: A look at the future. Workshop summary. Washington, DC: The National Academies Press, p. 2.

4 Cooke M, Irby DM, O'Brien BC. Educating Physicians: A Call for Reform of Medical School and Residency. San Francisco, CA: Jossey Bass; 2010, p. viii.

5 Cooke, M, Irby, DM, O'Brien, BC. Educating Physicians: A Call for Reform of Medical School and Residency. San Francisco, CA: Jossey Bass; 2010, p. ix.

6 Supercomputers Make Discoveries that Scientists Can't – Tech – 27 August 2014 – New Scientist. Available at: http://www.newscientist.com/article/mg22329844.000-supercomputers-make-discoveries-that-scientists-cant.html#.VDF9hucOtq4. Accessed October 5, 2014.

7 The National Library of Medicines Visible Human Project. Available at: http://www.nlm.nih.gov/research/visible/visible_human.html. Accessed October 8, 2014.

8 Kim J, Kang D-I, Soh K-S, Kim S. Analysis on postmortem tissues at acupuncture points in the image datasets of visible human project. *Journal of Alternative & Complementary Medicine*, 2012;18(2):120–129.

9 Robb RA. Virtual (Computed) Endoscopy. 1990. Available at: http://www.nlm.nih.gov/archive/20120612/research/visible/vhp_conf/robb/robb_pap.htm. Accessed September 12, 2014.

10 Robb RA. Virtual (Computed) Endoscopy. 1990. Available at: http://www.nlm.nih.gov/archive/20120612/research/visible/vhp_conf/robb/robb_pap.htm. Accessed September 12, 2014, p. 1.

11 Ward R, Pouchard L. Visual Interface to Human Medical Data. The Virtual Soldier Hotbox, 2005. Available at http://www.virtualsoldier.us/hbox.htm (accessed October 20, 2015).

12 The Virtual Soldier Project. Available at: http://www.virtualsoldier.us/. Accessed October 9, 2014.

13 Sokolowski JA, Banks CM. A proposed approach to modeling and simulation education for the medical and health sciences. In: Proceedings of the 2010 Summer Simulation Conference, July 11–15, 2010, Ottawa, Canada.

14 Hunter P, Robbins P, Noble D. The IUPS Human Physiome Project. *Pflugers Archives: European Journal of Physiology* 2002;445(1):1–9.

15 Coveney PV, Diaz-Zuccarini V, Graf N, Hunter P, Kohl P, Tegner J, Viceconti M. Integrative approaches to computational biomedicine. *Interface Focus* 2013;3(2):2.

16 Fenner JW, Brook B, Clapworthy G, Coveney PV, Feipel V, Gregersen H, et al. The EuroPhysiome, STEP and a roadmap for the virtual physiological human. *Philosophical Transactions of the Royal Society A.* 2008;366(1878):2979–2999. Available at: http://rsta.royalsocietypublishing.org/content/366/1878/2979. Accessed August 5, 2015.

17 Hunter P, Robbins P, Noble D. The IUPS human physiome project. *Pflugers Archives: European Journal of Physiology* 2002;445(1): 8.

18 Hunter P, Chapman T, Coveney PV, Bono B de, Diaz V, Fenner J, et al. A vision and strategy for the virtual physiological human: 2012 update. *Interface Focus.* 2013;3(2). Available at: http://rsfs.royalsocietypublishing.org/content/3/2/20130004. Accessed August 5, 2015.

19 Neuman B, Fawcett J. The Neuman Systems Model, Vol. 448, 5th edition. Boston, MA: Prentice Hall; 2010, p. 13.

20 Lawford PV, Narracott AV, McCormack K, Bisbal J, Martin C, Brook B, et al. Virtual physiological human: training challenges. *Philosophical Transactions of the Royal Society A.* 2010;368(1921): 2842.

21   Lawford PV, Narracott AV, McCormack K, Bisbal J, Martin C, Brook B, et al. Virtual physiological human: training challenges. *Philosophical Transactions of the Royal Society A.* 2010;368(1921): 2844.

22   Roadmap for the Digital Patient." (The Digital Patient Community and the DISCIPULUS Consortium). EU Project Discipulus. Vanessa Díaz-Zuccarini, Marco Viceconti, Veli Stroetmann, and Dipak Kalra (eds). 2013.

23   Cooke M, Irby DM, O'Brien BC, Shulman LS (foreword by). Educating Physicians: A Call for Reform of Medical School and Residency. San Francisco, CA: Jossey Bass; 2010, 320 pp.

24   Benner P, Sutphen M, Leonard V Day L. Educating Nurses: A Call for Radical Transformation. San Francisco, CA: Jossey Bass; 2009.

25   Engineering a Learning Healthcare System: A Look at the Future: Workshop Summary. Washington, DC: National Academies Press; 2011. 307 pp. Available at: http://www.nap.edu/catalog.php?record_id=12213. Accessed August 5, 2015, p. 4.

26   Engineering a Learning Healthcare System: A Look at the Future: Workshop Summary. Washington, DC: National Academies Press; 2011. 307 pp. Available at: http://www.nap.edu/catalog.php?record_id=12213. Accessed August 5, 2015, p. 2.

27   Engineering a Learning Healthcare System: A Look at the Future: Workshop Summary. Washington, DC: National Academies Press; 2011. 307 pp. Available at: http://www.nap.edu/catalog.php?record_id=12213. Accessed August 5, 2015, p. 7.

28   Engineering a Learning Healthcare System: A Look at the Future: Workshop Summary. Washington, DC: National Academies Press; 2011. 307 pp. Available at: http://www.nap.edu/catalog.php?record_id=12213. Accessed August 5, 2015, pp. 23–24.

29   Markel H. Abraham Flexner and his remarkable report on medical education: A century later. *JAMA.* 2010;303(9):888–890.

30   Cooke M, O'Brien BC. Educating Physicians: A Call for Reform of Medical School and Residency. San Francisco, CA: Jossey Bass; 2010, p. 304.

31   Cooke M, O'Brien BC. Educating Physicians: A Call for Reform of Medical School and Residency. San Francisco, CA: Jossey Bass; 2010, pp. v–vi.

32   Cooke M, O'Brien BC. Educating Physicians: A Call for Reform of Medical School and Residency. San Francisco, CA: Jossey Bass; 2010, p. vi.

33   Cooke M, O'Brien BC. Educating Physicians: A Call for Reform of Medical School and Residency. San Francisco, CA: Jossey Bass; 2010, p. 23.

34   Guskey TR. The Case Against Percentage Grades. *Educational Leadership.* 2013;71(1):68. Available at: http://proxy.lib.odu.edu/login?url=http://search.ebscohost.com/login.aspx?direct=true&db=f5h&AN=90068952&site=eds-live&scope=site. Accessed August 5, 2015.

35   McGaghie WC, Issenberg SB, Cohen ER, Barsuk JH, Wayne DB. Does simulation-based medical education with deliberate practice yield better results than traditional clinical education? A meta-analytic comparative review of the evidence. *Academic Medicine.* 2011;86(6):706–711. Available at: http://www.ncbi.nlm.nih.gov/pmc/articles/PMC3102783/. Accessed August 5, 2015.

36   Cooke M, O'Brien BC. Educating Physicians: A Call for Reform of Medical School and Residency. San Francisco, CA: Jossey Bass; 2010. 304 pp. 25–26.

37   Fenner JW, Brook B, Clapworthy G, Coveney PV, Feipel V, Gregersen H, et al. The EuroPhysiome, STEP and a roadmap for the virtual physiological human. *Philosophical Transactions of the Royal Society A.* 2008;366(1878):2979–2999. Available at: http://rsta.royalsocietypublishing.org/content/366/1878/2979. Accessed August 5, 2015, p. 2989.

20

THE DIGITAL PATIENT: A VISION FOR REVOLUTIONIZING THE ELECTRONIC MEDICAL RECORD AND FUTURE HEALTHCARE

RICHARD M. SATAVA

Department of Surgery, University of Washington, Seattle, WA, USA

INTRODUCTION

The electronic medical record (EMR) of today is literally an electronic version of the centuries-old paper medical record. Data are entered textually (or an image is pasted/linked to the record). Some EMRs contain "tools" that can automatically transform the data into a graph, a chart, or a report, for the purposes of comparison, trending of data, etc., as well as search for specific information nearly instantaneously. Likewise, the data (including the images) in the EMR can be immediately transported literally anywhere in the world. While these changes are a huge step beyond the printed record, they are simply an incremental improvement over the paper records. Instead of collecting together sheets of paper with exactly the same data, sending paper physically from one department (or place) to another, or picking up the x-ray film or video with the chart, these functions are being done (supposedly) cheaper, faster, and more efficiently—electronically. The truly disruptive technology that fundamentally changes record keeping is the "Digital Patient" as the EMR. The forerunner of the Digital Patient is the 'Visible Human Project' (1994 – the National Library of Medicine), the first total body scan (with accompanying photographs), under the direction of Dr. Michael Ackerman, MD, and performed by Dr. Victor Spitzer, PhD, and Dr. David Whitlock, MD, PhD [1]. A complementary project called the "Digital Anatomist Project" was performed by Cornelius Rosse, MD, DSc, and by James Brinkley, PhD at the University of Washington was building the software infrastructure, ontology, and taxonomy that would generate the image of the "Visible Human" [2]. Subsequently, researchers such as William E. Lorensen, PhD of General Electric Research Center (GERC) who developed

The Digital Patient: Advancing Healthcare, Research, and Education, First Edition.
Edited by C. Donald Combs, John A. Sokolowski, and Catherine M. Banks.
© 2016 John Wiley & Sons, Inc. Published 2016 by John Wiley & Sons, Inc.

the "marching cubes' algorithms that permitted automatic segmentation of CT and MRI image, and many others contributed over time to the Visualization Tool Kit (VTK) that provided the computational and analytic tools necessary to necessary to bring (three-dimensional) 3D patient images "to life" and presage the rise of the Digital Patient.

The **Digital Patient** is defined as a full 3D dynamic interactive model of a patient, based upon a reconstructed anatomical image (CT or MRI total body scan—preferably when the patient is well), into which is instantiated the mathematical algorithms that define the properties of the anatomy, physiology, genetics, behaviors, etc. from the macroscopic to nanoscopic levels. When the patient-specific data are added to the Digital Patient model, then an "information equivalent" of that patient results—in the most minute detail of every parameter that makes up that individual—as a visual representation of that patient. The term that refers to this image is frequently called an "avatar," which is defined as "manifestation in human form [3]" or in computer terms "graphical representation of the user or the user's alter ego or character" [4]. Initial research by the Defense Advanced Research Projects Agency (DARPA) Virtual Soldier Project [5] coined the term "HOLOMER" (holographic medical electronic representation) to explicitly designate the scientific use of such a virtual object (an avatar), specifically for medical purposes and to differentiate a holomer from many other uses of avatars. The holomer is simply the image (virtual object—which is the Digital Patient Avatar) and all its data and algorithms, whereas the *Digital Patient is the holistic term* that incorporates not only the holomer but also all the applications and the "personalization" of the holomer for a specific individual—the holomer looks and responds exactly like the person. The following section on "applications" will expand upon the critical aspect of the holistic approach, and the overall impact on the broad range of effects that the Digital Patient (and to a certain extent, the holomer) will have upon disrupting the approach to medical record keeping by going back to the most fundamental "first principles" of integrating patient care, education/training, and research to radically enhance the basic capabilities of the EMR.

Before leaving the Digital Patient, it is also essential to mention the "artificial medical organic representation" (ARTIMOR). This is an entirely new concept, based upon new research in tissue engineering, regenerative medicine and microelectromechanical systems (MEMS)—it is a physical compliment to the holomer. The DARPA microphysiologic system (MPS) research project defines it as a "human-body-on a-chip" [6], which is a "microfluidic chip with all the major different tissues and organs of the patient." Today, there are commercial generic "organs-on-a-chip" [7] that are grown from stem cells and differentiated into various cell types and microsized organs, and are used for toxicology, drug screening, basic science research, etc. The holomer and artimor are, respectively, information representations and living representations of the patient—and in the future the two chips could be on a single card, and although complimentary, they will provide different functions.

The **electronic medical record (EMR)** in its present form is a static dataset, in which each parameter is entered into the record without linking to or affecting any other parameter. Because of the underlying equations and algorithms (physiologic, biochemical, neuro-endocrine, behavioral, etc.) in the proposed Digital Patient, the EMR will become dynamic; and when one parameter changes, it will affect other parameters that are linked to it. In addition, the current EMR is viewed by reading text, or perhaps by looking at a static image, chart, graph, etc.; however, the Digital Patient is a *whole new interface*—it is an interactive, dynamic visual record (holomer) of the actual patient; when a parameter changes, the image may visually change. This is an intuitive interface—you actually see the image transform as affected by the data change. Thus, once the Digital Patient (with its imaging and algorithms) becomes the interface, then the full power of modeling and simulation can be employed—this will be elaborated later.

The EMR comprises two components: personal information (about the person) and healthcare information (about the provision of care to that person by a healthcare provider). In addition to what the current EMR provides in terms of personal and provision of care aspects, the Digital Patient will be able to provide prediction of outcomes, based upon evidence-based simulation. An example of this would be giving a patient a medication. It will be possible to input dozens of variations of the same medicine or many trials of different medications to the Digital Patient, with the simulation (nearly immediately) providing likely outcomes of the individual variations—with the opportunity to select the best medication with the greatest effect and least chance of complications. This use of simulation is standard practice in non-medical disciplines—creating dozens of virtual models of a new product, subjecting the virtual models to literally hundreds of various tests, and determining the best design and function of the various models—before building an actual product. Admittedly, the human body is much more complex that a sophisticated machine; however, the fundamental principle of the use of simulation to test, evaluate, and select highest quality with least complications is applicable.

Another aspect of the EMR is the acquisition of data to be entered into the record. At the moment, most information is entered in typographically, though everyday more data are being directly uploaded from the diagnostic machine (lab test, x-ray, etc.). In the immediate future, the automatic uploading of personal data will exponentially increase. A combination of the many new health sensors that are being worn and the "Internet of Things" ("smart," everyday appliances, devices, instruments, and even automobiles) will be sensing data (not only physiologic and biochemical but also behavioral and social interaction data) about every person, and transmitting the data back to their "personal record" on the Internet. The initial implementation is currently beginning with the elderly and "smart houses," which monitor the elder person's physical, behavioral, and emotional status from sensors throughout their home—allowing many persons to remain in their own home rather than be confined to a nursing home. While it will be nearly impossible to monitor all that data in the current EMR, the Digital Patient will be able to present that data in near real time in an easily understood visual form.

APPLICATIONS OF THE DIGITAL PATIENT AS THE EMR

The applications of the EMR are focused on clinical care; however, the real advantage is that the information in the EMR should be "repurposed" as de-identified data, for all aspects of healthcare—clinical care, education/training, and research—as well as for healthcare administration. It is true that all six aspects currently have some use of the EMR, including but not limited to the following applications:

1. clinical care;
2. as repository of information about the patient and progress of healthcare interventions;
3. infrequently as pre-operative planning (usually with x-ray, CT, or MRI images);
4. education/training, in the form of case presentations and case reports, yet very little in terms of training (i.e., procedures);

5. research, in terms of clinical trials and retrospective reviews; and
6. administration in terms of quality assurance, risk management, billing, etc.

However, the addition of the Digital Patient vastly opens up the opportunities in all four areas and opens new areas—the Digital Patient is an integrated "system of systems" record (e.g., a decrease in cardiac output will reflect changes in all the various organs, and neuro-endocrine pathways). The Digital Patient has inherent properties beyond those of the current EMR, such that there are common denominators for the expanded use of the EMR, which include the following:

- Intuitive (as above)—interacting visually with the image of the patient without searching through numerous menus, folders, hyperlinks, etc.;
- Dynamic and interactive—as information is added/changed by the healthcare provider or automatically downloaded from a device (e.g., lab report), the visual image is immediately updated, and the holomer visibly change;
- System of systems—due to the fact that all data are linked, the overall effect of a single change is translated through the various organs, tissues, etc.;
- Inter-operable—data from one patient can use the same holomer infrastructure to create a different patient specific Digital Patient; in doing so, huge databases of individual de-identified patients can be rapidly developed as well as integrated for meta-analyses;
- Three-dimensional image—allowing information can be seen intuitively by rotating, slicing, "fly-through," the image, providing perspectives not possible in the real patient;
- Predictive—by substituting different values for data, resulting in multiple outcomes from which to choose the best—personalized—result (see text).

One of the most important applications (and that is not currently in use) for the Digital Patient is the capability to develop "digital libraries," analogous to the various didactic educational tools such as case-based learning, etc. Of particular value is the use in training, where not only the skills to perform a generic procedure can be practiced, but also the numerous variations of disease presentations of that simple procedure (see the following text). It is the number of different variations of a specific activity (procedure) that allows a person to graduate from competent to expert.

In addition to the aforementioned clinical example of predictive analytics for clinical decision making in patient care, the following applications serve to illustrate the enormous opportunity of using the Digital Patient as the foundation for the EMR. Note that many of the applications provide advantages in more than a single area—for example, surgical rehearsal is valuable both for clinical care and education/training.

Surgical Rehearsal

One of the first reports of using a virtual model for surgical rehearsal was that of a lower extremity to predict outcomes of an orthopedic procedure (Achilles tendon transfer) by Scott Delp, PhD,and Joseph Rosen, MD, in 1990 [8], and although it was not a patient-specific image, the resulting gait was as predicted. Recently, Jacques Marescaux, MD, has begun using patient-specific images (from CT scan) of liver cancer to rehearse the surgical procedure in this very difficult procedure, resulting in a decrease in operating time by 25% and a decrease in blood loss from 5 units to 2 units per patient [9]. There are currently surgical rehearsal reports in numerous different surgical specialties. In addition, the first patient-specific surgical rehearsal simulator was for endovascular procedures, in which the angiogram of the patient was imported into the simulator, and the actual procedure was performed with exactly the catheters that were used during the simulation of the procedures. Today, there are a number of virtual reality simulators that are used for skills training (see the discussion later) that include the capability to import patient specific data (i.e., they are DICOM compatible). The use of such patient-specific surgical rehearsal is infrequent, and used principally for complicated procedures, mainly because the time spent rehearsing is significant (and is not reimbursable) and the realism of the images (and their responses) is still relatively simplistic. However, reports of preoperative surgical rehearsal had demonstrated reduced outcomes and fewer errors [10].

Virtual Autopsy

A "virtual autopsy," first described by Michael Thali, MD [11], is simply a total body scan on a deceased individual, to which specific computational tools are used (slicing, edge detection, fly through, etc.) to examine the image similar to performing a real autopsy. Due to numerous factors, clinical autopsy has decreased to only about 5–10% of all in-hospital deaths. Thus cause of death and final co-morbid diagnoses are deduced indirectly or from known pathology ante mortem in nearly all cases. While there is approximately 90% correlation of a virtual autopsy to a true autopsy, addition of virtual autopsy to the EMR would provide objective evidence on cause of death and comorbid conditions on all patients. An overlooked opportunity is the ability to "virtually exhume" the patient at a later time, when further forensic evidence or new research provides data that could change the final diagnoses.

In addition to the clinical and forensic applications, virtual autopsy provides a rich database for future research, especially in terms of meta-analyses of large populations for public health and objective evidence for critical national policies. By de-identifying the data from virtual autopsy, virtual cadavers (especially those with interesting diseases or anomalies) can be used for education in the anatomy laboratories at various levels from medical/nursing schools to residency and fellowship, as well as being available for surgical rehearsal for teaching specific surgical and other procedures. The virtual autopsy is yet one more source for developing "digital libraries." It has been proposed by Thali that imaging technologies will continue to greatly improve in resolution and fidelity, to a point where virtual histology will be available as well from scan [12], greatly enhancing the usefulness of a Digital Patient.

Virtual Education

The revolution in medical education is *objective assessment* and *training to proficiency*, both on real patients and on patient actors—this is an "evidence-based education," comparable to today's evidence-based clinical practice. The use of modeling and simulation can provide unique educational tools for teaching (cognitive), training (psychomotor skills), and assessing performance objectively and quantitatively. Virtual patients, derived from a digital library (database) of de-identified Digital Patients, can greatly enhance students' exposure to literally thousands of different "patient experiences," which is obviously not possible in the real world.

The Objective Structured Clinical Exam (OSCE) uses real actors who play roles of specific diseases for students to practice critical clinical skills and who are assessed with objective scoring tools that precisely score the student's performance. This is extremely costly in terms of paying actors, training both actors and evaluators, housing large educational centers, etc. Because of these costs, the number of "patients" that the student is exposed to is very limited. In addition, for complex diseases like diabetes, which has many different possible manifestations, the student is exposed to only one or two possibilities by real patients (actors). The use of virtual patients [13] (based upon real Digital Patient data and images) on a simulator or over the Internet can create the same educational value (including assessment of performance) as a patient actor [14]. Clearly, there are certain things that cannot be simulated (yet), and therefore the student must have exposure to some real patient actors. However, the student can be trained to a very large variation of the disease presentations using virtual patients, and improve performance (especially the cognitive, perceptual, psychomotor skills, and patient-interactive components) to a high level of proficiency at a fraction of the cost, as a prelude to an encounter with a patient actor.

A very expensive and high-risk patient experience for surgical training is performing complex surgical procedures, where errors (even simple errors), could result in fatal outcomes. The practice on animals, the see-one, do-one, teach-one method, or even mentoring on a live patient has unacceptably high risks. In addition, the assessment of an individual resident's performance under these conditions is extremely subjective and variable. The introduction of psychomotor skills and procedural simulators offers the opportunity to "practice" surgery in a safe environment with no harm to a patient when errors occur. In addition, assessment can be quantitative (the simulator measures precisely psychomotor skill performance), and the training to proficiency (i.e., correctly performed with absolutely no errors) can be achieved before the resident is permitted to operate upon a patient. This is accomplished by beginning with simple basic skills and incrementally progressing in complexity until full procedures are completed to a proficiency benchmark that has been determined by performance of experts. This is proficiency-based progression of surgical technical skills [15].

Surgical simulators are now constructed to accept patient-specific data (CT, MRI, etc.). As mentioned earlier, using data (specifically, the holomer) from a library of de-identified Digital Patients, would allow the resident to gain proficiency through a large experience of the many variations in which a surgical disease or injury could present. While surgical procedural simulation using virtual reality (VR) has been in use for over 20 years, the additional use of a vast repository of Digital Patient holomers that can be imported into the simulators represents a huge improvement in not only gaining proficiency but also gaining enough (virtual) experience to achieve expert status.

Virtual Clinical Trials

The challenges to conducting clinical trials are numerous—practical issues such as patient accrual (enough patients with consistency of inclusion criteria), scheduling both patient and researcher times, loss of follow-up before the end of the trial, etc.), and study design issues (enough patients to randomize to the necessary experimental groups, insuring all the patients have all the data collected, long duration needed for clinical outcomes, etc.) to mention a few. The de-identified database of Digital Patients (either centralized national registry or individual institution registries) provides the opportunity to perform virtual clinical trials, referred to as "randomized registry trials" [16]. Registries of Digital Patients would have uniform datasets, providing access to hundreds, thousands, or even millions of similar patients (with identical datasets, but every patient would have a unique set values for the each of the data points) with massive numbers of variables and follow-up over decades. Once the "clinical" trial is designed and the specific parameters to be included/excluded as the criteria are chosen, the registry(ies) could be searched for all patients meeting precisely all the criteria (including outcomes over decades of time) and simulate (computational analytics) the results over a weekend on a super-computer. This is accomplished by data-mining using Big Data (discussed later), which includes not only the precise patient specific data but also powerful analytical and computational tools. The data can be displayed not only by using typical tables, graphs, charts diagrams, etc. but also by using a composite holomer that intuitively displays results through visual representations of the various tissues, organs, or systems using 2D, 3D, or 4D visualization and cartographic techniques. Such visualization techniques not only instantly bring recognition of complex results but also prompt recognition of novel inter-relationships not possible with simple text or abstract charts and graphs. In addition, the variable parameters in the holomer can be interactively manipulated to immediately demonstrate the alternative outcomes possible as various parameters are changed (i.e., drug choice/dose, and tissue removal).

Personalized EMR—The Quantified Self

The personalized aspect of the EMR is the patient-specific database of an individual's health status. By definition, the personalized EMR contains all the information *about* the person, but not the care provided to the person. This is also referred to as the "quantified self" [17]. Currently, these data are available (usually) on a commercial password-protected website, and/or on a hospital EMR server as simple data in text, graphs, charts, etc. Often, there are "normal values" or simple interpretations as to what the values mean; however, for most persons, such information is difficult to interpret. With the holomer as the interface and the biologic/social/behavioral algorithms to generate the holomer, it would be easier (obvious) for the person to understand the meaning, since it is a visual image relative to their own body. Other applications include the personalized de-dentified dataset being made available (with the patient's permission) to various researchers for clinical trials, or to educators to increase their "digital libraries" in educating and training various learners (see section "Virtual Education"). Today, patients are paid to participate in clinical trials; perhaps, persons could "sell" their personalized EMR, without the risk of taking medications, undergoing "experimental" surgery, etc.

Hospital Enterprise Integration

The EMR, at the hospital level, is an enterprise investment. Currently, it is static, though it is updated as new information is acquired. There are search capabilities and some analytic/ reporting capabilities as well. Unfortunately, there are only the beginnings of integrating all the different databases such as, personal demographics, medical history, laboratory information, radiologic reports and images, operative reports, clinical notes, and a myriad of other independent (and usually noncompatible) datasets into a single system-of-systems repository. In addition to the personalized data and the data on the provision of healthcare to the patient (clinical notes, etc.), the Digital Patient (as an application of Big Data) will leverage the most powerful analytic/reporting tools to integrate the EMR as a unified system-of-systems asset of the entire hospital enterprise.

Big Data, Social and Behavioral Issues, and Politics

New technologies mentioned earlier have logarithmically increased the amount of data that are acquired about patients (personal) and the healthcare administered to them (patient care). This is Big Data [18, 19]—the amount of information that is massively accumulating daily. There will be enormous changes, especially socially and politically, because of the ubiquity of such data, and the instant access to that data (unless protected via password, etc.). The biggest opportunity is that patients, and especially healthcare providers, can immediately find out the answer to almost any question on their cell phone apps, tablets, watches, and numerous other devices, or through social media such as twitter, instant messaging, etc.—thus, the emphasis will be on being able to ask the right question. It will become less important to have memorized the information, so education needs to begin placing emphasis on how to ask questions and where to find the information you need. Equally important is how to convey (display) the information—and here the new social technologies and media will demand a format that is intuitive and yet imparts huge amounts of information on portable devices—"a picture is worth a thousand words." From a political standpoint, already we are seeing how instant access, sharing, and distributing information has placed immense pressure upon politicians to be absolutely correct before making statements, including healthcare issues. Immediate access to the type of Big Data, that is the Digital Patient, will hopefully assist in making more evidence-based decisions. Also, it will be interesting to see if the government agencies responsible for healthcare can promulgate information based upon healthy lifestyles: using visual documentation with tools such as the Digital Patient can bring relevance, intimacy, and immediacy of such messages to improve compliance for healthy life styles. And most important, the new technologies that define the Digital Patient are bringing new hope and therapies to sufferers of psychological disorders of Alzheimer's disease, degenerative neurologic diseases, and traumatic brain injury and post-traumatic stress disorder (TBI/PTSD) [19].

DISCUSSION

The concept of a Digital Patient has been around for more than 20 years, and evidenced by the quality scientific research described in the other chapters, there is a growing opportunity to solve some of our impending challenges, of which Big Data will become one of the most difficult. We are a victim of success; our technological discoveries have overcome our ability to understand and use the massive amounts of data that are being generated everyday. As little as 10 years ago, a terabyte of data (10^{12}) was virtually unknown, and today more than an exabyte (10^{18}) of data (a million terabytes) is being created everyday [18, 19], much of it in biomedical research and healthcare. The Digital Patient is just one of the early attempts to harness the power of this wealth of knowledge, and the incorporation of the technologies and applications of the Digital Patient as the EMR may well be the first steps into a most extraordinary healthcare future. The challenges in developing the Digital Patient are huge, but bootstrapping current successes in modeling/simulation, biologically based algorithms, predictive analytics, data visualization, intuitive interfaces, and other emerging tools will redirect the social, cultural, behavioral, and political landscape for the future of healthcare.

CONCLUSION

As massive volume, variety, and rate of generating information threatens to overwhelm our ability to use this information to improve healthcare, a new paradigm needs to be developed. The Digital Patient as the medical record provides one positive step to exploit the underlying technologies to manage our patients with higher quality and safety. The barriers are high, the amount of work needed is extraordinary, and the cost is not inconsequential. However, continuing on the same old pathway of tweaking the EMR with minimal incremental improvements is not an option. The concepts herein, derived from the evidence in the chapters of this book, will signal at least one important solution (of the many needed) to create the next generation of healthcare.

REFERENCES

1 Ackerman MJ, Spitzer VM, Scherzinger AL, Whitlock DG. The Visible Human data set: an image resource for anatomical visualization. *Medinfo*. 1995;8 Pt 2:1195–8.

2 Rosse C, Mejino JL, Modayur BR, Jakobovits R, Hinshaw KP, Brinkley JF. Motivation and organizational principles for anatomical knowledge representation: the digital anatomist symbolic knowledge base. *J Am Med Inform Assoc*. 1998;5(1):17–40.

3 Oxford English Dictionary. Available at: http://www.oed.com (accessed February 21, 2015).

4 Wikipedia. Available at: http://en.wikipedia.org/wiki/Avatar_(computing) (accessed February 22, 2015).

5 Virtual Soldier Project. Available at: http://www.virtualsoldier.us (accessed February 22, 2015).

6 Pallotta B. DARPA/DSO Micro-Physiological System. Available at: http://www.darpa.mil/program/microphysiological-systems (accessed October 20, 2015).

7 Bhatia SN, Ingber DE. Microfluidic organs-on-chips. *Nat Biotechnol*. 2014;32(8):760–72.

8 Delp SL, Loan JP, Hoy MG, Zajac FE, Topp EL, Rosen JM. An interactive graphics-based model of the lower extremity to study orthopaedic surgical procedures. *IEEE Trans Biomed Eng*. 1990;37(8):757–67.

9 Soler L, Marescaux J. Patient-specific surgical simulation. *World J Surg*. 2008;32(2):208–12.

10 Fried MP, Satava R, Weghorst S, Gallagher AG, Sasaki C, Ross D, Sinanan M, Uribe JI, Zeltsan M, Arora H, Cuellar H. Identifying and reducing errors with surgical simulation. *Qual Saf Health Care*. 2004;13 Suppl 1:i19–26.

11 Thali MJ, Yen K, Schweitzer W, Vock P, Boesch C, Ozdoba C, Schroth G, Ith M, Sonnenschein M, Doernhoefer T, Scheurer E, Plattner T, Dirnhofer R. Virtopsy, a new imaging horizon in forensic pathology: virtual autopsy by postmortem multislice computed tomography (MSCT) and magnetic resonance imaging (MRI)—a feasibility study. *J Forensic Sci*. 2003;48(2): 386–403.

12 Thali MJ, Dirnhofer R, Becker R, Oliver W, Potter K. Is 'virtual histology' the next step after the 'virtual autopsy'? Magnetic resonance microscopy in forensic medicine. *Magn Reson Imaging*. 2004;22(8):1131–8.

13 Thalmann NM, Thalmann D. Towards virtual humans in medicine: a prospective view. *Comput Med Imaging Graph*. 1994;18(2):97–106.

14 Oliven A, Nave R, Gilad D, Barch A. Implementation of a web-based interactive virtual patient case simulation as a training and assessment tool for medical students. *Stud Health Technol Inform*. 2011;169:233–7.

15 Gallagher AG. Metric-based simulation training to proficiency in medical education: what it is and how to do it. *Ulster Med J.* 2012;81(3):107–13.

16 Lauer MS, D'Agostino RB Sr. The randomized registry trial—the next disruptive technology in clinical research? *N Engl J Med.* 2013;369(17):1579–81.

17 Smarr L. Quantifying your body: a how-to guide from a systems biology perspective. *Biotechnol J.* 2012;7(8):980–91.

18 Big Data. Available at: http://en.wikipedia.org/wiki/Big_data (accessed March 3, 2015).

19 Rothbaum BO, Rizzo AS, Difede J. Virtual reality exposure therapy for combat-related post-traumatic stress disorder. *Ann N Y Acad Sci.* 2010;1208:126–32.

21

REALIZING THE DIGITAL PATIENT

C. Donald Combs[1] and John A. Sokolowski[2]
[1] *School of Health Professions, Eastern Virginia Medical School, Norfolk, VA, USA*
[2] *Virginia Modeling, Analysis and Simulation Center, Old Dominion University, Suffolk, VA, USA*

> *The past turns out to be oddly reassuring because a pattern emerges. Each time we're faced with bewildering new thinking tools, we panic—then quickly set about deducting how they can be used to help us work, meditate, and create.*
> —Clive Thompson, *Smarter Than You Think*

Data are everywhere now, being aggregated, analyzed, and repackaged. We are in an era of Big Data, living with the recognition that almost everything we do is being captured as one or another type of data, with the hope that all that data can be used to help us become smarter, healthier, safer, and richer, and with the fear that our privacy is being invaded and that our risk for harm is increasing. It is in this broader context that this book addresses one of the more hopeful Big Data undertakings—that is, the construction and deployment of the Digital Patient.

The capacity to measure one's personal physiological and social metrics, compare those metrics with the metrics of millions of other humans, personalize needed therapeutic interventions, and measure the resulting changes will ultimately realize the vision of personalized medicine—wherein patients and their providers will be able to detect disease at an earlier age, provide optimal therapy based on the characteristics of each individual, and reduce adverse responses to therapy; where pharmaceutical companies can improve the process of drug discovery and clinical trials and where the healthcare industry's emphasis truly shifts from reaction to disease to prevention of disease and promotion of wellness. Implicit in this vision is the integration of a sustained focus on improving the outcome measures of healthcare—safety, effectiveness, patient-centered, timeliness, efficiency, and equity—into clinical practice.

Having the goal of improved outcomes for patients in mind helps to frame the importance of the Digital Patient: *it is among the most powerful tools that we can develop and*

The Digital Patient: Advancing Healthcare, Research, and Education, First Edition.
Edited by C. Donald Combs, John A. Sokolowski, and Catherine M. Banks.
© 2016 John Wiley & Sons, Inc. Published 2016 by John Wiley & Sons, Inc.

deploy to improve health. The most commonly referenced definition of the Digital Patient is that provided through the European Union's DISCIPULUS project: *a technological framework that, once fully developed, will make it possible to create a computer representation of the health status of each citizen that is descriptive, interpretive, integrative and predictive.* Not explicitly stated, but implied, is that this framework will include behavioral, social, temporal, and spatial dimensions in addition to the biological. An illustration outlining the stages involved in developing the Digital Patient framework is shown in Figure 21.1 (and described in more detail in Chapter 2).

Biologists have traditionally sought to understand living things largely by examining their constituent parts. For example, they studied individual genes, proteins, or signaling molecules to learn everything they could about the structure and function of a single biological entity. The emerging scientific strategies of system-of-systems analysis and convergence add a new dimension to this traditional approach. Researchers seek to understand both each constituent of a biological network and how all of a network's constituents function together. They use cutting-edge technologies to gather as much information as they could about a biological system. They then use this information to build mathematical and graphical models that account for the behavior of the system. They test these models by gathering additional data, often by perturbing a system through genetic or environmental changes. In this way, they build an understanding of biological systems that can be used, for example, to explore what goes wrong when a biological system becomes diseased and how to treat or prevent that disease. Increasingly, they also take into account the influence of behavior and social context on the biological system (see Chapters 7, 9, and 10).

The concept of a fully integrated Digital Patient, maintained with each person's current healthcare data, is powerful and compelling. Yet, the range of applications means the complexities are significant, not least in the areas of privacy and security. A few examples from the perspective of a patient expose some of this complexity (see also Chapter 9).

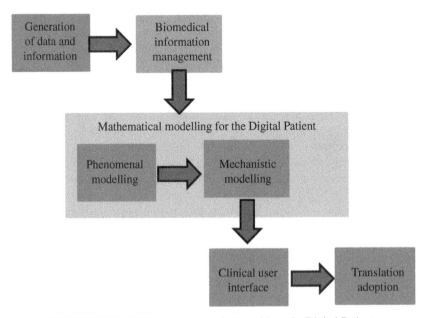

FIGURE 21.1   Different areas needed to achieve the Digital Patient.

Biomedical professionals require approved secure access to my personal data, routinely and in emergencies; my wearable and implanted technology must update my Digital Patient routinely with current status data; an alarming event, detected by a sensing device or Digital Patient computation, must inform me, my family and friends, and my trusted healthcare providers of the need for an intervention; the infrastructure must support the collaboration of multiple specialists around my complex, interacting diseases; models must be able to access a wealth of anonymized reference data, routinely amassed from patients.

Thus, privacy, synchronicity (the timeliness with which models produce actionable information) and clarity of data organization and analysis are fundamental challenges that must be addressed in completing the Digital Patient.

Further complicating the construction of the Digital Patient is the current lack of agreement on how we categorize patient information. As shown in Figure 21.2, an individual's patient data include molecular data and clinical data, and the two data sets are not often integrated in a manner that is understandable or easily usable by patients or healthcare providers. Developing a consistent terminology and aggregation methodology for this disparate data is therefore a fundamental challenge to the Digital Patient.

Figure 21.2 illustrates the breadth of the data that needs to be integrated in the Digital Patient. It also foreshadows yet another challenge—the development and consistent use of a common taxonomy and the evolution of useful ontologies.

Medical research comprises many disciplines and therefore many ways of describing data. During his research on constructing a concise medical taxonomy, McGregor identified 53 general topics derived from established medical specialties, recognized diseases, therapies, and general medical topics. He then subdivided the information into 374 topics and subtopics. When he compared the results of this subdivision with the MEDLINE Medical Subject Headings used to categorize research topics in medical journals, he was able to demonstrate that straightforward conceptual mapping is possible. Therefore, there is an existing basis for the more rigorous taxonomy of data required in an effective Digital

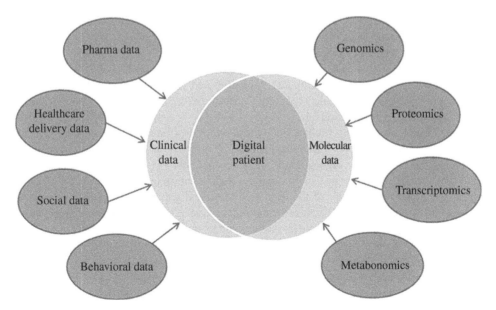

FIGURE 21.2   A sampling of data sources for the Digital Patient.

Patient. This insight is important for the contextualization and reliability of models and simulations supporting medical research and clinical practice (see Chapter 15).

Biomedical systems, as has been demonstrated throughout this book, are highly complex. Modeling this complexity accurately is, of course, essential to the Digital Patient. Therein lies another fundamental challenge—the integration of models operating at different temporal and spatial scales and, collectively, possessing some formidable characteristics:

Non-linearities: Many responses have upper and lower boundaries with different levels of physiological sensitivity in between.

Redundancy: Many physiological states are the result of multiple mechanisms pushing and pulling on the observable response. Redundancy makes it difficult for a researcher or clinician to identify important causal mechanisms.

Disparate time constants: The importance of an observation often depends on the timing of the protocol. (For instance, the control of arterial blood pressure is a mix of fast-acting neural mechanisms, slow-acting hormonal mechanisms, and long-term effects of body fluid volume and compositions.)

Individual variation: Physiological responses are a qualitative and quantitative function of sex, age, body composition, and other individualities.

Emergence: Many high-level integrative behaviors of the biological system cannot be described solely by the sum of the respective inputs from basic processes (see Chapter 10).

There are many collaborative efforts underway that address some of the issues important to building out the Digital Patient. For example, the challenges of maximizing value from Big Data are being addressed the US National Institutes of Health's (NIH) BD2K program, through the European Union's Horizon 2020 initiative, through the European Big Data Value Association and through various Chinese Ministry of Science and Technology (MoST) initiatives. The challenge of encouraging consistency in terminology, ontology, and registries is being addressed through International Health Terminology Standards Development Organization (IHTSDO), the Simulation Industry Standards Organization (SISO), and the NIH Data Discovery Index Consortium. Model construction and interoperability are foci of the Physiome Project, the European Virtual Physiological Human Institute (VPH), and the US Interagency Modeling and Analysis Group (IMAG) and its companion group, the Multiscale Modeling Consortium (MSM).

Having clinical information in electronic form that is computable has been a great challenge for biomedical informatics since the dawn of the discipline. Unfortunately, most health information still sits in silos today, and health information exchange for the purpose of supporting care between organizations and levels of care (e.g., hospital to primary care), until very recently, has been an exception rather than the norm (see Chapters 9, 10, 15, and 16). The size and complexity of the domain and ethical and medico-legal requirements coupled with the variability of healthcare practice as often encountered render most traditional IT approaches to e-Health unfit, including standardization activities to date. The Connecting for Health Program in the United Kingdom, for example, is considered one of the largest IT project failures in history. It is fair to say that, to a large extent, health information has been the weakest link in the chain when we consider other related domains like bioinformatics, pharmaceutical research and development, and medical device technology in the quest for integrated biomedicine.

An important rule of thumb in capturing structured and computable clinical data is to obtain them as part of routine clinical practice. Post hoc data collection has been shown to be very expensive and error-prone. At times, it is impossible to capture the clinical context in which the data were collected. Data sources can be very diverse and range from operational electronic health record (EHR) systems to well-structured longitudinal disease registries and bio-banks. Patient contributions to health records, increasingly using mobile devices and sensors, are also important and can add valuable insights about environmental and behavioral factors as well (e.g., food, air quality, exercise, and mood).

Being able to make health information linkable and computable requires standardization at several levels (see Figure 21.3 and Chapter 9). Both data and terminology standards are reasonably mature, although there is considerable overlap among certain terminology and ontology systems such as SNOMED CT and LOINC. It is the content standards that have to tackle most of the difficulties arising from breadth, depth, complexity, variability, changeability, and longevity aspects of health information management. Indeed, much of the current debate is focused on such standards, and there are considerable efforts within the ICT disciplines to develop fit-for-purpose standards and specifications. Exchange standards (e.g., HL7 v2 messaging or the FHIR-based API) further tackle the dynamic aspects of health information flow, and ideally they should use the same or a compatible model of information. They clearly should leverage representational aspects from content standards (e.g., use the same definition for laboratory results or drugs and adverse reactions). Collectively, the need for a variety of standards represents another fundamental challenge to completing the Digital Patient.

Finally, the Digital Patient will not be constructed based solely on new information from all the "omics" fields, from the various efforts to model the human physiome and represent it virtually, from systems analysis, or from Big Data. It will only be realized through the purposeful collaboration of researchers (whether they are patients or scientific, clinical, or policy researchers) on both their own research and the framework into which their research

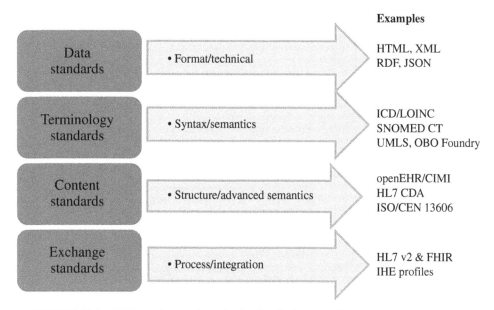

FIGURE 21.3   Different layers of standardization for health information (from Chapter 9).

will fit. The Digital Patient will continue to depend on the efforts of a wide variety of individual researchers and modelers across many disciplines worldwide. It is inevitably an emergent phenomenon, governable only by sustained cooperation among those with an interest in its development and with guiding principles of openness, flexibility, rigorous validation and reliability processes, and respect for patient privacy.

Realizing the tremendous potential of the Digital Patient is, as this concluding discussion has shown, going to be difficult, requiring us, as Thompson implies, to quickly set about deducing how the Digital Patient can be completed and used to help us work, meditate, and create health as envisioned by the World Health Organization. The chapters in this book collectively serve as the basis for our understanding of the collaborative research agenda for constructing the Digital Patient:

> The Digital Patient research agenda requires the establishment of an enduring, voluntary collaborative mechanism, much like the W3 Consortium governing the web, that involves an academically broad, international cadre of researchers, patients and clinicians capable, over time, of addressing the fundamental challenges identified in this chapter: taxonomic clarity, useable ontologies, protection of privacy, integration of data and models with differing temporal and spatial characteristics, standards, and a process for accrediting the validity and reliability of the constituent models of the Digital Patient.

INDEX

Wiley Series in
Modeling and Simulation

Mission Statement

The *Wiley Series in Modeling and Simulation* provides an interdisciplinary and global approach to the numerous real-world applications of modeling and simulation (M&S) that are vital to business professionals, researchers, policymakers, program managers, and academics alike. Written by recognized international experts in the field, the books present the best practices in the applications of M&S as well as bridge the gap between innovative and scientifically sound approaches to solving real-world problems and the underlying technical language of M&S research. The series successfully expands the way readers view and approach problem solving in addition to the design, implementation, and evaluation of interventions to change behavior. Featuring broad coverage of theory, concepts, and approaches along with clear, intuitive, and insightful illustrations of the applications, the Series contains books within five main topical areas: Public and Population Health; Training and Education; Operations Research, Logistics, Supply Chains, and Transportation; Homeland Security, Emergency Management, and Risk Analysis; and Interoperability, Composability, and Formalism.

Advisory Editors • Training and Education

Thiago Brito, University of Sao Paulo

Founding Series Editors

Joshua G. Behr, Old Dominion University
Rafael Diaz, Old Dominion University

Homeland Security, Emergency Management, and Risk Analysis

Forthcoming Titles

Zedda • *Risk and Stability of Banking Systems*

Interoperability, Composability, and Formalism

Operations Research, Logistics, Supply Chains, and Transportation

Public and Population Health

Arifin, Madey, and Collins • *Spatial Agent-Based Simulation Modeling in Public Health: Design, Implementation, and Applications for Malaria Epidemiology*

Forthcoming Titles

Hovmand • *Modeling Social Determinants of Health*
Kim and Hammon • *Modeling and Simulation for Social Epidemiology and Public Health*

Training and Education

Combs, Sokolowski, and Banks • *The Digital Patient: Advancing Healthcare, Research, and Education*